MENTAL HEALTH
Psycho-Social Perspectives

VOLUME THREE: Strength of Human Resources

The details of the forthcoming volumes

Volume 1: Issues and Interventions
Volume 2: Multigroup Analysis
Volume 3: Strength of Human Resources
Volume 4: Therapeutic Applications

About the Editors

Aradhana Shukla is Prof. and Head, Department of Psychology, Kumaun University Campus, Almora, Uttarakhand. Currently she is Campus Dean (Arts) at Kumaun University Campus, Almora. She has served in Department of Pediatrics of Banaras Hindu University, Post Doctoral Fellow (U.G.C.) at University of Gorakhpur and has been serving here for last 27 years. She has published 100 research papers of national and international repute, ten books in which nine are published by national agencies and one from Germany (LAP). She has carried out 4 major projects from ICSSR and UGC and co-worked in UNICEF and GFATM-Round 7 projects. She has guided 45 Ph.D. students and prepared 26 psychological tests. Moreover, she has attended 40 Seminars of national and international repute and organized 4 seminars in her department. Her major thrust areas are: developmental psychology, personality psychology, cultural psychology, environmental psychology and mental health care system.

Anubhuti Dubey is Associate Professor of Psychology at Department of Psychology, DDU Gorakhpur University, Gorakhpur. Her research interest includes Health Psychology, Applied Social Psychology, Gender and Health and Counselling. She had published a book entitled "Psychological Perspectives on Chronic Illness". She had also completed a research project sponsored by ICSSR on "Psychological Dynamics of Health and Illness in Women of Eastern Uttar Pradesh." She had published 25 research papers in journals of national and international repute and also contributed 11 chapters in different edited volumes. Four students had been awarded their Ph.D. thesis under her supervision. She had received university gold medals at under-graduate and post-graduate levels. She is also a Master Trainer and Supportive Supervisor for Training HIV/AIDS counsellors under GFATM-Round 7 programmes.

MENTAL HEALTH
Psycho-Social Perspective

Volume Three
Strength of Human Resources

Edited by
Aradhana Shukla
Anubhuti Dubey

CONCEPT PUBLISHING COMPANY PVT. LTD.
NEW DELHI-110059

ISBN-13: 978-93-5125-173-6 (Series)
ISBN-13: 978-93-5125-171-2 (Vol. III)

First Published 2017

Published and Printed by

Concept Since 1974

Concept Publishing Company Pvt. Ltd.
Regd. Office:
A/15-16, Commercial Block, Mohan Garden,
New Delhi-110059 (INDIA)
Phones : 25351460, 25351794, *Fax* : 091-11-25357109
E-mail : publishing@conceptpub.com
Website: www.conceptpub.com

Editorial Office: H-13, Bali Nagar, New Delhi-110 015, India.

Cataloging in Publication Data—DK Courtesy: D.K. Agencies (P) Ltd. <docinfo@dkagencies.com>

Mental health : psycho-social perspectives / edited by Aradhana Shukla, Anubhuti Dubey.
pages cm
Contributed articles.
Includes bibliographical references and index.
Contents: volume three. Strength of human resources — volume four. Therapeutic applications
ISBN 9789351251712 (vol. III)
ISBN 9789351251729 (vol. IV)
ISBN 9789351251736 (series)

1. Mental health—Social aspects—India. 2. Mental health—India. I. Shukla, Aradhana, editor. II. Dubey, Anubhuti, editor.

RA790.7.I5M46 2017 DDC 362.20954 23

Preface

We desire to live a healthy and happy life. It is a common and well accepted fact that everyone desires to live a healthy life. The mind and bodily functions are closely embedded hence, the relative significance of mental health along with physical wellness cannot be denied. As mind and bodily functions are closely embedded we cannot deny the relative significances of mental health along with physical wellness. Mental health is an integral part of health, mental health is more than the absence of mental illness, and mental health is intimately connected with physical health and behaviour. Mental health is the foundation for well-being and effective functioning for an individual and for a community. Good mental health is a sense of well-being, confidence and self-esteem. It enables us to fully enjoy and appreciate other people, day-to-day life and our environment.

Mental health is the sheer responsibility of a person himself. The mental health field aims to deal with (1) mentally ill people, (2) people at risk, and (3) promoting mental health of normal people so that their normality can be sustained.

If we go back into the history of mental health we can see that it was treated either as "boon of God" (good or positive mental health) or "curse of God" (bad or negative mental health). Both the Eastern and Western evidences support the notion. Not only in abroad but our ancient evidences also support this notion. The Western literatures on mental health were seen hallucinations as communication of humans with bad souls, ghosts and witches. Moreover, in the ancient Indian literature of Ayurveda, Mental disorders are represented as various forms. The aetio-genesis of these disorders was thought to be endogenous because of provoked humours like *Vat*, *Pitta* and *Kaph*. Exogenously the causes were attributed to sudden fear or association with ill influence of certain mythological gods or demon. *Charak Samhita* listed Psychiatry as *'Bhuta Vidya'*. Psychotherapy was known as *Ilaj-I-Nafsani* in Unani Medicine. But time never remains stable. Years and years were passed and the outlook of people towards mentally ill people become more and more aversive and they were treated like an undesirable social being for whom only such behaviour was required that was only meant for animals or criminals. Even with the advent of modern scientific methods and practical thoughts, the stigma and discrimination against mentally illnesses prevail the society. However, the advocates of Psychology started a soft touch and healing approach for the mentally ill people. Again it took decades to develop behaviour and psycho-therapies against tying mentally ill people with iron chain, and treat them like prisoners. A complete soft and medico-human environment under single roof was constructed for them and it was termed as asylum or mental hospital. Psychologists attempted such patients to get out from the boundaries and from the trap of *ojhas, neem-hakims* and other such traditional healers and placed them at asylum. The patients were properly medicated along with different psychotherapies and many of them got complete recovery. At first the asylums were established in abroad but in India the first asylum was established in 1787 by Surgeon Kenderline in Calcutta and thereafter many asylums were made. This period was relatively longer but it opened the doors of a new era for the support and care of mental ill-health. They not only paid attention to treat the mentally ill people but also concentrated on maintaining and nurturing public health, and trying to eradicate the stigma and discrimination faced by people with mental disorders. Psychologists and mental health care professionals are still trying to launch innovative programmes for the same. The focal theme of these developmental programmes are the utilization of community resources for mental health care. These programmes have given new vision to the mental health care professionals to prevent mental disorders and promote mental health. This also needs a greater role for the non-medical mental health care professionals and better utilization of cultural resources in terms of belief, practice and important social institutions like family and community groups. The contemporary world's realization about mental health and mental illness has come to a point where we find passionate discussions and caring mental health professionals to deal with mental disorder and promote well-being.

Keeping these views into consideration, the innovative thought of this series appeared in our mind and we decided to pool the thoughts of psychologists and healthcare professionals regarding various concerns of mental health. The basic aim of this series was: (i) to bring concepts, issues, strengths and treatment in a single jacket, (ii) bring a sense of mental health awareness in people so that they can make their health safe with additional attention on social health, (iii) to carve the research competence in young researchers, and (iv) to put forth the mental health policies before the readers, so that a better understanding of mental health can be developed.

About the series Mental Health: Psycho Social Perspectives

It is a series on the psychology of mental health and we have tried to cover as many areas as possible and we could justify its name, i.e. rethinking. Many traditional notions of mental health have been reconceptualised and many concepts in a new framework have been introduced. Initially we planned to bring out only four volumes in this series, as detailed below:

1. ***Mental Health: Psychological Issues and Interventions:*** In this volume we have covered various issues that foster or hamper mental health. Also, strategies to minimize negative mental health and improve positive mental health are discussed.
2. ***Mental Health: Multigroup Analysis:*** This volume covers the conceptual background and psycho-social perspective of mental health in various social settings.
3. ***Mental Health: Strength of Human Resources:*** In this volume we have tried to throw light on the promotional strategies of mental health following which a person can be relieved from negative mental health.
4. ***Mental Health: Therapeutic Applications:*** This volume covers a range of behavioural therapies which were found effective to minimize or overcome mental ill-health.

The first two volumes, after publication, were well received among the scholars and students. Just afterwards we started receiving encouraging responses from the intellectuals and the research scholars to continue this series. Now, we have decided to make this project "an ongoing series" and we invite the academic world to contribute their words of knowledge to share with the next generation.

We have exercised our best attempt to seek out as many experiences as possible and we also anticipate that this will open new foresight for the researchers. However, we will be highly blessed to obtain the healthy and critical comments from our colleagues, seniors and friends and we will appreciate them from the bottom of our hearts.

Aradhana Shukla
Anubhuti Dubey

Acknowledgements

We, the editors, feel immense pleasure to present our series on mental health before the august readers. We hope that it will be admired by you all and the comments will be highly appreciated.

We feel our deep sense of gratitude and thankfulness to our respected contributors. It was only their support that the volumes came in the shape. We are thankful to Mr. Abhishek and Mr. Pankaj Tewari for computer task.

Last but not least, we are thankful to Mr. Ashok Kumar Mittal, M/s. Concept Publishing Company Pvt. Ltd., New Delhi to shape our dreams in concrete form.

Aradhana Shukla
Anubhuti Dubey

Acknowledgements

Contents

List of Contributors

Anubhuti Dubey is Associate Professor, Department of Psychology, DDU Gorakhpur University, Gorakhpur, U.P., India.
Email: anubhutiddu@rediffmail.com

A. Shanmugiah is Associate Professor of Psychiatry, Institute of Mental Health, Kilpauk, Chennai, Tamil Nadu, India.

Prof. Aradhana Shukla is Professor, Department of Psychology, SSJ Campus, Kumaun University, Almora, Uttarakhand, India.
Email: aradhana.shukla5@gmail.com

Archana Shukla is Assistant Professor, Department of Psychology, University of Lucknow. Lucknow (India).
Email: archana.kshitish@gmail.com

Prof. Bharat H. Mimrot, Head, Department of Psychology, NKSPT's Arts, Science and Commerce College, Badnapur, Jalna, Maharashtra, India.
Email: bharat.mimrot@rediffmail.com

Deepti Mehrotra is Faculty at Navayuga Radiance Senior Secondary School, Lucknow (India). Email: deepti1991.edu@gmail.com

Dhananjay Kumar is Associated Professor, Department of Psychology, DDU Gorakhpur University, Up, India

Garima Singh is Research Scholar, Department of Psychology, DDU Gorakhpur University, Gorakhpur (U.P.), India.
Email: garima_alwaysyours@rediffmail.com

Harshita Shukla is Research Scholar, Department of Psychology, DDU Gorakhpur University, Gorakhpur (U.P.), India.
Email: h1234.shukla@gmail.com

Megha Kharkwal is Research Scholar, Department of Psychology, Kumaun University Campus, Almora.

Mohammad Ali Khalid is Director, Academic Programmes Professional Institute of Business and Visiting Faculty Ahsanullah University of Science and Technology, Bangladesh. Email: md_khalid@live.com

Pankaj Bharti is Associate Professor, Entrepreneurship Development Institute of India, New Delhi, India.

Purnima Awasthi is Assistant Professor in Department of Psychology, Banaras Hindu University, Varanasi, Uttar Pradesh, India.
Email: awasthip9@gmail.com

R. Jeyaprakash is Director, Institute of Mental Health, Kilpauk, Chennai, Tamil Nadu, India.

Ram Kalap Tiwari is Associate Professor, Department of Psychology, K.S. Saket P.G. College, Ayodhya, Faizabad, Uttar Pradesh, India.
Email: tiwarirk111@gmail.com

Ravi P. Pandey is Research Scholar, Department of Psychology, Faculty of Social Sciences, B.H.U., Varanasi (U.P.), India.

Reeta Chauhan is Research Scholar in Department of Psychology, Banaras Hindu University, Varanasi, Uttar Pradesh, India.

Prof. Rita Rani Talukdar is Associate Professor, Department of Psychology, Gauhati University, Guwahati, Assam-781014, India.
Email: rrtalukdar@yahoo.co.in

Saroj Verma is Professor, Department of Psychology, Banaras Hindu University, Varanasi, Uttar Pradesh, India.
Email: saroj_vrma@rediffmail.com

Shaimaa E. Basha is Faculty in Psychology Department, Faculty of Arts, Helwan University.

Shilpa Singh is Counsellor Psychology (IGNOU), Dronacharya Government Degree College, Gurgaon (Haryana), India.
Email: shilpaasingh@gmail.com

Subhash Meena is Research Scholar, Department of Psychology, Jai Narain Vyas University, Jodhpur (Rajasthan), India.
Email: sbhshmeena@yahoo.com

Suhas Shetgovekar is Associate Professor, Discipline of Psychology, SOSS, IGNOU, New Delhi, India. Email: sshetgovekar@ignou.ac.in

Sunil K. Verma is Assistant Professor, Department of Psychological Science, Vivekananda College, Delhi University, New Delhi, India.
Email: verma.sunil77@gmail.com

V. Smitha Ruckmani is Assistant Professor of Psychology-*cum*-Clinical Psychologist, Institute of Mental Health, Kilpauk, Chennai, Tamil Nadu.
Email: ruckmani1968@yahoo.com

Introduction

Aradhana Shukla & Anubhuti Dubey

Health is a broader concept including physical, social and mental health. Mental health has been reported as an important focus influencing individual and various behaviour, activities, happiness and performance.

Mental health is not just a state of happiness or contentment that one achieves and it can be retained for life. Further, it involves a continuous adaptation to changing circumstances; a dynamic process where living, reacting being strives to achieve a balance between internal demands and the requirements of a changing environment as defined in the annual report of the *"World Federation of Mental Health"*. It is not merely the absence of mental disorder but a state in which the individual lives harmoniously with himself and others adopting to and participating in an ever-changing social setting and with the sense that he is achieving self-realization through satisfaction of his basic needs.

Similarly, the expert committee in mental health of the World Health Organization defined mental health as *"a condition subject to biological and social factor, which enable the individual to achieve the satisfactory systems of his own potentially conflicting, instinctive dreams to form and maintain harmonious relations with other, and to participate in constructive change in his social and physical environment."*

The concept of positive mental health is basically related to one's concept of the nature of man. Fornom (1955) states in his book that "the approach of normative humanism is based on the assumption that, as in any other problem there are right and wrong, satisfactory and unsatisfactory solution to the problems of human existence. Mental health is achieved if man develops in to full maturity according to the characteristics and laws of human nature; mental illness exists in the features of such development. From this premise, the criterion of mental health is not one of in the virtual adjustment to a given social orders but a universal one valid for all men of giving a satisfactory answer to the problem of human existence.

Another life of thought relates mental health to the competence with which an individual lies in his environment and the competence of social institution *(home, school, work, reservation etc.)* to make this living as effective as possible. This approach considers mental health in term of the quality of interaction between an individual and his environment rather that in intra psychic manifestation (Bower 1966).

Clearly, all these qualities of mental health are fundamental importance to good adjustment. Reaction to environment, work, marriage and to other interpersonal are constantly affected by our state of mind. A sense of well efficiency is of inestimable values in the resolution of personal difficulty and conflicts. Mental health or ill-health, therefore, permeates the adjustment process and may be regarded both as condition and as an integral part of adjustment part (Jahoda 1958).

Keeping these views in consideration third volume of *"Mental Health: Psychological Perspective"* was planned and this volume was captioned as. *"Mental Health: Strength of Human Resources"*. There are twenty one articles in this volume and they are well organized and thoughtful. The first chapter written by *Aradhana Shukla,* explains the relative importance of human strength and the ways of its exploration. *Mohammed Khalid* narrated the branch of positive psychology and enhancement of human resources in organizations through it. *Dhananjay Kumar* has discussed self-regulation in terms of human strength. *Reeta Chauhan, Poornima Awasthi* and *Saroj Verma* have overviewed the notion of meaningfulness in life while *Ramkalap Tiwari* has explained the concept of spiritual psychology. The conception of mindfulness has been explained by *Aradhana Shukla* in global perspective, e.g. Structure, function and consequences and *Anubhuti Dubey* has made an Indo-Western comparison of positivism. Similarly, the notion of optimism and pessimism in positive psychology are discussed by *Shaaima E. Basha* and promoting devices for positive mental health is discussed by *V. Smitha, Ruckmani, A. Shanmugiah* and *P. Jeyaprakash* and *Garima Singh* and *Anubhuti Dubey* presented a detailed account of mental health.

There are some more chapters which discuss the applied aspects of human strength. *Sunil K. Verma* and *Pankaj Bharti* discussed values beyond boundaries in a theoretical perspective and *Suhas Shetgovekar* narrated the application of positive psychology among employees in India. *Subhash Meena* explored the concept of positive and *Archana Shukla* and *Shilpa Singh* presented the notion of wellness among elderly.

Older people have also been considered in this volume and *Bharat H. Mimrot* has stated the relationship between mental health and death anxiety in them. In this sequence *Harshita Shukla* and *Anubhuti Dubey* have shed light on the pattern of mental health, well-being and quality of life as correlates of successful ageing.

In addition, there are some other papers of multi-social and cutline segment. A very thoughtful and interesting chapter is presented by *Archana Shukla* and *Deepti Mehrotra* in which they have shed light on the life of Female Sex Workers (FSW). Modern life style of adolescents and impact of peer pressure and parental behaviour on their smoking tendency is narrated by *Purnima Awasthi, Ravi P. Pandey* and *Saroj Verma. Rita Rani Talukdar* described tribal children and their cognitive competence and married life of women of capital/non-capital region is described by *Megha Kharkwal* and *Aradhana Shukla.*

In the concluding chapter *Aradhana Shukla* has provided some skills to strengthen human life. We, hope that these chapters will satisfy the quench of researches and teaching professionals. Even though, it is a humble endeavour, we hope this volume will be able to promote new vision.

Aradhana Shukla
Anubhuti Dubey

1
Searching Strength in Human Life

Aradhana Shukla and *Anubhuti Dubey*

"Let us examine that one could set up a kind of scope or yardstick to measure the success of life—the satisfactoriness to the individual and in the environment in his mutual attempts to adopt with each other. Towards the end of such yardstick, positive adjunctures like *"peaceful"*, *"constructive"*, *"productive"* might appear and at other end such words as, *"confusive"*, *"destructive"*, and *"chaotic"*. These would describe the situation, in general for the individual himself. There might be at one hand of the *"yardstick"* such terms as, *"healthy"*, *"happy"*, *"creative"* and at the other hand, *"miserable"*, *"criminal"*, *"delirious"* (Menninger, Mayman and Pruyser, 1963).

These days clinical psychologists and healthcare professionals are taking serious interest in deep concentration on the problem, etiology, diagnosis and treatment of people and they try their best to make them normal and enable them to join the mainstream of society. They treat the clients in such a way that he could make a holistic change in his personality and can prove himself before the society as a normal fellow. This collaborative endeavour of clinician, healthcare professionals and client results in terms of positive feedback and the client feels a sense of holistic self-satisfaction and self-fulfilment. These senses work as a power, energy and a force to build a person and they feed positive characteristics in the person and turn him towards the positive side of life.

This force is termed as, *"strength"* which in abstract mode always help a person to lead a normal and positive life. These strengths may be either society based or individual based or both (basically situational). They can be seen as positive traits of personality and reflect positive mental health. This idea had shaped a movement in psychology which was named as positive psychology (Wood and Tarrier, 2010).

The aim of positive psychology is to cure the dysfunction in humans and promote optimal functioning in them. It provides the ways and resources to understand human living, achievements and potentialities (Linley, Joseph, Harrington & Wood, 2006; Seligman & Cikszentmihalyi, 2000). The agenda of positive psychology is basically based on human strength. It helps a person to search his own inner strength to build an acceptable and favourable ground of his personality. Peterson and Seligman (2004) have stated that the use of personal and/or psychological strengths energizes human experiences and alleviate well-being. It can be truly said that strength is the power of the "sublime expression of the life instinct" (Menninger *et al.*, 1963). It can be defined as a "capacity for feeling, thinking and behaving a way that allow optimal functioning in the pursuit of valued outcome" (Linley and Harrington, 2006).

Peterson and Seligman (2004) have noted that strengths are the consequences of well-being and they lead to beneficial outcomes. The benefits may not be in terms of financial gain but provide mental satisfaction. They are intrinsically valued irrespective of goal directed behaviour.

Dealing with the concept of personal strength Wood and associates (2011) have stated that personal strengths are the characteristics of person that allow them to perform well at their best. Peterson and Seligman (2004) have specified that strengths are:

- Intrinsically considered as a moral quality, irrespective of benefits,
- Stable traits,
- Enhances of other people when exposed, and
- Focus of individual development.

Peterson (2004) has given a small but broad list of human strength and stated them as, "possible criteria for significant strength". They are as follows:

- Identifying the real self and feeling a sense of ownership and authenticity.
- Curiosity and a thrust to know.
- Rapid learning.
- Spontaneous and continuous learning in accordance with the strength.
- Discovering of own strength.

- Epiphany invigoration rather than exhaustion while using the strength.
- Art of creation and pursuit.
- Intrinsic motivation.

Searching human strength as the "rightness" in humans Hodges and Clifton (2004) also defined it and stated it as a spontaneous pattern of thought, feeling and behaviour that must be productive. They narrated strength as the extent on latent and they are very near to perfection in task. Moreover, twenty four Character strengths are placed in six categories of virtues. They can be clubbed in six categories as follows:

1. **Strength of Wisdom and Knowledge**: It can be defined as cognitive power and it is comprised creativity, curiosity, open mindedness, love of learning and wisdom.
2. **Strength of Courage:** It has been made with bravery, persistence integrity and vitality.
3. **Strength of Humanity:** It promotes interpersonal strength and involves interpersonal love, kindness and social intelligence.
4. **Strength of Justice:** It protects against excess of everything and comprises citizenship, fairness and leadership.
5. **Strength for Temperance:** It is the most important human value and comprises forgiveness, mercy, humility and modesty, prudence and self-regulation.
6. **Strength of Transcendence:** This strength makes a connection (link) of the person to the universe. It deals with appreciation of beauty and excellence, gratitude, hope, humour and spirituality.

These strengths make a person aware about him and the whole world and they generate a sense of well-being. Govindji and Linley (2007) have also reported that reports of strength use are positively correlated with the reports of well-being. On the ground of these notions, it can be said that:

- *Strength is a great capacity of facing challenges:* Strength is such a powerful energy that provides mental skills and physical capabilities to meet the challenges of life.
- *Strength can never allow aggression:* Strength is the consequence of resilience. Resilience gives a positive energy and makes a person more active. A person in complete psycho-physical health does not found in aggressive mode because he

knows his envy and capabilities and is confident that any situation can be faced by him successfully.

- *Mental and physical health is the two sides of a coin:* Mental and physical health can never be separated. They are the two sides of a coin. Physical and mental health work in synergy and feed each other to form a strong individual. In order to make a person strong, medical professionals stress on the equivalence of psychological wellness and strength. To build inner strength we must build both, i.e. physical endurance and mental mode.
- *Identification of natural health is the basic step:* The first and foremost thing is to make a significant identification of strength and their use is required. We can see the Clifton's list of strengths or the strength list of the VIA Institute and check our own strength. In addition, we can go through the qualities of a self-actualizer proposed by Abraham Maslow and make our own check.

It is not so easy to check our own strength. It is very easy for us to get our views about own physical health and strength because changes concurring it can easily be noticed, but mental strength, as it is the fostering agent of our behaviour and work indirectly so, it cannot be identified easily. Not only it is a complex process of self-evaluation, but also the others cannot be evaluated in a single situation and in a single response. Although building and then maintaining inner strength is a lifelong process yet it pays throughout the life. Thus, it is sure that it is the psychological capital that is connected with individual's strength, perceptions, attitudes towards work and the most important the general outlook of life (Luthans, *et al.*, 2007). It has been noticed that it fosters human flourishing and optimal functioning (Cole, Daly & Mal, 2009).

Explanation of Strength in Hindu Tradition

Hindu tradition focuses on interconnectedness, i.e. harmonious union. This harmonious union may be presented as, single, unifying principle underlying all of earth (Stevenson & Haberman, 1998).

Upanishads stress on personal improvement and lifelong progression. It stresses the fact that the aim *(quest)* of life is to attain ultimate self-knowledge and to strive for the betterment of oneself. The Hindu tradition solely focuses on individuals. Upanishad states that, *"a man turns into something good by good actions and something bad by bad actions"* (Stevenson and Haberman, 1998).

Satkarma (good action) has always been encouraged in Upanishads. It has always been opined in Indian system that in case a person takes rebirth the *satkarma* of his previous birth *(purva janma)* pay their cost. These *satkarma* help him for self-betterment. The good life in Hindu tradition, therefore, encompasses individuals who are continually achieving knowledge and continually working towards good actions (Dashelgaurd, Paterson and Seligman, 2005; Paterson, 2004).

Some Basic Human Strengths

Bensen (1998) has classified human strength in two basic types, i.e. internal strength (that a person develops by ownself) and external strength *(that is fostered by the society)*. When these two types meet together, they form the ground of human strength.

Internal Forces	*External Forces*
➢ Constructive use of time Creative activities youth programmes religiosity time at home	➢ Support It deals with scholastic support and child-adult relation and parental involvement in schooling
➢ Commitment to learning Achievement motivation, school engagement, homework bounding to school reading for pleasure	➢ Boundaries and expectation Boundaries related to family, school, peer group, adult role and positive expectation
➢ Positive values Caring equality and social note integrity honesty responsibility restraint	➢ Social competence Planning and decision make-up interpersonal competence, resistance and conflict management
➢ Social competencies Planning and decision-making interpersonal competencies, resistance, peaceful conflict resolution	➢ Empowerment Community value youth as resources safeties and service to others
➢ Positive identity Personal power shameful purpose positive future oriented	

In general, if we compile the apparent attributes of strength we will put gratitude, wisdom, curiosity, hope, optimism, mindfulness, positive future orientation, zest, enthuses, vigour, energy, humanity, justice, temperance and transcendence at one place. Thus, it is apparent that it comprises psychological, social and emotional well-being.

Knowing and Nurturing Personal Strength through Self-experiment

It is common fact that an individual cannot evaluate or at least know about the personal strength. He may watch them very frequently, but considers them as the basic element of his behaviour. But it is possible to know and understand more about our strength and share it with others. Some tips are as follows:

- *Searching the weaknesses and strengths of friends:* We can ask our friends to describe their weaknesses and strengths and then make a self-preparation, i.e. do we have these weaknesses or strengthes.
- *Discovering our own strength:* Same process as done before can also be implemented on us.
- *Searching parental strength:* After searching our own strengths we can classify them and use them in group as desired by the circumstance.

References

Benson, P.L.; Leffett. N., Scales, P.C. and Blyth, D.A. (1988). Creating Healthy Communities for Children and Adolescents. *Applied Developmental Science.* 2, 138, 159.

Chen, D.J., and Lim, V.K. (2012). Strength in Adversity: The Influence of Psychological Capital on Job Search. *Journal of Organizational Behaviour, 33*(6), 811-839.

Cole, K., Saley, A. and Mak, A. (2009). Good for the Soul Relationship between Work Well-being and Psychological Capital. *Journal of Socio-Economics.* 38, 464-474.

Hodges, T.D. and Cliflon, D.O. (2004). Strength based Development in Practice. In P.A. Linley and S. Joseph (Eds.). *Positive Psychology in Practice* (pp. 256-268). Hoboken N.J.: Wiley.

Linley, P.A., Joseph, S., Harrington, S., and Wood, A.M. (2006). Positive Psychology: Past, Present, and (possible) Future. *The Journal of Positive Psychology,* 1(1), 3-16.

Linley, P.A. and Harrington, S. (2006). Playing to your Strengths. *Psychologist,* 19(2), 86-89.

Luthans, F., Yusuf, C.M. and Avolio, B. (2007). *Psychological Capital Developing the Human Competitive Age.* New York: Oxford University Press.

Meeninger, K., Mayman, M. and Pruyser, P.W. (1963). *The Vital Balance.* New York: Viking Press.

Peterson, C. and Seligman, M.C.P. (2004). *Character Strength and Virtues: A Hand Book and Classification.* Washington DC: American Psychological Association.

Seligman, M.E.P. and Csikszentmihalyi, M. (2000) Positive Psychology: An Introduction. *American Psychologist,* 55, 5-14.

Stevenson, L., and Haberman, D.L. (1998). *Ten Theories of Human Nature.* Oxford: Oxford University Press.

Wood, A.M. and Tarrier, N. (2010). Positive Clinical Psychology: A New Vision and Strategy for Integrated Research and Practice. *Clinical Psychology Review, 30*(7), 819-829.

Wood, A.M., Linley, P.A., Maltby, J., Kashdan, T.B. and Hurling, R. (2011). Using Personal and Psychological Strengths leads to increases in well-being over time: A Longitudinal Study and the Development of the Strengths use Questionnaire. *Personality and Individual Differences,* 50, 15-19.

2

Enhancing Human Resource in Organizations Through Positive Psychology

Mohammad Ali Khalid

With growing demands in the organizational world and a greater requirement for knowledge work, creativity, innovation and, organizational settings will need to find ways to facilitate their employees to do and be their best. Positive psychology is emerging as an essential contributor to the success in the workplace because of its unique focus on flourishing and transform-good-into-great angle on many of the factors that contribute to organizational performance. First of all the aim of this chapter is to review and know essential modern HRM (Human Resource Management) challenges in India, secondly, to argue that the underlying weakness is the way organizations and employees respond to these challenges, and lastly to talk about how positive psychology can play an important role. This chapter also discusses the major issues which are faced by Human Resource (HR) managers and that can be introduced by adopting the view of positive psychology to support HR with the changes that are occurring in the organizations and the financial system. Moreover, positive psychology emphasizes that subjective well-being, resilience, optimism and hope would be able to reveal as an effective competence to contain rising trends. The main concern of this chapter is to recommend a basic rethink to HRM issues and propose function of positive psychology as a possible explanation. In this way, it could be helpful to plan HR strategies and involvements in a more considerate way.

Empirical research is suggested that positive psychology has the possibility to make a significant difference in the workplace. During the last two decades positive psychology has received increased attention. Various researchers have visited positive source facility to investigate their affiliation with employees' workplace outcomes (Youssef & Luthans, 2007; Vohra & Goel, 2009; Richez, 2009; Gu & Day, 2007; Chahal & Mehta, 2010). The appearance of positive resource abilities like subjective well-being, resilience, optimism and hope encourage the achievement probability of interventions to deal with various HRM challenges.

Human Resource Management today speaks of organizing and successfully surviving the ever transforming circumstances. Though, India and other developing countries are manifest by their unpredictable political and financial circumstances; there are indecisive surroundings for HRM in particular and for the organizations in general. India is a land of different religions, languages, castes, typical rich culture and ancient traditions. In India, HRM is greatly influenced by community and cultural norms. Sparrow and Budhwar (1997) approved that these norms establish the manner of employees and also form the job climate. Researchers had not only recognized variety of particular features of Indian management but identified Indian HR. Compliance to superiors, fear of taking autonomous decisions, confrontation to change, reluctance to accept right and unmanageable etc. are some of these (Sharma, 1984; Sparrow and Budhwar, 1997). Similarly, Tayeb (1996) also illustrated that Indians are industrial, inventive, meticulous, motivated and money-oriented. While working in Indian context such distinctiveness have to be taken into reflection by strategy makers and HR professionals. Nonetheless, Budhwar and Varma (2011) after analyzing the literature, acknowledged the existence of both "culture-bound" (e.g. national culture and national institutions) and 'culture-free' (e.g. age, size and nature of the firm) determinants of HRM in India.

Human Resource Management

Human Resource Management is the procedure of appropriate and maximize consumption of existing limited experienced personnel. The core function of the human resource management is to make well-organized use of accessible human resource in the organization. One of the best examples at current situation is production business that has been facing severe deficiency of skilled personnel. Therefore, it would be a great attempt to operate the skills optimistically to increase the organizational behaviour. Each organization aspires to have experienced and proficient people to make the organization more successful than their competitors. Without human resources (humans) no action in the organization can be done and HR is the most significant property for the organization rather than land and buildings. Torrington and Hall (1987) revealed that "A series of an activity which first enables working people and their employing organizations to agree about the objectives and nature of their working relationship and, secondly, ensures that the agreement is fulfilled". While Miller (1987) recommends that HRM relates to those decisions and actions which concern the management of employees at all levels in the business and which are related to the implementation of strategies directed towards creating and sustaining competitive advantage.

The construction of every creation or service depends upon human mind, attempt and their working hours. It is not possible that any service or product can be formed without the help of human being. For producing or constructing anything human being is the primary source. At present time, various experts assert that technology and machinery are replacing human resource and decreasing their function or attempt. But still technology and machinery have been allocated by the individual support and besides companies have been constantly investigate for brilliant, expert and competent professionals to further develop most recent technology and machinery, which yet again have to be controlled or used by individuals to bring out products. For every workplace to function successfully, it must have source of men, funds, resources and technology. The resources by themselves cannot accomplish the goals of associations that they require to be composed, harmonized and utilized through human resources. Furthermore, the successful management of human resources is also essential. Therefore, human resource management has appeared as a main purpose in organizations. Human resource management is the executive function that deals with issues linked to people such as profit, employee inspiration, compensation, presentation, administration, association, improvement, protection, wellness contact, hiring management, and supervision.

The entire human resource actions are contained by human resource management. While these actions are discharged efficiently and they will result in a knowledgeable and enthusiastic personnel who will assist, comprehend executive aims. Human Resource Management assists the supervisors to hire, choose, guide and increase members for an organizational setting so in this way HRM is an executive function.

Positive Psychology in Milieu

Increasing special focus on pathology the discipline of psychology in the previous decade has witnessed a rising consideration to so far ignored positive aspects of life. This is made promising during the prominent positive psychology movements which suggest that a non-negative approach can be taken to study people (Seligman and Csikszentmihalyi, 2000). Seligman (1998a: 4) has advocated positive psychology as the logical and practical approach to reveal people's strengths and encourageing their positive performance. Though, whether positive psychology is culture-free or culturally-rooted that is still a subject of argument among psychologists, but however, researchers have always tried to determine and recognize the complication of cultural influences.

At the time while assessing the role of positive psychology on human resource management, Indian culture focuses on subjective well-being, hope, optimism and resilience. These four resource abilities are also called positive psychological qualities. But, a big debate always remains on their 'trait' *versus* 'state' nature. The literature has revealed that these constructs are relevant and linked to occupational presentation (Youssef & Luthans, 2007; Adams *et al.*, 2002; Luthans *et al.*, 2005; Coutu, 2002), social adjustments and universal employment (Klohnen, 1996), well-being and life satisfaction and (Klohnen, Vandewater, and Young, 1996). These capabilities are briefly depicted below:

1. ***Resilience:*** Resilience is usually defined as the ability of people to hold out suffering and to recover from harsh conditions (Garmezy, 1991; Turner, 2001; Luthans, 2002). Paul and Garg (2012a) in a review of literature widely concluded that resilience as it applies to individual employees of an organization can be defined as a psychological capability to face, locate and respond to the unnecessary circumstances, generally unpredicted, formed by some harsh conditions, work-related pressure or even by an alteration in roles and responsibilities or operational atmosphere, in such a manner so as to maintain performing in an improved method.
2. ***Subjective Well-being:*** Subjective well-being (SWB) is generally used to indicate the 'good life' that is a scientific term. It can be defined as the self-assessment of one's emotional condition. In simplest way it refers to how people understand the quality of their lives and comprise both affective responses and cognitive decisions (Diener, 1984). It consists of the affective element and a cognitive element. Diener (1984) also articulated SWB in terms of feelings and confirmed SWB to be the understanding of high levels of pleasant feelings and dispositions, low levels

of negative feelings and dispositions, and high life satisfaction. Farid and Lazarus (2008) describe it as the overall approving appraisal of one's own life and effort and domain contentment such as those interrelated to physiological, psychological and sociological.

3. ***Hope:*** Hope is conceptualized as consisting of pathways and organization (Snyder, 1994). Pathways are the apparent abilities to generate ways to preferred objectives. Organization reveals the apparent inspiration to utilize those ways. The amount of pathways and organization assists group to attain their ambitions. Further, Snyder, Irving and Anderson (1991: 287) state it as a positive motivational situation that is based on an interactively consequent sense of unbeaten organization and pathways.
4. ***Optimism:*** Optimism is a universal faith of human being that in the future good things will occur more than the terrible things (Scheier and Carver, 1985). Seligman (1998b) declared optimism as an acknowledgment technique that give details about positive actions in terms of individual, everlasting, and persistent causes and negative actions in terms of outside, momentary, and situation-specific ones. A person's conviction that a target is reasonable assists one to defeat harsh conditions faced in accomplishment of their aim (Utsey *et al.*, 2008).

RANGE OF HUMAN RESOURCE MANAGEMENT

The range of human resource management involves every action that come under the standard of human resource management. These actions are as follows:

1. **Human Resources Preparation:** Human resource preparation refers to a course of action by which the company to recognize the amount of jobs vacant that whether the company has a large amount of staff or lack of staff and to deal with this large amount or lack of staff.
2. **Job Analysis Plan:** Job analysis plan is another significant part of human resource management. Job analysis helps to give a comprehensive clarification about each and every job in the company.
3. **Recruitment and Selection:** Organization prepares advertisements and publishes them in the newspapers that are

based on information collected from job analysis. This is called recruitment. Recruitment and selection are yet another vital area of human resource management because a number of applications are acknowledged after the advertisement is published further, interviews are conducted and the right employee is selected.

4. **Orientation and Induction:** This is another essential area of human resource management. Once the employees have been preferred an orientation or induction curriculum is conducted. The employees are knowledgeable about the conditions of the company they explain about the managerial background, ethics, work principles and initiate to the other employees.
5. **Training and Development:** Each employee goes undertraining programme which facilitates him to put up a superior presentation on the job. Training curriculum is also conducted for accessible staffs that have a lot of knowledge and this process is called refresher training.
6. **Performance Evaluation:** Performance evaluation is conducted by organizations time to time. The human resource department checks the performance of the employee. Based on these evaluation future incentives, promotions, increments in income are determined.
7. **Compensation Arrangement and Reimbursement:** There are different policies regarding compensation and other profits. It is the duty of the human resource department to look into remuneration and compensation arrangement.
8. **Inspiration, Well-being, Security and Happiness:** Inspiration becomes essential to maintain the amount of employees in the organization. It is the work of the human resource department to look into the special ways of inspiration. Apart from this certain well-being and security rules have to be followed for the profits of the employees. This is also handled by the HR department.
9. **Industrial Relations:** Maintaining co-ordinal associations with the union members is another significant area of human resource management. This will assist the company to stop strikes, lockouts and make sure flat functioning in the company. The human resource officer is accountable for given that support in the different human resource purposes that contain training, recruitment, staffing and improvement, performance monitoring and employee analysis.

Importance of Human Resource Management

Human Resource Management becomes important for workplace due to the following motives:

1. ***Objective***: Human resource management assists a workplace to accomplish its objective from time-to-time by generating a positive outlook among workforce. Therefore, its main concern is dropping consumption and building greatest utilization of resources etc.
2. ***Facilitates Professional Growth***: Appropriate human resource policies prepare well-trained employees and makes them prepared for future promotions. Their ability can be utilized in the existing company in which they are at present working and also for the other companies which the workforce may join in the future.
3. ***Healthier Relationships between Union and Management***: Further, effective human resource management practices can facilitate the company to sustain co-ordinal association with the unions.
4. ***Facilitates an Individual to Work in a Team***: Individuals team work and tuning can be achieved through healthy human resource practices. These types of practices make individuals very relaxed while they work in team and it also improves the team work.
5. ***Recognizes Individual for the Future***: While employees are frequently trained, so, they are prepared to meet the job necessities. The organization is also capable to recognize potential workforce who can be promoted in the future for the top rank jobs. Therefore, HRM prepare people for the future.

Positive Psychology Lending a Hand

Black and Ulrich (1999) clarified the two-fold functions of HR professionals as initial, to increase, describe, and explain the capacities essential and subsequent, to devote, plan, and distribute HR practices that make sure these capacities. They suggest that view of positive psychology can play a major role while HR professional execute their subsequent role. The challenges regarding to HRM cannot be determined on their own. It involves hard work in the form of appropriately calculated interventions and their appropriate release or execution. The results would be amazing if these interventions are applied along with the amount of different constructs of positive psychology as per the conditions. Since, it is clearly said that before sowing one has to arrange the land, as well, before addressing the human resources to any interventions, it is very significant to get ready them first. It would assist recruits to build up an approach towards overcoming the troubles and challenges. In this way, resilience, which is one of the positive resource ability, is an ability that allows persons to endure adversity, in facing hardship, to continue primary efficient and fit lives (Bolton, 2004). In the multifaceted communication between the human being and the surroundings, resilience not only provides for the positive psychological capability to recover from job-related pressure and crisis but also for structure an outlook to deal with the realities of the organizational world. Masten, Best, and Garmezy (1990) stated that resilience is the procedure of flourishing adjustment towards challenging or hostile conditions. The research evidence advocates that resilience has hopeful connotations for workplaces (Richez, 2009; Vohra & Goel, 2009; Youssef & Luthans, 2007; Chahal & Mehta, 2010). Resilience can assist people adapt to changes more profitably. This positive aptitude can assist those people who naturally refuse to accept transform. Resilience can also come to the release of professionals who abjectly give up to superiors by making them more perseverant and self-sufficient. It can facilitate them build positive outlooks to not only stay alive in a complicated condition but also to expand competencies. Masten (2001) in resiliency theory declared that most people will do well regardless of disclosure to immense hardship. It has extensive connotation for workplaces struggling to resist various challenges posed by the energetic atmosphere as resilience is a theory that identifies the significance of defensive factors and proficiencies. Leadbeater (2004) mentioned that resilience can assist persons construct crucial features of strength-building procedures. Additionally, resilience leads to workplace dedication and an increase in exhibit of residency behaviours (Paul and Garg, 2012b; Luthar *et al.*, 2000; Campbell-Sills *et al.*, 2006) and therefore, assists to decrease income and enhance contentment.

Another positive ability that is subjective well-being (SWB) is generally known as pleasure. Between a variety of positive constructs considered under the domain of positive psychology, pleasure is disputed to be the complete plan and conclusion of human survival (Aristotle, 1974) and the foremost appreciated aims in the life of people (Diener & Oishi, 2000). In reality, pleasure is fundamentally the treatment for all human tribulations. In the organization also many troubles take place due to the fact that people are not pleased. Work stress, time limits, and pressure have made people's life further dreadful. SWB can assist people to energize and take concern in the occupation. It is necessary for most favourable implementation of the human being. It acts as a defence to many challenging actions that a human being faces though at job and assist him/her increase on ethics as well. These ethics then allow persons to not only scrutinize rituals but also to perform them. SWB is reflected through positive knowledge at job which in turn increases employment contentment (Kiziah, 2009). Additional happy workers will be more accessible to the diverse interventions designed to addressing unusual issues. Carleton (2009) has recommended a variety of interventions to enhance worker contentment. Well-being and employee dedication is positively linked to each other (Meyer and Maltin, 2010) and work-life equilibrium (Gröpel and Kuhl, 2009), and disapprovingly connected to pressure and suffer exhaustion. It is extreme and further significant in the case of conditional workers. Therefore, if well-being is concerned, then manageing agreement labours would not be much of a problem for HR professionals. Moreover, a comprehensive sense of contentment which defines SWB, make human resources more occupied (Myers and Diener, 1995).

Hope is always related to objective achievement and positive emotions. People high in hope execute better performance at the organization. It is also found to be associated to positive outcomes like elevated contentment, condensed earnings and be exhausted etc. (Vohra & Goel, 2009). Further, hopefulness may also repeat a sense of accommodating the ability with a feeling of being nurtured. Hopeful workforce would have an encourageing power making them to enlarge labours to attain goals. It is consequently planned here that a sense of hope would allow persons to make excellent career choices and assist them in charting out their career strategies. Moreover, hopefulness would also assist managers to take autonomous decisions and develop as leaders.

Optimism refers to a universal belief that the future will generate good outcomes. Several studies have found that every constructs of positive psychology are connected and precede each other. Hope has been found to impact well-being of human resources (Scheier & Carver, 1985) and consequently add to all the conclusion of well-being. Optimism would also assist to decrease the fear of taking autonomous decisions among executives. Additionally, being optimistic, companies can work on progression development also. This would definitely help in filling the management void.

Implications and Conclusion

This work highlights that even though all HR actions require being deliberately associated with the organization's overall planned ideas but at the same time it has to be seen that the HRM challenges and the fundamental troubles are not left unattended. On the whole, positive psychology can offer HRM a sufficient method to deal with these troubles by providing a support to HR involvement. While, each and every challenges and troubles are eventually related with the humans so, it is must first set-up these humans before addressing them to any involvements. The belief of positive psychology conversed in this study may not frankly undertake the HRM challenges, but absolutely supply by making workforce prepared for advance dealing. These positive source capabilities can be considered as harmonizing medicines given to patients along with the other specific medicines to treat a particular ailment. Therefore, it is sensible to HR practitioners to think about these source capabilities while scheming HR intrusions so as to guarantee their achievement.

References

Adams, V.H., Snyder, C.R., Rand, K.L., King, E.A., Sigmon, D.R., and Pulvers, K.M. (2002). Hope in the workplace. In R. Giacolone and C. Jurkiewicz (Eds.), *Handbook of Workplace Spirituality and Organizational Performance*: 367-377.

Aristotle. (1974). *The Nichomacean Ethics* (J.A.K. Thomson, Trans.). Penguin, Harmondsworth, NY.

Black, J.S., and Ulrich, D. (1999). The new frontier of global HR. In P. Joynt and P. Morton (Eds), *The Global HR Manager*, Institute of Personnel and Development, London.

Bolton D. (2004). Change, coping and context in the resilient organization. *Mt Eliza Business Review, 7*(1), 57-66.

Budhwar, P.S., and Varma, A. (2011). Emerging HR management trends in India and the way forward. *Organizational Dynamics*, 40, 317-325.

Campbell-Sills, L., Cohan, S.L., Stein, M.B. (2006). Relationship of resilience to personality, coping, and psychiatric symptoms in young adults. *Behaviour Research and Therapy, 44*(4), 585-599.

Carleton, E.L. (2009). Happiness at work: Using positive psychology interventions to increase worker well-being. Thesis published by ProQuest Dissertations and Theses, Canada.

Chahal, H., and Mehta, S. (2010). Antecedents and Consequences of

Organizational Citizenship Behaviour (OCB): A Conceptual Framework in Reference to Healthcare Sector. *Journal of Service Research, 10*(2), 25-44.

Coutu, D.L. (2002). How resilience works. *Harvard Business Review,* 80(5), 46-55.

Diener, E. (1984). Subjective well-being. *Psychological Bulletin*, 95, 542–575.

Diener, E., and Oishi, S. (2000). Money and Happiness: Income and subjective well-being across nations. In E. Diener and E.M. Suh (Eds.), *Culture and Subjective Well-being* (pp. 185-218).

Farid, M. and Lazarus, H. (2008). Subjective well-being in rich and poor countries. *Journal of Management Development*, *27* (10), 1053-1065.

Garmezy, N. (1991). Resilience in children's adaptation to negative life events and stressed environments. *Pediatric Annals*, 20, 459-466.

Gröpel, P. and Kuhl, J. (2009). Work-life balance and subjective well-being: The mediating role of need fulfilment. *British Journal of Psychology*, 100, 365-375.

Gu, Q., and Day, C. (2007). Teachers resilience: A necessary condition for effectiveness. *Teaching and Teacher Education*, 23, 1302-1316.

Kiziah, J.E. (2009). Job Satisfaction *vs*. Work Fulfilment: Exploring positive experience at work. Thesis published by ProQuest Dissertations and Theses, Canada.

Klohnen, E.C. (1996). Conceptual analysis and measurement of the construct of ego-resiliency. *Journal of Personality and Social Psychology,* 70, 1067-1079.

Klohnen, E.C., Vandewater, E.A., and Young, A. (1996). Negotiating the middle years: Ego-resiliency and successful midlife adjustment in women. *Psychology and Ageing*, 11, 431-442.

Leadbeater, B.J., Schellenbach, C.J., Maton, K.I. and Dodgen, D.W. (2004). Research and policy for building strengths: Processes and contexts of individual, family, and community development. In K.I. Maton, C.J. Schellenbach, B.J. Leadbeater, and A.L. Solarz (Eds.), *Investing in Children, Youth, Families and Communities: Strengths-based Research and Policy*. Washington DC: American Psychological Association.

Luthans, F. (2002). The need for and meaning of positive organizational behaviour. *Journal of Organizational Behaviour*, 23, 695-706.

Luthans, F., Avolio, B.J., Walumbwa, F.O., and Li, W. (2005). The psychological capital of Chinese workers: Exploring the relationship with performance. *Management and Organization Review,* 1, 249-271.

Luthar, S.S., Cicchetti, D., and Becker B. (2000). The construct of resilience: A critical evaluation and guidelines for future work. *Child Development*, 71(3), 543-562.

Masten, A.S., Best, K.M., and Garmezy, N. (1990). Resilience and development: Contributions from the study of children who overcame adversity. *Developmental Psychopathology*, 2, 425-44.

Masten, A.S. (2001). Ordinary Magic: Resilience Processes in Development. *American Psychologist*, 56(3), 227-238.

Meyer, J.P., and Maltin, E.R. (2010). Employee commitment and well-being: A critical review, theoretical framework and research agenda. *Journal of Vocational Behaviour,* 77, 323-337.

Miller, P. (1987) Strategic Industrial Relations and Human Resource Management: Distinction, Definitions and Recognition. *Journal of Management Studies,* Vol. 24(4), 347-361.

Myers, D.G., and Diener, E. (1995). Who is Happy? *Psychological Science,* 6(1), 10-19.

Paul, H., and Garg, P. (2012a). Revisiting Resilience in Indian Context. In conference proceeding of International Conference on Management in New World Order: Concepts and Practices from India (pp. 380-397).

Paul, H., and Garg, P. (2012b). Elevating organizational consequences through employee resilience. In conference proceeding of National Conference on Emerging Challenges for Sustainable Business held at IIT Roorkee during June 1-2, 2012.

Richez, M.M. (2009). Resilience, Job Stress and Organizational Commitment of Staff Nurses, Ohio, USA: Case Western Reserve University.

Scheier, M.F., and Carver, C.S. (1985). Optimism, coping, and health: Assessment and implications of generalized outcome expectancies. *Health Psychology,* 4, 219-247.

Seligman, M. (1998a). *Learned optimism.* Pocket Books, New York.

Seligman, M. (1998b). Building Human Strength: Psychology's forgotten mission. In C.R. 34. Snyder., and S.J. Lopez. (2007) (Eds.). *Positive Psychology: The Scientific and Practical Explorations of Human Strengths.* Sage, New Delhi.

Seligman, M.E.P., and Csikszentmihalyi, M. (2000). Positive psychology: An introduction. *American Psychologist,* 55, 5-14.

Sharma, I.J. (1984). The culture context of Indian Managers. *Management and Labour Studies,* 9(2), 72-80.

Snyder, C.R. (1994). *The Psychology of Hope: You can get to there from here.* New York: Free Press.

Snyder, C.R., Irving, L., and Anderson, J. (1991). Hope and Health: Measuring the will and the ways. In C.R. Snyder and D.R. Forsyth (Eds.), *Handbook of Social and Clinical Psychology* (pp. 285-305).

Sparrow, P.R., and Budhwar, P. (1997). Competition and Change: Mapping the Indian HRM recipe against the world wide patterns. *Journal of World Business,* 32, 224-242.

Tayeb, M. (1996). India: A Non Tiger of Asia. *International Business Review,* 5(5), 425-445.

Torrington, D., and Hall, L. (1987) *Personnel Management: A New Approach,* New York: Prentice Hall.

Turner, S.G (2001). Resilience and Social Work Practice: Three Case Studies. *Families in Society: The Journal of Contemporary Human Services,* 82 (5), 441-448.

Utsey, S.O., Hook, J.N., Fischer, N. and Belvet, B. (2008). Cultural orientation, ego resilience, and optimism as predictors of subjective well-being in African-Americans. *Journal of Positive Psychology,* 3(3), 202-210.

Vohra, N., and Goel, A. (2009). Influence of positive characteristics on organizational commitment and job satisfaction of Indian middle managers. *Working paper series WPS No. 63 of IIM*, Calcutta.

Youssef, C.M., and Luthans, F. (2007). Positive Organizational Behaviour in the Workplace: The Impact of Hope, Optimism, and Resilience. *Journal of Management*, 33(5), 774-800.

3

Human Strength

Self-Regulation

Dhananjay Kumar

The urge of psychologists to take a more open and appreciative perspective regarding human potentials, motives, and capacities had led to the initiation of positive psychology which is an attempt to relook on the issue of the imbalance. However, such an effort is difficult within the present reductionist epistemological traditions, which trains us to view "positivity" with suspicion. And it is right that we receive such training, because we tend to be taken in, at least at times, by our own delusions and wishes. However, such skepticism, taken too far, may itself constitute a "negativity bias" which thwarts a clear understanding of reality.

Positive psychology is the study of the conditions and processes that contribute to the flourishing or optimal functioning of people, groups, and institutions. Defined in this way, positive psychology has a long history, dating back to William James's writings on what he termed "healthy mindedness" in 1902, to Allport's interest in positive human characteristics in 1958, to Maslow's advocacy for the study of healthy people in lieu of sick people in 1968, and to Cowan's research on resilience in children and adolescents (e.g., Cowan, 2000).

Positive psychology is the study of how human beings prosper in the face of adversity (Seligman & Csikszentmihalyi, 2000). Its goals are to identify and enhance the human strengths and virtues that make life worth living, and allow individuals and communities to thrive. Seligman realized that psychology had largely neglected the latter two of its three pre-World War II missions: curing mental illness, helping all people to lead more productive and fulfilling lives, and identifying and nurturing high talent. The advent of the Veterans Administration (in 1946) and the National Institute of Mental Health (in 1947) had largely rendered psychology a healing discipline based upon a disease model and illness ideology. With this realization, Seligman resolved to use his APA presidency to initiate a shift in psychology's focus towards a more positive psychology (Seligman, 1999).

Sheldon and King (2001) defined positive psychology as "nothing more than the scientific study of *ordinary* human strengths and virtues", one that "revisits the *average* person". In this definition is the acknowledgement that our field as a whole is relatively silent regarding what is typical, because what is typical is positive. Despite the very real impact of the negative aspects of life documented in the past few decades of psychological research, most people are doing well, and we, as psychologists, tend to overlook the greater part of human experience and the majority of people, families, groups, and institutions" (Myers, 2000; Diener and Diener, 1996; Biswas-Diener and Diener, 2001).

Positive Psychology is also the study of positive emotion, positive character, and positive institutions (Seligman and Csikszentmihalyi, 2000). Drawing on methods effectively used to advance the science of mental disorders, positive psychologists have been studying mental health and well-being. Building on pioneering work by Rogers (1951), Maslow (1954, 1962), Jahoda (1958), Erikson (1963, 1982), Vaillant (1977), Deci and Ryan (1985), and Ryff and Singer (1996)—among many others—positive psychologists have enhanced our understanding of how, why, and under what conditions positive emotions, positive character, and the institutions that enable them flourish (e.g., Cameron, Dutton, and Quinn, 2003; Easterbrook, 2003; Gardner, Csikszentmihalyi, and Damon, 2001; Kahneman, Diener, and Schwarz, 1999; Murray, 2003; Vaillant, 2000).

Positive psychologists do not claim to have invented the good life or to have ushered in its scientific study, but the value of the overarching term *positive psychology* lies in its uniting of what had been scattered and desparate lines of theory and research about what makes life most worth living (Peterson and Park, 2003).

Human Strength

In positive psychology, strengths are built-in capacities for certain thoughts, feelings, and behaviours. Everyone possesses all the character strengths associated with the six virtues of wisdom, courage, humanity, justice, temperance, and transcendence, to a greater and lesser extent. One can be particularly gifted in one area and weak in another, but if he is like most people, he will be often somewhere in between. The particular pattern of strengths is part of what makes anyone unique. One can probably enjoy using his strengths and do it well naturally. When someone plays from his strengths, he is likely to feel more energetic and perform better than when trying to use a capacity that comes less naturally. Knowing your strengths is helpful only if you use them. Positive psychology is an umbrella term for theories and research about what makes life most worth living (Seligman and Csikszentmihalyi, 2000).

Strengths of character and positive experiences such as a satisfied life are among the central concerns of positive psychology (McCullough and Snyder, 2000; Seligman, 2002). Character strengths can be defined as positive traits reflected in thoughts, feelings, and behaviours. They exist in degrees and can be measured as individual differences. They are grounded in biology through an evolutionary process that selected for these predispositions towards moral excellence.

Character strength is "a disposition to act, desire, and feel that involves the exercise of judgement and leads to a recognizable human excellence or instance of human flourishing" (Yearley, 1990: 13). Character strengths are plural—that is, good character comprises a family of positive traits. Character strengths are *not* segregated mechanisms with automatic effects on behaviour. People can reflect on their own strengths of character and talk about them to others. Indeed, research appears to confirm that strengths are associated with a wide range of desirable psychological and behavioural outcomes. In research on individuals, Govindji and Linley (2007) found that people who used strengths more frequently experienced greater subjective and psychological well-being. Longitudinal research by Wood, Linley, Maltby, Kashdan, and Hurling (2011) confirmed that people who use their strengths experience less stress. Similar research by Linley, Nielsen, Wood, Gillett, and Biswas-Diener (2010) found that people who used their strengths were more likely to achieve their goals. Seligman, Steen, Park, and Peterson (2005) found that people who identify and use their strengths experienced higher levels of happiness and lower depression levels, even as much as 6 months after the intervention was concluded. These results were replicated in a small sample of university administrators in a study by Minhas (2010) who found that people who actively developed their strengths experienced increased well-being and elevated levels of self-esteem.

One of the most influential and ambitious projects undertaken in this field was the development of the Values in Action Classification of Strengths and Virtues (VIA-CSV; Peterson and Seligman, 2004). The VIA-CSV is intended to be a "manual of the sanities" by describing 24 character strengths that enable human flourishing, subsumed within six overarching virtues that are valued across cultures (wisdom, courage, humanity, justice, temperance, and transcendence).

Classification of 6 Virtues and 24 Strengths (Peterson and Seligman, 2004)

1. ***Wisdom and Knowledge*: Cognitive strengths that entail the acquisition and use of knowledge:**

   Creativity—Thinking of novel and productive ways to do things.

   Curiosity—Taking an interest in all of ongoing experience.

   Open-mindedness—Thinking things through and examining them from all sides.

   Love of learning—Mastering new skills, topics, and bodies of knowledge. Perspective being able to provide wise counsel to others.

2. ***Courage Emotional Strengths*:** That involves the exercise of will to accomplish goals in the face of opposition, external or internal:

   Authenticity—Speaking the truth and presenting oneself in a genuine way.

   Bravery—Not shrinking from threat, challenge, difficulty, or pain.

   Persistence—Finishing what one starts.

   Zest—Approaching life with excitement and energy.

3. ***Humanity*:** Interpersonal strengths that involve "tending and befriending" others:

   Kindness—Doing favours and good deeds for others.

   Love—Valuing close relations with others.

   Social intelligence—Being aware of the motives and feelings of self and others.

4. ***Justice*:** Civic strengths that underlie healthy community life:

   Fairness—Treating all people the same according to notions of fairness and justice.

   Leadership—Organizing group activities and seeing that they happen.

   Teamwork—Working well as member of a group or team.

5. ***Temperance*:** Strengths that protect against excess:

   Forgiveness—Forgiving those who have done wrong.

Modesty—Letting one's accomplishments, speak for themeselves.
Prudence—Being careful about one's choices; not saying or doing things that might later be regretted.
Self-regulation—Regulating what one feels and does.

6. ***Transcendence***: Strengths that forge connections to the larger universe and provide meaning:
Appreciation of beauty and excellence—Noticing and appreciating beauty, excellence, and/or skilled performance in all domains of life.
Gratitude—Being aware of and thankful for the good things that happen.
Hope—Expecting the best and working to achieve it.
Humour—Liking to laugh and tease; bringing smiles to other people.
Religiousness—Having coherent beliefs about the higher purpose and meaning of life.

Self-Regulation

The term "self-regulation" has many possible meanings, and definitions vary across authors and research areas. While the existence of multiple definitions can be confusing, the different kinds of self-regulation described in the literature can be easily understood as regions along a continuum going from comparatively simple and mindless control mechanisms to complex, hierarchical, and deliberate mental processes.

In the broadest sense, the concept of self-regulation applies to all forms of goal-directed behaviour (Carver and Scheier, 2011; Hofmann *et al*., 2012; Tops *et al*., 2010). It is important to realize that, by this definition, self-regulation does not require goals to be explicitly represented by the individual organism, even if the goal may be clearly observable by an outside observer.

Dennett (2009) has explained it clearly. He said that in very simple organisms, natural selection tracks the causal regularities that affect survival and reproduction, since those organisms that are better at utilizing the causal structure of their environment are also proved to be good at surviving and reproducing. As a result of this selection process, evolution equips organisms with machinery that supports effective goal-directed performance with no need for the individual organism to possess any representation of the underlying goals and causal properties. As organisms evolve more sophisticated nervous systems, however, goals and reasons may begin to be actively represented, even if only partially and implicitly. Evolution has provided humans with a remarkable ability to explicitly represent their goals (or at least some of them), communicate them and employ those representations to build detailed plans.

Self-regulation in the narrow sense defines it as a subset of behaviours—broadly defined to include cognitive operations in addition to body movements—whose main function is to change the probability of later behaviours by the same organism (Barkley, 2001). Some scholars refer to narrow-sense self-regulation as *self-control* (Carver and Scheier, 2011; Hofmann *et al.*, 2012). The most important component of narrow-sense self-regulation is *inhibition*, ability to override behaviours and responses that are not aligned with existing goals. Defined in this way, inhibition does not require explicit goal representations, although it requires the presence of multiple interacting control systems within the same organism. Simple forms of inhibition can take place in absence of a control hierarchy; when self-regulation processes become hierarchically organized whereas higher-order systems may acquire the ability to flexibly inhibit lower-order systems in the service of higher-order goals (Carver and Scheier, 2011; Filevich *et al.*, 2012; Kopp, 2012).

The human capacity for self-regulation appears to be much more extensive than what is found in other animals, which may suggest that the evolutionary pressures that guided the selection of traits that make up human nature, such as participation in cultural groups, found self-regulation to be especially adaptive and powerful (Baumeister, 2005). If so, then self-regulation may be one of the most distinctively human traits. Although human beings are capable of more self-regulation than other animals, however, their capacity is far less than the perceived ideal. Self-regulation failures can produce personal and social problems that will plague citizens in modern societies (Baumeister, Heatherton, and Tice, 1994).

In other words, self-regulation set the extent that alter the self's responses to achieve a desired state or outcome that otherwise would not arise naturally.

Self-regulation can be explained from various perspectives. One model of self-regulation describes this capacity in terms of *feedback loops* popularly known as TOTE loops, (test–operate–test–exit) (Carver and Scheier, 1981, 1998). According to this model, people test their current state in relation to internal standards. When an incongruity between the desired and current states is detected, people initiate actions to eliminate this discrepancy. Once the discrepancy is reduced, the self-regulation process enters the exit phase and is terminated. Competing models of self-regulation have been proposed. For example, one model views the capacity for self-regulation as a skill that remains constant and unchanged across consecutive attempts at self-control, and that can be increased gradually over time through practice. An alternative model conceptualizes self-regulation as a knowledge structure or schema that, when activated or primed, makes available other information that supports self-regulatory goals through the process of spreading activation.

Contrary to the skill and cognitive schema models, findings have confirmed that self-regulation suffers after an initial attempt at self-control, suggesting that an act of self-control consumes some limited resource.

The construct of *self-regulatory strength* is relevant at the stage, when a person detects a discrepancy and is ready to initiate actions to reduce it. The person must have the inner psychological resources (i.e., self-regulatory strength) to alter behaviour in a way that will bring him or her closer to internal standards or goals. This form of self-regulation is one important function of the executive system, which also subsumes other forms of volitional and active capabilities of the self, including planning and problem solving, goal-directed behaviour, decision making, as well as logical and intelligent thought. According to the strength model, depletion of limited self-regulatory resources should selectively undermine the controlled and deliberate operations of the executive system. In brief, the depletion of self-regulatory resources is contingent upon the operations of the active, but not upon the passive self.

Self-regulation theorists agree upon the major distinction of self-regulation into two broad components that capture the numerous cognitive, emotional, and behavioural challenges that must be resolved in goal pursuit: goal setting and goal striving (Carver and Scheier, 1982; Mischel, Cantor, and Feldman, 1996). Goal setting involves determining which goals one wants to pursue and the criteria for judging success. Depending on the setting and the individual, goal setting may be a fairly effortless and quick process or one that involves extensive deliberation and resource use.

Goal striving refers to planning and executing actions that promote goal attainment and shielding those goals from distraction or disruption. Although goal striving typically follows goal setting, there may be times when goal setting follows goal striving. Regardless of their temporal order, both goal setting and goal striving are necessary for successful self-regulation.

Interpersonal Processes

Various evidences suggest that the depletion of limited resources can have debilitating personal consequences. Interpersonal processes and behaviours that support social life also require self-regulatory resources and can be affected by depletion. People transform selfish impulses into behaviours that support group interests, pro-social behaviours, and adhere to rules and laws governing social life.

Accumulating research suggests that pro-social behaviours require a great deal of self-control. In a study, depleted participants were less willing to help. As evidenced by their responses to hypothetical scenarios and their unwillingness to volunteer their time to assist the victim of a tragedy (DeWall, Baumeister, Gailliot, and Maner, 2008). It is evinced that choosing pro-social over selfish motivations consumes resources.

Research from the other areas of psychology suggests that acts of benevolence can actually increase as a result of depletion. The self-regulatory depletion in turn mediated compliance with further requests for charitable acts (e.g. donating money or volunteering) due to a greater reliance on heuristic principles, such as likability or reciprocity (Fennis, Janssen, and Vohs, 2009). It can be concluded that performing charitable actions are dependent on the availability of limited self-regulatory resources.

Another study examined the effect of self-control on the emergence of anti-social behaviours and found that depleted participants were more likely to misrepresent their performance by falsely reporting fewer errors on a task and claiming a greater monetary reward for their performance (Mead, Baumeister, Gino, Schweitzer, and Ariely, 2009). Other socially damageing behaviours have also been shown to be affected by the depletion of resources. In a study, in comparison with non-depleted participants, depleted participants were more likely to aggress against others (DeWall, Baumeister, Stillman, and Gailliot, 2007).

Self-regulatory challenges of social and cultural life stem from the tendency to favour in group over outgroup members against the need to tolerate inter-individual and intergroup diversity. In this respect, in order to coexist peacefully, people must inhibit biases and stereotypes (e.g. those related to ethnicity, race, religion, or sexual orientation).

Processes that can facilitate effective interpersonal exchanges require self-control, confirmed by further researches. They showed that attempts to manage impressions or to present oneself in a manner that runs counter to one's natural tendencies is effortful and depletes limited self-regulation resources (Vohs, Baumeister, and Ciarocco, 2005). Studies have also shown that social interactions between people who share different features can entail self-regulatory costs. One study found that white participants who interacted with someone of a different race performed more poorly on a subsequent measure of executive attentional capacity in comparison to participants who engaged in a same-race interaction. It suggests that attempt to negotiate interracial exchanges effectively depletes self-regulation resources (Richeson and Shelton, 2003).

Other studies showed that different approaches to interracial interactions can augment these self-regulatory costs. One study found that participant instructed to avoid expressing prejudice during an interracial exchange performed worse on the Stroop colour-naming task than did participants instructed to focus on having a positive interracial exchange (Trawalter and Richeson, 2006). These findings suggest that resource depletion is not an inevitable consequence of interracial interactions, but that the goal to inhibit or suppress prejudices rather than to enhance the quality of the interaction can have self-regulatory costs.

Other studies has shown that suppressing stereotypes draws on limited self-regulation resources and can thus be undermined by depletion (Govorun and Payne, 2006), as well as interfere with subsequent attempts at self-control (Gordijn, Hindriks, Koomen, Dijksterhuis, and Van Knippenberg, 2004). The suppression of stereotypes has been shown to undermine self-control particularly among people with a low motivation to suppress stereotypes (Gailliot, Plant, Butz, and Baumeister, 2007). Interpersonal interactions can require high or low social coordination, depending on whether the interaction is characterized by high or low maintenance, respectively. In contrast to low-maintenance interactions, high-maintenance interactions require considerable effort to achieve social coordination. Given the effortful and challenging nature of high-maintenance interactions, people may, therefore, be tempted to withdraw from such interactions or to express their impatience or frustration (Finkel *et al.*, 2006). In brief, high maintenance interpersonal encounters depleted self-regulation resources. These findings suggest that prosocial or relationship enhancing behaviours heavily rely on a limited resource, and a depleted state can interfere with capacity to override selfish and anti-social responses in favour of socially desirable responses. In can be concluded that self-regulatory strength is necessary if people are to use their inner restraints in the service of elevating prosocial goals over selfish impulses and desires.

Regulation of Interpersonal Behaviour

In addition to the general-purpose non-specific self-regulatory systems, people also possess mechanisms that are dedicated to particular functions. Such mechanisms operate in a specific range of situations and handle only limited kind of regulatory problem. One such mechanism, the *socio-meter* appears to be involved in the control of interpersonal behaviour. Previous writings and research related to socio-meter have clearly demonstrated its connection to self-esteem, but, its functions go far beyond simply affecting how people feel about themselves (Leary and Baumeister, 2000). The fundamental prerequisite of interpersonal life is that a person be minimally accepted by other people and avoid wholesale rejection. Virtually all social relationship such as friendship, group memberships, and pair-bonds—require the individual to be accepted by others. Because of the adaptive advantages of being accepted by other people, human beings possess a strong need for acceptance and belonging (Baumeister and Leary, 1995). Since social acceptance and rejection have vital importance throughout evolution, human beings have developed a psychological system that monitors and responds to events that are relevant to interpersonal acceptance and rejection. Thus, a module that evolved to facilitate acceptance and avoid rejection would be expected to respond to cues indicating real or potential rejection, evoke feelings that alert the individual to the threat, and motivate the person to behave in ways that minimize the probability of rejection and promote acceptance.

According to socio-meter theory, people possess a socio-meter that monitors the interpersonal environment for cues that are relevant to a person's relational value in the eyes of other people—the degree to which other people regard their relationships with the individual as valuable or important (Leary, 2002). Rejection and acceptance are the end points on a continuum of relational value.

People are exceptionally sensitive to events that have implications for their relational value (Weisbuch, Sinclair, Skorinko, and Eccleston, 2009). People monitor the environment for cues relevant to their relational value on a preattentive level. For example, the cocktail party effect, in which a person orients towards his or her name in the noisy hubbub of a party or Cherry's (1953) demonstration about non-conscious vigilance for indications of how one is regarded by others. Furthermore, people think a good deal about other people's perceptions and evaluations of them and try to anticipate how others will react to them in future situations.

The affective output of the socio-meter serves accurately these functions. Indications about being approved or that one's relational value is high, lead to positive affect. Indications that one is disapproved of or that one's relational value is low, lead to negative affect. Studies in this regard have shown that perceived rejection (i.e., low relational value) is associated with negative emotions such as hurt feelings, jealousy, and sadness, with increased attention to the problematic interpersonal situation (Leary, Koch, and Hechenbleikner, 2001).

Typically, whenever people experience acceptance and rejection, they also feel good or bad about themselves. Socio-meter theory suggests that these self-relevant feelings—state self-esteem—are part of this regulatory system (Leary, 2006). When the socio-meter detects cues that have unacceptably low relational value, it not only triggers negative affect but also started a process to assess whether one's low relational value is due to some personal action, shortcomings, or deficiency. People are generally vigilant about the possibility that their low relational value is at least partly their own fault, which leads them to feel bad about themselves. However, when people are certain that their exclusion by other people does not reflect on them personally, their state self-esteem is unaffected (Leary, Tambor, Terdal, and Downs, 1995). These effects on self-esteem have been demonstrated cross-culturally. Countries in which people have frequent interactions with friends found to be higher nationwide self-esteem than countries without strong social practices, even when researchers control for happiness, individualism, neuroticism, and economic factors (Denissen, Penke, Schmitt, and van Aken, 2008).

Research supports the idea that people possess a regulatory mechanism that responds to changes in relational value, and the concept of a socio-meter provides a framework for conceptualizing a variety of phenomena, such as self-esteem, interpersonal emotions, and reactions to rejection.

Social Relationship

Over the past decade, a growing body of research has emerged to support the idea that social relationships have strong and wide-ranging effects on people's self-regulatory success (see Vohs and Finkel, 2006).

The fact that many acts of self-regulation occur within social contexts, the consequences of self-regulation likely extend beyond self-directed accomplishments to social and interpersonal relationships.

In a situation of high rate of everyday interdependence of most close relationship partners, the self-regulation abilities of one partner have also implications for the other partner (Kelley, 1979). If one partner struggles with self-control, the other partner also suffers. Low levels of self-regulatory strength are likely a major vulnerability in a close relationship partner, while high levels are likely a major asset.

Individuals vary in the degree to which they can self-regulate successfully in everyday life. According to one influential model, exertions of self-regulation depend upon a limited, unitary resource, *self-regulatory strength* (Baumeister, Vohs, and Tice, 2007; Muraven and Baumeister, 2000). Just as some individuals have more physical strength than others, in the similar way some individuals have more self-regulatory strength, more reserves of this limited capacity to engage in self-control efforts than others.

Many researchers have demonstrated that individual differences in self-regulatory strength have important implications for interpersonal relationships. Scholars have measured these individual differences to assess the degree to which individuals are successful at regulating their thoughts, feelings, or behaviours in a goal-directed manner with various approaches. In researches employing self-reports, participants indicate their agreement with items assessing general self-regulatory success. Such research demonstrates that individuals who report greater (or lesser) self-regulatory success in general also report superior relationship functioning. They respond to partner offenses more constructively and less violently, experience less family conflict and less anger, and have better communication skills (Finkel and Campbell, 2001; Finkel, DeWall, Slotter, Oaten, and Foshee, 2009; Tangney, Baumeister, and Boone, 2004).

In some researches assessing individual differences in self-regulatory strength with cognitive tasks, participants perform a computer-based task assessing their facility at overriding automatic cognitive responses. Research demonstrates that individuals who exhibit strong (or weak) self-regulatory ability on these cognitive tasks tend to be more polite and less interpersonally offensive (von Hippel and Gonsalkorale, 2005).

In researches assessing individual differences in self-regulatory strength with behavioural tasks, participants are exposed to laboratory-based task assessing their success at resisting the urge to enact a tempting behaviour that is counter-productive to their longer term self goal. In some approaches researchers presented a dilemma to young children (Mischel, 1974). In one study, the number of seconds children delayed gratification, predicted their parents' assessments of their ability to maintain friendships 10 years later (Mischel, Shoda, and Peake, 1988). In another research, the length of time the children delayed gratification predicted their teacher's positive assessments of their interpersonal functioning (Ayduk *et al.*, 2000). The ability to delay gratification did not predict interpersonal functioning among socially secure children.

Behaviour Change

Models of health behaviour, for example, Social Cognitive Theory (SCT), Bandura (1986); the Theory of Planned Behaviour (TPB), Ajzen (1991), the Theory of Reasoned Action (TRA), Ajzen and Fishbein (1980), have focused on demonstrating how people determine whether to adopt a given behaviour. The decision to adopt a new behaviour is dependent upon an analysis of the relative costs and benefits associated with different courses of action. These theoretical perspectives have primarily been used to explain why people engage in a particular unhealthy or healthy behavioural practice. Limited consideration has been given to an ongoing sequence of behaviours. For example, TRA (Ajzen and Fishbein, 1980) and TPB (Ajzen, 1991) make no distinction between decisions regarding the initiation of a behaviour and in those regarding the maintenance of that behaviour over time. Investigators have used these approaches to examine long-term behavioural outcomes, but focused narrowly on whether people's behavioural practices become sufficiently stable, as if behaviour is a function of itself and not contingent on a set of mediating variables (Ajzen, 2002; Wood, Quinn, and Kashy, 2002).

According to SCT (Bandura, 1986), self-efficacy beliefs are principle determinant of both the initiation and the maintenance of a change in behaviour. Confidence in one's ability to take decisions serves to sustain effort in the presence of challenges. The successful implementation of changes in behaviour boosts people's confidence, which in turn facilitates further action, whereas experiences of failure serve to undermine personal feelings of efficacy.

But behaviour change involves not only adopting a new pattern of behaviour, but also curbing a prior pattern of behaviour. Several researchers have argued (Baumeister, Heatherton, and Tice, 1994; Muraven and Baumeister, 2000) that to override, inhibit, or alter a dominant response tendency, people must possess a sufficient degree of self-regulatory strength, conceptualized as a limited, but renewable, cognitive resource that is drained whenever someone attempts to regulate his or her emotions, thoughts, or behaviour. Since deficits in self-regulatory strength are seem to be a primary determinant of self-regulatory failure, relapses are predicted to be more likely when people are faced with repeated demands to manage their thoughts, feelings, or behaviour. Support for this position has been obtained from a series of empirical investigations across a range of domains (e.g. Baumeister, Bratslavsky, Muraven, and Tice, 1998; Muraven, Tice, and Baumeister, 1998).

References

Allport, G.W. (1958). *Becoming: Basic Considerations for a Psychology of Personality.* Oxford, England: Verlag.

Ayduk, O., Mendoza-Denton, R., Mischel, W., Downey, G., Peake, P.K., and Rodriguez, M. (2000). Regulating the interpersonal self: Strategic self-regulation for coping with rejection sensitivity. *Journal of Personality and Social Psychology, 79*, 776-792.

Ajzen, I. (1991). The theory of planned behaviour. *Orgcnizational Behaviour and Human Decision Processes, 50*, 179-211.

Ajzen, I. (2002). Residual effects of past on later behaviour: Habituation and reasoned action perspectives. *Personality and Social Psychology Review, 6*, 107-122.

Azjen, I., and Fishbein, M. (1980). *Understanding Attitudes and Predicting Social Behaviour.* Englewood Cliffs, NJ: Prentice Hall.

Bandura, A. (1986). *Social Foundations of Thought and Action: A Social Cognitive Theory*. Englewood Cliffs, NJ: Prentice Hall.

Barkley, R.A. (2001). The executive functions and self-regulation: An evolutionary neuropsychological perspective. *Neuropsychology Review, 11*, 1-29.doi:10.1023/A:1009085417776.

Baumeister, R.F., Bratslavsky, E., Muraven, M., and Tice, D.M. (1998). Ego depletion: Is the active self a limited resource? *Journal of Personality and Social Psychology, 74*, 1152-1265.

Baumeister, R.F., Heatherton, T.F., and Tice, D.M. (1994). *Losing Control: How and why People Fail at Self-regulation.* San Diego, CA: Academic Press.

Baumeister, R.F., and Leary, M.R. (1995). The need to belong: Desire for interpersonal attachments as a fundamental human motivation. *Psychological Bulletin, 117*, 497-529.

Baumeister, R.F., Vohs, K.D., and Tice, D.M. (2007): The strength model of self-control. *Current Directions in Psychological Science, 16*, 351-355.

Biswas-Diener, R., and Diener, E. (2001). Making the best of a bad situation: Satisfaction in the slums of Calcutta. *Social Indicators Research, 55*, 329-352.

Cameron, K.S., Dutton, J.E., and Quinn, R.E. (Eds.). (2003). *Positive Organizational Scholarship: Foundations of a New Discipline.* San Francisco: Berrett-Koehler.

Carver, C.S., and Scheier, M.F. (1981). *Attention and Self-regulation: A control theory approach to Human Behaviour*. New York: Springer.

Carver, C.S., and Scheier, M.F. (1982). Control Theory: A Useful Conceptual Framework for Personality—Social, Clinical, and Health Psychology. *Psychological Bulletin, 92*, 111-135.

Carver, C.S., and Scheier, M.F. (1998). *On the Self-regulation of Behaviour.* New York, NY: Cambridge University Press.

Carver, C.S., and Scheier, M.F. (2011). Self-regulation of action and affect. In K.D. Vohs and R.F. Baumeister (Eds.), *Handbook of Self-Regulation: Research, Theory, and Applications*—2nd edition (pp. 3-21). New York: Guilford.

Cherry, E.C. (1953). Some experiments on the recognition of speech, with one and with two ears. *Journal of Acoustical Society of America, 25*, 975-979.

Cowan, E. (2000). Psychological Wellness: Some hopes for the future. In D. Cicchetti, J. Rappaport, I. Sandler, and R.P. Weissberg (Eds.), *The Promotion of Wellness in Adolescents* (pp. 477-503).

Deci, E.L., and Ryan, R.M. (1985). *Intrinsic Motivation and Self-determination in Human Behaviour.* New York: Plenum Press.

Denissen, J.J.A., Penke, L., Schmitt, D.P., and van Aken, M.A.G. (2008). Self-esteem reactions to social interactions: Evidence for socio-meter mechanisms across days, people, and nations. *Journal of Personality and Social Psychology, 95*, 181-196.

Dennett, D. (2009). Darwin's "strange inversion of reasoning". *Proceedings of the National Academy of Sciences USA, 106*, 10061-10065. doi:10.1073/pnas.0904433106.

DeWall, C.N., Baumeister, R.F., Gailliot, M.T., and Maner, J.K. (2008). Depletion makes the heart grow less helpful: Helping as a function of self-regulatory energy and genetic relatedness. *Personality and Social Psychology Bulletin, 34*, 1653-1662.

DeWall, C.N., Baumeister, R.F., Stillman, T.F., and Gailliot, M.T. (2007). Violence restrained: Effects of self-regulatory capacity and its depletion on aggressive behaviour. *Journal of Experimental Social Psychology, 43*, 62-76.

Easterbrook (2003). *The Progress Paradox: How Life Gets Better while People Feel Worse.* New York: Random House.

Erikson, E. (1963). *Childhood and Society* (2nd ed.). New York: Norton. Erikson, E. (1982). *The Life Cycle Completed.* New York: Norton.

Fennis, B.M., Janssen, L., and Vohs, K.D. (2009). Acts of benevolence: A limited-resource account of compliance with charitable requests. *Journal of Consumer Research, 35*, 906-924.

Filevich, E., Kühn, S., and Haggard, P. (2012). Intentional inhibition in human action: The power of 'no'. *Neuroscience and Biobehavioural Reviews, 36*, 1107-1118.doi:10.1016/j.neubiorev.2012.01.006.

Finkel, E.J., and Campbell, W.K. (2001). Self-control and accommodation in close relationships: An interdependence analysis. *Journal of Personality and Social Psychology, 81*, 263-277.

Finkel, E.J., Campbell, W.K., Brunell, A.B., Dalton, A.N., Scarbeck, S.J., and Chartrand, T.L. (2006). High-maintenance interaction: Inefficient social coordination impairs self-regulation. *Journal of Personality and Social Psychology, 91*, 456-475.

Finkel, E.J., DeWall, C.N., Slotter, E.B., Oaten, M., and Foshee, V.A. (2009). Self-regulatory failure and intimate partner violence perpetration. *Journal of Personality and Social Psychology, 97*, 483-499.

Gailliot, M.T., Plant, E.A., Butz, D.A., and Baumeister, R.F. (2007). Increasing self-regulatory strength can reduce the depleting effect of suppressing stereotypes. *Personality and Social Psychology Bulletin, 33*, 281-294.

Gardner, H., Csikszentmihalyi, M., and Damon, W. (2001). *Good Work: When Excellence and Ethics Meet*. New York: Basic Books.

Gordijn, E.H., Hindriks, I., Koomen, W., Dijksterhuis, A., and Van Knippenberg, A. (2004). Consequences of stereotype suppression and internal suppression motivation: A self-regulation approach. *Personality and Social Psychology Bulletin, 30*, 212-224.

Govindji, R., and Linley, A. (2007). Strengths use, self-concordance and well-being: Implications for strengths coaching and coaching psychologists. *International Coaching Psychology Review, 2*, 143-153.

Govorun, O., and Payne, K.B. (2006). Ego-depletion and prejudice: Separating automatic and controlled components. *Social Cognition, 24*, 111-136.

Hofmann, W., Schmeichel, B.J., and Baddeley, A.D. (2012). Executive functions and self-regulation. *Trends in Cognitive Sciences, 16*, 174-180. doi:10.1016/j.tics.2012.01.006

Jahoda, M. (1958). *Current Concepts of Positive Mental Health*. New York: Basic Books.

Kahneman, D., Diener, E., and Schwarz, N. (Eds.). (1999). *Well-being: The Foundations of Hedonic Psychology*. New York: Russell Sage Foundation.

Kelley, H.H. (1979). *Personal Relationships: Their Structure and Processes*. Hillsdale, NJ: Erlbaum.

Kopp, B. (2012). A simple hypothesis of executive function. *Frontiers in Human Neuroscience, 6*, 159. doi:10.3389/fnhum.2012.00159.

Linley, P.A., Nielsen, K.M., Wood, A.M., Gillett, R., and Biswas-Diener, R. (2010). Using signature strengths in pursuit of goals: Effects on goal progress, need satisfaction, and well-being, and implications for coaching psychologists. *International Coaching Psychology Review, 5*, 6-15.

Leary, M.R. (2002). The interpersonal basis of self-esteem: Death, devaluation, or deference? In J. Forgas and K.D. Williams (Eds.), *The Social Self: Cognitive, Interpersonal, and Intergroup Perspectives* (pp. 143-159). New York: Psychology Press.

Leary, M.R. (2006). Socio-meter theory and the pursuit of relational value: Getting to the root of self-esteem. *European Review of Social Psychology, 16*, 75-111.

Leary, M.R., and Baumeister, R.F. (2000). The nature and function of self-esteem:

Socio-meter theory. In M.P. Zanna (Ed.), *Advances in Experimental Social Psychology* (Vol. 32, pp. 1-62). San Diego, CA: Academic Press.

Leary, M.R., Koch, E., and Hechenbleikner, N. (2001). Emotional responses to interpersonal rejection. In M.R. Leary (Ed.), *Interpersonal Rejection* (pp. 145-166). New York: Oxford University Press.

Leary, M.R., Tambor, E., Terdal, S., and Downs, D.L. (1995). Self-esteem as an interpersonal monitor: The Socio-meter Hypothesis. *Journal of Personality and Social Psychology, 68*, 518-530.

Maslow, A.H. (1954). *Motivation and Personality.* New York: Harper & Row.

Maslow, A.H. (1962). *Toward a Psychology of Being.* Princeton, NJ: Van Nostrand.

Maslow, A.H. (1968). *Toward a Psychology of Being.* New York: Van Nostrand.

McCullough, M.E., and Snyder, C.R. (2000). Classical sources of human strength: Revisiting an old home and building a new one. *Journal of Social and Clinical Psychology, 19*, 1-10.

Minhas, G (2010). Developing realised and unrealized strengths: Implications for engagement, self-esteem, life satisfaction and well-being. *Assessment and Development Matters, 2*, 12-16.

Mischel, W. (1974). Processes in delay of gratification. Berkowitz, L. (Ed.), *Advances in Experimental Social Psychology* (Vol. 7, pp. 249-292). New York: Academic Press.

Mischel, W., Shoda, Y., and Peake, P.K. (1988). The nature of adolescent competencies predicted by preschool delay of gratification. *Journal of Personality and Social Psychology, 54*, 687-696.

Mischel, W., Cantor, N., and Feldman, S. (1996). Principles of Self-regulation: The nature of willpower and self-control. In E.T. Higgins and A. Kruglanski (Eds.), *Social Psychology: Handbook of Basic Principles,* (pp. 329-360). New York, NY: Guilford.

Muraven, M.R., and Baumeister, R.F. (2000). Self-regulation and depletion of limited resources: Does self-control resemble a muscle? *Psychological Bulletin, 126*, 247-259.

Muraven, M., Tice, D.M., and Baumeister, R. (1998). Self-control as limited resource: Regulatory depletion patterns. *Journal of Personality and Social Psychology, 74*, 774-789.

Murray, C. (2003). *Human accomplishment: The Pursuit of Excellence in the Arts and Sciences, 800 B.C. to 1950.* New York: Harper Collins.

Myers, D.G (2000). The funds, friends, and faith of happy people. *American Psychologist, 55*, 56-67.

Peterson, C., and Park, N. (2003). Positive psychology as the even handed positive psychologist views it. *Psychological Inquiry, 14*, 141-146.

Peterson, C., and Seligman, M.E.P. (2004). *Character Strengths and Virtues: A Handbook and Classification.* Oxford, England: Oxford University Press.

Peterson, C., Park, N., and Seligman, M.E.P. (2005a). Assessment of character strengths. In G.P. Koocher, J.C. Norcross, and S.S. Hill III (Eds.),

Psychologists' Desk Reference (2nd ed., pp. 93-98). New York, NY: Oxford University Press.

Proctor, C., Maltby, J., and Linley, P.A. (2009). Strengths use as a predictor of well-being and health-related quality of life. *Journal of Happiness Studies, 10*, 583-630.

Richeson, J.A., and Shelton, J.N. (2003). When prejudice does not pay: Effects of interracial contact on executive function. *Psychological Science, 14*, 287-290.

Rogers, C.R. (1951). *Client-centered Therapy: Its Current Practice, Implications, and Theory.* Boston: Houghton Mifflin.

Ryff, C.D., and Singer, B. (1996). Psychological well-being: Meaning, measurement, and implications for psychotherapy research. *Psychotherapy and Psychosomatics, 65*, 14-23.

Seligman, M.E.P. (1999). The President's address. *American Psychologist, 54*, 559-562.

Seligman, M.E.P., and Csikszentmihalyi, M. (2000). Positive Psychology: An introduction. *American Psychologist, 55*, 5-14.

Seligman, M., Steen, T., Park, N., and Peterson, C. (2005). Positive Psychology Progress: Empirical Validation of Interventions. *American Psychologist, 60*, 410-421.

Sheldon, K.M., and King, L. (2001). Why Positive Psychology is necessary. *American Psychologist, 56*, 216-217.

Tangney, J.P., Baumeister, R.F., and Boone, A.L. (2004). High self-control predicts good adjustment, less pathology, better grades, and interpersonal success. *Journal of Personality, 72*, 271-322.

Tops, M., Boksem, M.A.S., Luu, P., and Tucker, D.M. (2010). Brain substrates of behavioural programmes associated with self-regulation. *Frontiers in Psychology, 1*, 152. doi:10.3389/fpsyg.2010.00152.

Trawalter, S., and Richeson, J.A. (2006). Regulatory focus and executive function after interracial interactions. *Journal of Experimental Social Psychology, 42*, 406-412.

Vaillant, G.E. (1977). *Adaptation to Life.* Boston: Little, Brown.

Vaillant, G.E. (2000). Adaptive Mental Mechanisms: Their role in a positive psychology. *American Psychologist, 55*, 89-98.

Vohs, K.D., Baumeister, R.F., and Ciarocco, N. (2005). Self-regulation and Self-presentation: Regulatory resource depletion impairs impression management and effortful self-presentation depletes regulatory resources. *Journal of Personality and Social Psychology, 88*, 632-657.

Vohs, K.D., and Finkel, E.J. (Eds.). (2006). Self and Relationships: Connecting intrapersonal and interpersonal processes. New York: Guilford Press. *Journal of Personality and Social Psychology, 79*, 776-792.

von Hippel, W., and Gonsalkorale, K. (2005). "That is bloody revolting!": Inhibitory control of thoughts better left unsaid. *Psychological Science, 16*, 497-500.

Washington, DC: Child Welfare League of America Press. Diener, E., and Diener, C. (1996). Most people are happy. *Psychological Science, 7*, 181-185.

Wood, A.M., Linley, P.A., Maltby, J., Kashdan, T.B., and Hurling, R. (2011). Using psychological strengths leads to less stress and greater self-esteem, vitality, and positive affect: Longitudinal examination of the strengths use questionnaire. *Personality and Individual Differences, 50*, 15-19.

Wood, W., and Neal, D.T. (2007). A new look at habits and the habit–goal interface. *Psychological Review, 114*, 843-863.

Wood, W., Quinn, J.M., and Kashy, D.A. (2002). Habits in everyday life: Thought, emotion, and action. *Journal of Personality and Social Psychology, 83*, 1281-1297.

Yearley, L.H. (1990). *Mencius and Aquinas: Theories of Virtue and Conceptions of Courage.* Albany, NY: State University of New York Press.

4

Meaning in Life

An Overview

Reeta Chauhan, Purnima Awasthi and *Saroj Verma*

Recent years have been recognized for growing concern about youths' health and psychological well-being in relation to goal or purpose in their life. Studies considering the concept of meaning in life have investigated it as an indicator of health and well-being. The concept of meaning in life describes the significance of one's life. It represents the natural need for people to draw conscious meaning in their lives to live a healthy and well-adapted life and efforts to generate a sense of significance and purpose in life. Studies reveal that meaning in life is an important construct for both clinical and normal population. It plays a significant role in the development of life's goal of an individual and plays its crucial role during crisis. Meaning in life works as resource for individuals, which help them in adopting appropriate coping processes in adverse conditions that may come in their lives. Studies regarding presence and search of meaning in life indicate that in most of the studies higher search of meaning in life is associated with maladaptive psychosocial functioning of individuals while higher presence of meaning in life contributes to adaptive psychosocial functioning and associated with greater sense of well-being. Studies that cover the patients suffering from chronic illness show that meaning in life acts as a buffer during stressful situations.

During last few decades several books have presented the description about the construct of meaning in life. Some of them such as *Man's Search for Meaning* (Frankl, 1976), *Meaning and Void: Inner Experience and the Incentives in People's Lives* (Klinger, 1977), *Meaning of Life* (Baumeister, 1991), *The Search for Meaning* (Naylor, Willimon & Naylor, 1994), and *The Human Quest for Meaning: Theories, Research, and Applications* (Wong, 2013) etc. provide detailed information for the concept of meaning in life. Meaning of life is a broad term about the ultimate purpose of life which has its root in philosophy. Most of the books centred to this ultimate quest for life's meaning. Meaning in life is about the significance of one's life. Authors explain meaning in life with the help of external and internal motivational factors in terms of individuals' behaviour they exhibit in crucial life circumstances. The studies carried out during the last decade were tremendous and related to diverse spheres and different strata of human life such as religion, health, work, education, mental health and life satisfaction and indicate the importance of meaning in life in enhancing health and well-being of people.

Methodology

This chapter focuses on the empirical work carried out during the last ten years (2004-2014) in the field of health and well-being describing the relationship between meaning in life and health and well-being. Science Direct, Springer, Jstor and Google Scholar were searched for studies related to meaning in life and its association with individuals' mental health and well-being.

Search keys such as meaning in life, sense of coherence, purpose in life, sense of meaning in life, meaningfulness, presence and search of meaning in life, meaning in life and well-being/mental health/physical health/psychosocial functioning/life satisfaction/adolescents/cancer/smoking/internalizing and externalizing problem/suicide/personality/mediator/moderator/attachment etc. are used to search the relevant articles. The studies associated with gerontology and organizational psychology is excluded from this review.

Meaning in Life

The construct of meaning in life has been defined by several researchers in terms of belief in a purposeful pattern of the universe, which in turn can be defined from religion and/or spirituality (Yalom, 1980). According to Frankl (1984) it represents the natural need for people to find conscious meaning in their lives to live a healthy and well-adapted life and includes the main motivational principle that describes struggle for a sense of significance and purpose in life. It deals with the cognizance of order, the pursuit and attainment of worthwhile goals, an accompanying sense of fulfilment coherence, and purpose in one's existence (Reker and Wong,

1988: 221). Purpose in life can be considered as a feeling of people for their meaning to present and past life goals in life with a sense of directedness and upholding a belief that gives purpose to the life (Ryff, 1989). The pursuit and achievement of meaningful goals is commonly associated with the attainment of meaning in life (Baumeister, 1991; Reker, 2000). Meaning in life can be considered as a positively balanced framework of beliefs about the coherence of the world and one's own life which bring a sense of wonder and joy in living (Shwartzberg and Janoff-Bulman, 1991). Meaning in life can be considered as the belief and sense that life is meaningful (Ryff and Keyes, 1995), and "....at its heart it refers to people's beliefs that their lives are significant and that they transcend the ephemeral present" (Steger, 2009: 680).

By looking above definitions of meaning in life one can assume the diversity of conceptualization. All definitions are indicating towards a single construct, i.e. meaning in life. Its emergence in intellectual world can be traced with emergence of existential philosophy. Existential philosophers and psychologists have long argued that the experience of meaning lies at the heart of human existence. Every individual has own philosophy of life and perceptions regarding the meaningfulness of his/her life. Frankl (1959/2006: 110-113) emphasized that meaning in life differs from individual to individual and it always changes but never ceases. He asserts that a will-to-meaning is the basic sustenance of existence (Frankl, 1967, 1969), i.e. a primary motivation in an individual's life.

Human being has two aspects of life, one is biological and the other is cultural. In cultural domain language play a key linking role in sharing and communicating thoughts and feelings of individuals. One of the most integral part and ultimate goals of language is to convey the right meaning which is intended. Higher cognitive processes such as thinking involve meaning, symbols and connections between concepts. Meaning means the same thing, i.e. mental representations of expected relationships. These mental representations include anything that one may expect to be related to anything as well as people, places, objects, events in any way that they can interpret as related to concerned phenomena. It may be causally, spatial temporally as well as teleologically (teleos means complete or a meaningful life is a purpose-driven life). When individuals meet something that is not presently related to an existing frame of meaningful associations, it will be meaningless. It becomes meaningful once an association is revealed or forced (Proulex and Heine, 2006).

Well-being phenomena cover two approaches within self such as hedonic and eudiamonic approach of well-being. It is well known that hedonic approach focuses on the subjective happiness or positive mood, while eudiamonic approach focuses on a deeper sense of flourishing. Meaning in life has been recognized as a basic dimension of eudiamonic well-being. From this perspective, Ryff and Keyes (1995) anticipated meaning in life as a critical component of mental health and personal growth.

Stress and coping literature considers meaning in life as a person's belief about meaningfulness and purposefulness of one's own life. Reker and Wong (1988) proposed meaning in life as cognitive phenomenon with motivational and affective consequences which regulates the impact of stress on health or act as a buffer. Park and Folkman (1997) discriminate meaning as global and situational. Global meaning refers to individuals' general orienting system (Pargament, 1997), which allows them to observe their current reality, imagine alternative realities, interpret the past, anticipate the future and then direct their behaviour accordingly. Situational meaning is related to specific experiences of life events.

As such global meaning has potent impact on health and emotional well-being in both ordinary times and times of crisis. In stressful encounters, global meaning informs the ways people appraise the significance of situations in terms of their relevance and implications (Lazarus and Folkman, 1984). Global meaning system includes beliefs, goals and subjective feelings of purpose or meaning in life (Dittman-Kohli and Westerhof, 2000; Park and Folkman, 1997). These are the core schemas through which people interpret their experiences including beliefs. Goals may be desired future states or states already possessed that one desires to maintain (Karoly, 1999; Klinger, 1998). Global goals are internal representations of ultimate concerns (Emmons, 2005). The last part of this system, i.e. subjective sense of meaning refers to feeling of meaningfulness, direction or purpose in life.

Need of Meaning

Need of Meaning is underpinned with developmental phenomenon. As in infancy humans do not individuate self from other. The attendant "oceanic feeling" (Freud, 1930/1991: 252) is thus linked with security and well-being, and constitutes a state that people implicitly and eternally long to re-experience. Meaning frameworks begin as prelinguistic networks of related propositions (Bruner, 1990), and the cognitive mechanism that establishes systems of expected association that actives from the moment of birth (Walton and Bower, 1993). Infants are innately capable of differentiating different visual pattern (pattern recognition), and auditory stimuli, with time these observed regularities in our environment form the basis for complex systems for relations that we subsequently come to implicitly expect. As the cognitive ability enhances, the innate associative mechanism is applied to gradually more complex elements of our internal and external environments, resulting in mental representations of expected relations that become broader and abstract (Murphy and Medin, 1985). The emergence of self-concept (Harter, 1996) and development of theory of mind (Tomasello, Kruger, and Ratner, 1993) in childhood are the consequent of such type of processes. Inconsistent or incoherent (away from expected relation) novel experience becomes meaningless for an individual.

Sources of Meaning in Life

Sources of meaning are derived from activities and experiences that further can enhance meaning pertaining to particular events. It does not constitute meaning but provide a sense of meaning. Sources of meaning may comprise of family, one's capacities, carrier, personal relationships, social activism, religion and many more depends on an individual lives. In older adults, it is well documented that sense of meaning is significantly associated with worship service attendance. The association of religious belief and social support in such activities provide a sense of identity which may cause better mental health (Elliot and Hayward, 2007; Krause, 2003). Study indicates that loving God (images of loving God) enhances the sense of purpose in life (Stroop, Draper and Whitehead, 2013). Similarly, in another study on Muslim students, religion emerged as an important source of meaning. Mohamad, Abd Razak, and Mutiu (2011) investigated about meaning in life with the help of semi-structured interview comprised different themes (Meaning is to serve God's purpose, Life as a test, Meaning as a virtue etc.). They reported that meaning in life is an external factor for them and religion is an important source of meaning in their life.

Among these sources of meaning, experiences in nature/nature connectedness, i.e. "individual's experiential sense of oneness with natural world" has been emerged as a significant source of meaning especially for middle and older adults (Mayer and Frantz, 2004: 504; Reker and Woo, 2011). It is argued that nature connectedness is directly related to search for meaning and happiness. The extent to which nature provides feeling of connectedness and continuity in this temporary world can enhance one's sense of meaning and this in turn provides greater satisfaction and well-being. Nature connectedness enhances meaning in life and those who feel highly connected with nature extract greater sense of well-being. Meaning in life also act as a mediator between nature connectedness and well-being (Cervinka, Roderer and Hefler, 2012; Howell, Passmore and Buro, 2013; Nisbet, Zelenski and Murphy, 2011).

Development and Maintenance of Meaning

Different psychologists propose different notions of development and maintenance of meaning of people. Viktor Frankl (1988, 1992) developed Logotherapy as a theoretical system of understanding the way people develop and maintain meaning in their lives. Frankl (1992) emphasized three types of values such as experiential values, creative values and attitudinal values through which a person can find meaning. What a person learns through the experience of life comes under the experiential values (e.g. enjoying music, scenery or building positive relationship), what a person creates and contributes to life have creative values (e.g. building home, defending belief) and attitudinal values, through what an individual decides freely to do, when confronted with inevitable suffering or an irreversible situation (Frankl, 1988). Even if suffering inhibits an individual from experiencing meaning, s/he can always turn to an ultimate value and draw meaning from it. Frankl (1992) emphasized the importance of attitudinal values, considering that people are ready and willing to sustain suffering, as long as they can find a meaning in it. According to Battista and Almond (1973), a sense of coherence in life can provide meaning in life. Concept of sense of coherence includes a meaningfulness dimension, which is a significant factor regulating the impact of stress on health (Zika and Chamberlain, 1992: 134).

On the other hand, Reker and Wong (1988) affirm that the pursuit and attainment of worthwhile goals can cause meaning in life. They systematically define meaning in terms of the PURE model (Wong, 2010). PURE model underline the four crucial components that refer to Purpose, Understanding, Responsible action, and Enjoyment/Evaluation. It is assumed that absent or lack of any of these components may lead to a meaningless life. These components entail the four major psychological processes for living the good life such as motivational (purpose, life goals, needs), cognitive (understanding, making sense of life, life framework), social/moral (responsibility, accountability, commitment), and affective (enjoyment/evaluation, positive emotions, feeling of fulfilment).

Ryff and Singer (1998) assume that goal directedness can lead to meaning in one's life. Ryff (1989; Ryff and Keyes, 1995) proposed and tested a theoretical model of psychological well-being that includes six dimensions of wellness, one of which is purpose in life. Baumeister (1991) has proposed that there are four needs for meaning that human seek to fullfil in order to view their lives meaningful. Through the need for self-efficacy, values in life, purpose in life, and self-worth people can achieve meaning in life. The need for purpose is concerned with goals. The framework of goals provides a readymade template for the creation of meaningful life narratives. This need of purpose causally connects temporally distal events with each other and this causal interpretive approache is used as means of coping by chronic illness patients (Baumeister and Newman, 1994; Taylor, 1983).

Meaning in Life and Well-being

Meaning in life is a positive psychological variable. Martin Seligman defines the meaningful life as "using your signature strengths and virtues in the service of something much larger than you are." He comments that authentic is meant "as preface to the meaningful life". Meaning in life as suggested by several studies, is a substantial component of well-being" (Ryff and Keyes, 1995; Zika and Chamberlain, 1992).

García-Alandete, Soucase, Nohales, and Martinez (2013) conducted study on Spanish undergraduate (N = 226, 87 men; 139 women) to examine the predictive role of meaning in life and gender differences on psychological well-being. They pointed out that meaning in life was a strong predictor of psychological well-being and women were significantly higher on psychological well-being than men. The scale Purpose-in-Life Test-10 item form ($\alpha = .85$) used in this study was based on logotheraputic postulate. It measures life satisfaction (retrospective and current) and meaning in life, and personal purpose and goals (prospective).

Rathi and Rastogi (2007) investigated meaning in life among Indian students. They assessed meaning in life among preadolescent (12-15 yrs.) and adolescent (16-18 yrs.) sample of 104 students from class 9th and 12th of different schools. The measure used for assessment of meaning in life was Personal Meaning Profile (P.T.P., Wong, 1998), a 57-item scale with seven sub-scales (i.e. achievement, relationship, religion, self-transcendence, self-acceptance, intimacy, and fair treatment). The scale has high reliability and validity with overall Cronbach's alpha coefficient of 0.93 and 0.94 respectively. The result of the study revealed female participants scored higher on relationship, self-acceptance, intimacy, and fair treatment of the subscale of PMP than their male counterparts, but there was no difference on achievement, religion and self-transcendence subscale. The overall result indicates that meaning in life was highly correlated with psychological well-being of students.

It is concluded by psychologists that meaning arises happiness, which in turn provides sense of well-being. A study in similar line was conducted by Santos and Magramo (2012) to find out the relationship between meaning in life and subjective well-being. The sample consisted of college students (N = 969, 469 males, 500 females) and their age ranged from 15-21 years. The Meaning in Life Questionnaire (MLQ; Steger, Frazier, Oishi and Keler, 2006) that assess two dimensions, namely presence and search of meaning in life was used in the study. The presence items assessed individuals' perception of how meaningful life is and search items focused to the individuals' active search for meaning in life. Meaning in life was found to be positively related to subjective well-being. Gender differences regarding presence and search subscale were also observed. Females reported higher search for meaning in life while their male counter-parts reported higher levels of presence of meaning in their life. There were also differences regarding age and meaning in life. Younger students scored lower on meaning in life than older students.

Another study with similar conceptualization was carried out on students of Turkish University. The sample size was relatively small (N = 232, 171 female and 61 male) and a wider age range were used (18-26 years) in this study. The findings were also quite similar as scores on both subscales of meaning in life significantly predicted subjective well-being. Regression showed that presence of meaning in life predicted greater subjective well-being while search of meaning in life gave negative predictions (Dogan, Sapmaz, Tel, Sapmaz and Temizel, 2012).

Researchers are trying to explore presence of meaning in life and search for meaning in life as separate construct. As concluded by Park, Park, and Peterson (2010) that presence of meaning acts as buffer. On the other hand, search of meaning in life may associate with depression and meaninglessness. On the contrary, many psychologists believe that it is a primary motivation of mankind which further contributes in psychological well-being and an inner tension for search of meaning in life is a crucial condition of mental health (Frankl, 1959/2006; Maddi, 1970). Cohen and Cairns (2010) investigated search of meaning in life and its association with subjective well-being on a heterogeneous sample (N = 106, 63 males, 43 females with minimum 18 yrs. and maximum

60 + yrs. of age) drawn from Australian population. Meaning in life questionnaire (MLQ) was used to assess the presence and search of meaning in life. They reported that high level of search of meaning in life (with low level of presence of meaning in life) was associated with clinical levels of depression. On the other hand, high level of presence of meaning in life was found to be associated with higher subjective well-being.

Cohen and Cairns (2012) further studied the search for meaning in life and its effect on well-being of male and female Australian adults with relatively larger sample size (Mean Age = 29, N = 500). Findings reveal that search of meaning in life, which focuses on the individuals' motivation for seeking meaning in their life is found to be important for the understanding the mechanism through which a person achieve well-being. The MLQ (Steger, Frazier, Oishi & Keler, 2006) was used in the study. The Chronbach's alpha for presence subscale was .88 and for search subscale was .90 for this study. Ultimately, the result of the study revealed that higher level of searching for meaning was associated with lower value of well-being while higher level of presence was associated with higher well-being of individuals. Steger, Oishi, and Kashdan (2009) reported that presence of meaning was associated with greater well-being among all age groups and older people have more meaning in their life. Result also revealed that search for meaning was associated with lower well-being especially in older people.

Dezutter *et al.* (2014) investigated a person-oriented approach of meaning in life in emerging adulthood. The study included American emerging adults (N = 8492, 72.5% women, 27.5% men). Both presence and search for meaning in life (MLQ; Steger, Frazier, Oishi and Keler, 2006) was found to be positively associated with psychosocial functioning. They reported that presence of meaning showed the most adaptive psycho-social functioning while search for meaning was associated with maladaptive psychosocial functioning.

The above mentioned findings clearly indicate meaning in life to be a positive psychological variable that is positively related to positive psychological variables such as psychological well-being and mental health and negatively correlated mental health problems such as depression, and maladaptive psychological functioning.

Schnell and Becker (2006) reported that meaningfulness can be predicted significantly, but moderately by personality factors in which Extraversion/Openness is significantly and positively related to meaningfulness while disagreeableness and conscientiousness associated significantly and negatively to meaningfulness. In his study Halama and

Dedova (2007) investigated the relationships between personality traits, level of meaning in life, hope and some aspects of positive mental health (self-esteem, satisfaction with life). The sample consisted of adolescents, age ranged from 16 to 19 years of age. For the assessment of sense of experiencing meaning in life, The Life Meaningfulness Scale was used. The scale comprises 18-items and is based on three component theory of meaning, i.e. cognitive, motivational and affective component (Reker and Wong, 1988). They reported that meaning in life was found to be highly correlated with positive mental health (self-esteem and satisfaction with life). Meaning in life and hope are related with personality traits (NEO-FFI), but cannot be fully explained by personality traits.

The researchers have observed qualitative and quantitative research methods to assess the concept of meaning in life. Qualitative approach provides an in-depth analysis of the particular construct and releases to the other influencing factors that may help in understanding the psychological, social, and transcendental mechanisms in the positive growth of human being. On the basis of findings, psychological interventions may be proposed. Only some researchers have taken the pain to assess this construct qualitatively. As humanistic psychologists focus on the individuals' subjective experiences, therefore, the importance of qualitative methods in assessment of such type of construct which have individual specific value cannot be ignored.

In qualitative studies researchers focus on the meaning in life of an individual with the help of cultural prophecy. Meaning can be considered as a culture bound phenomenon. Individuals associated with a particular culture have the similar thought expression medium, i.e. language which is further associated with religious teachings (i.e. Hindu philosophy) and mode of acquiring meaning in life.

Bhattacharya (2011) explores the association between meaning in life and subjective well-being qualitatively among Indian youth (N=10, Age 23-28 years). Study attempted to cull out the meaning in life as perceived by the youth in the Indian scenario. A semi-structured interview with Life Regard Index (LRI-28 item) was used to collect the responses and findings were interpreted with the help of Grounded theory. Different themes related with the construct of meaning in life, meaninglessness, happiness and unhappiness were used. For example, the themes of meaning in life focused on sense of worth and self-efficacy, fulfilment of aims and goals, self-growth, beliefs in Indian philosophy, life having inherent meaning, attainment of peace, hope as giving meaning in life etc. Themes of meaning in life were related to ups and downs in life that generally lead to meaninglessness, uncertainty about the future, loss in relationship. Themes of happiness shed light on feeling of peace, time spent with loved one, achievement in carrier and having a purpose in life etc., on the other hand, themes related to unhappiness were emotional turmoil, sense of loss, feeling of loneliness, unhappy memories and feeling of failures. The results revealed that meaning in life spans a huge time space in which not only individuals' past experiences, but also their future plans effect the way he provides meaning to his life. Study emphasized the cultural context in which the meaning in life emerges. The participants who reported clear meaning and purpose in life were found to be happier in life than participants who were experiencing meaninglessness from the uncertainty about future was found to be related to meaninglessness in the life. Findings indicate that individual' lives experiences and present life situations influence their interpretations regarding the meaning in life.

Meaning in Life and Health

Researches in the area of health psychology provide the evidence for the impact of meaning in life on health related outcomes and add the evidences in understanding of the probable mechanism through which meaning in life may influence health and well-being of individuals. Skrabaski, Kopp, Rozsa, Rethelyi and Rahe (2005) assessed the meaning in life and its relation to demographic characteristics, coping measures and health status among middle-aged people residing in Hungary (N = 12,640, 45-64 years). To assess meaning in life, Hungarian version subscale of Brief Stress and Coping Inventory consisted of eight items (Rahe and Tolles, 2002; Rahe, Veach, Tolles, and Murakami, 2000) was used. The results revealed meaning in life to be most closely associated with well-being, self-rated absence of depression, self-rated health, and self-rated absence of disability. Meaning in life was inversely related to premature total and oncological mortality for both men and women. For cardiovascular mortality, meaning in life was inversely related only for the women. Male total premature mortality and male cardiovascular mortality were found to be consistent with females' experience of meaning in life. Meaning in life also enhanced the self-efficacious beliefs, importance of religion, problem focused coping, and the reception of social support of these people.

The role of stress in perceived health outcomes of people suffering from chronic illness are well studied by the investigations under the transactional approach of coping. Lazarus and Folkman (1987) indicate that people's stress appraisal processes affect the health related outcomes. Meaning in life is equated with the sense of coherence which is considered as an important factor for regulating the effect of stress on health. Meaning in life is considered as a cognitive phenomenon with motivational and affective consequences. Park and Folkman (1997) in their meaning-making model of coping have given the probable mechanism of role of meaning in stressful situations. Meaning-making model has two levels of meaning, i.e. global meaning and situational meaning. The three aspects of global meaning, i.e. beliefs, goals, and subjective sense of purpose, are associated to general indices of health and well-being. They assert that the meaning-making model is a discrepancy based model in which discrepancy between appraised meaning (individuals' perception of a particular situation) and global meaning (i.e. what they believe and desire) creates distress. Generally, this discrepancy can be reduced by problem-focused coping and emotion focused coping or with the help of approach oriented intrapsychic efforts. In this process, meaning-making involves changing either the meaning of the stressor (appraised meaning) in a process of assimilation or in the processes of accommodation changing one's global beliefs and goals to improve the fit between the appraised meaning of the stressor and global meaning (Park, 2010b). Meaning making typically involves searching for a more constructive understanding of the situation and its implications. It also involves reconsidering global beliefs and revising goals (Wrosch, 2010) and questioning or revising one's sense of meaning in life (Park, 2010a).

Halama and Bakosova (2009) investigated the role of meaning in life between perceived stress and coping on general population. They drawn the sample (N = 204; 44 males, 160 females) from Slovakian university students. The Life Meaningfulness Scale was used to assess the meaning in life. The result of the study indicates that meaning in life act as a moderator of the relationship between perceived stress and avoidant coping, but not for emotion based coping. Higher meaning in life was associated with less avoidant coping while in the case of higher avoidant coping meaning becomes less useful against coping with stress among individuals.

Park, Malone, Suresh, Bliss and Rosen (2008) conducted a study on congestive heart failure patients (N = 155) for the assessment of quality of life and the role of meaning in life in coping processes. They assessed meaning in life with Perceived Personal Meaning Scale (PPMS-5 items, Wong, 1998). Internal consistency reliability was reported .92. They reported that the participant, who adopted the ways of coping through their faith and through accepting the situations and trying to understand their illness in a more positive way, reported higher levels of meaning over time. Meaning in life was found to be strongly associated with better physical and mental health.

Studies associated with adolescents suggested that meaning in life played a role in protecting adolescents from risking behaviours that harm their health. Meaning in life was found to be negatively associated with health drug use (Addad and Himi, 2008), sedative use (Koushede and Holstein, 2009) and positively associated with health enhancing behaviours, such as physical activity and diet control (Oztekin and Tezer, 2009; Myrin and Lagerstrom, 2006). Studies regarding gender showed meaning in life to be higher among males than females (Moksens, Espnes, & Lillefjell, 2012).

Steger, Fitch-Martin, Donnely and Rickard (2014) assessed the association between meaning in life and risking behaviours (i.e. substance use), of European American undergraduate students (N = 571, 75% female; M_{age}=20.83 years). For meaning in life only MLQ-presence subscale (Steger, Frazier, Oishi, and Keler, 2006) having Cronbach's α = .86, was used. The study explored an alternative explanation about the facilitative role of meaning in life towards a more positive health orientation which in turn might inhibit health-risking behaviours and increase health-promoting behaviours and ultimately health. Higher meaning in life reduced engagement in health risking behaviours that further enhanced physical health. Mediation analysis revealed meaning in life to be associated with more beneficial health orientation and less with health information denial.

Thege, Urban, and Kopp (2013) conducted a four-year prospective evaluation of the relationship between meaning in life and smoking status among Hungarian adults (N = 4,294, M_{age} = 54.7 + –16.5). The aim of the study was to assess the predictive power of life meaning construct concerning changes in smoking status. For assessing the meaning in Life, Meaning Subscale from the Brief Stress and Coping Inventory (BSCI-LM, Rahe and Tolles, 2002) was used. The result unfold that both baseline and follow-up meaning in life scores were found to be higher in stable non-smokers in comparison to stable smokers. On the other side, quitters and starters differed from stable non-smokers in their baseline, but not in follow-up life meaning scores. Study also indicated some other demographic factors, i.e. gender and education to have importance in context of smoking behaviour.

Krause and Hayward (2012) conducted a nation-wide longitudinal survey of older adults including six wave of data collection from 1992-2007 for assessing the role of religion and meaning in life in physical functioning. The scales, which were used for the assessment of meaning in life comprised four dimensions such as value, purpose, goals and reflections on the past (Battista and Almond, 1973; Wong, 1998) as well as indicators developed by Krause (2004) were used for data collection. The study revealed that older adults, who attended church more often, feel closer relationship with God and they provided emotional support to their social network members. Providing support to others was found to be very important factor because attitude of providing emotional support tended to bolster the sense of meaning in life, which in turn reduced the functional disability over time.

Pasarra and Kleftaras (2013) assessed the role of meaning in life and depression in adaptation to physical disability. The sample (N = 511) was quite heterogeneous having various types of physical disability (paraplegia 34.3%, quadriplegia 16.9%, amputation 24.3%, poliomyelitis 20.9%, multiple sclerosis 2.3% and hemiplegia 1.3%) and also with wide age range from 19-78 years. For measurement of meaning in life, the Greek version of Revised Life Attitude Profile consisted of 48 items was used (Reker, 1992). Reported Cronbach's alpha for adopted version was .89. Results indicated that meaning in life reduced the physical disability and made people easy with adaptation towards physical disability.

Studies carried out in the area of oncology have well explored the impact of meaning in life on the lives of people suffering from cancer. A review of 44 studies by Lee, Cohen, Edgar, Lainzner and Gagnon (2004) based on cancer patients reported a relationship between meaning as an outcome of cancer and meaning as an psychosocial adjustment to cancer. Another study revealed that perceptions of meaning in life and vulnerability of breast cancer co-occur and the factors that increase the disruptiveness of the cancer experience provide an opportunity for both responses. Meaning in life and vulnerability of breast cancer were found to be positively correlated. Demographic variables such as income and age, and physical symptoms and occurrence of other stressful life events also predicted meaning in life and vulnerability of breast cancer. Younger women reported both increased meaning and increased vulnerability as a result of their cancer experience as compared to older women. Women having higher income had reported significantly higher levels of meaning in life and vulnerability towards breast cancer than did those with lower income. Women who endorsed more physical symptoms after the diagnosis and who experienced a higher number of other stressors reported higher levels of meaning in life and vulnerability. Overall results indicated that perceptions of meaning in life increased positive affect of cancer patients (Bower, Meyerowitz, Desmond, Bernaards, Rowland, and Ganz, 2005).

Jim and Anderson (2007) conducted two studies while assessed meaning in life of cancer patients as a mediator between their physical and social functioning and distress. The first one was cross-sectional with heterogeneous sample (more than seven sites of disease, N = 420) of cancer patients with an average of five years since patients had been diagnosed. Eighty per cent of them reported being currently disease free. The second study was planned longitudinally for a homogeneous sample (N = 167) of breast cancer patients. The patients of this group were assessed at three occasions (18, 24 and 30 months post diagnosis). The Meaning in Life Scale (Jim, Purnell, Richardson, Golden-Kreutz and Anderson, 2006) having 21 items that represented four dimensions such as Harmony and Peace (4 items), Life Perspective, Purpose and Goals (7 items), Confusion and Lessened meaning (7 items) and Benefits of Spirituality (3 item) was used to assess the meaning in life of these patients. The coefficient alpha reliability was .93 for the first study and .90 for the second study. The result of the first study revealed that meaning in life partially mediated between physical and social functioning, and distress. In the second study, the result showed that the effect of impairment in social functioning on distress was fully mediated by meaning in life, while the effect of social functioning on distress was fully mediated through meaning in life. The results showed a special mechanism, i.e. meaning in life as potentially important in the adjustment process to the impaired physical and social functioning common among cancer survivors.

Similarly, some other studies with cancer patients also carried out to assess the mechanism through which meaning in life played a significant role between physical symptoms and depression. Meaning in life acted as a mediator (Simonelli, Fower, Maxwell, Barbara and Andersen, 2008). A longitudinal study on women (N = 72) primarily diagnosed with breast cancer, revealed that at base-line level a higher level of search for meaning in life was found to be associated with a higher level of negative affect. Women who engaged in an ongoing, unresolved search for meaning from baseline to follow-up also had a significantly higher level of negative affect at follow-up than women who infrequently or never engaged in a search for meaning over time (Kernan and Lepore, 2009).

Using narrative analysis, Saraf, Singh and Khurana (2013) conducted a study on Indian sample of cervical cancer patients to assess the association of meaning in life with long-term treatment recovery and survivorship of women patients (N = 10, age 35-60 years) belonged to post-treatment stage. They planned a semi-structured interview to assess the meaning in life before the diagnosis of cancer, meaning in life in current situation, experiences and significant others that influenced the patients since the diagnosis of cancer, change in perception of life since cancer diagnosis and their recovery, role of spirituality since cancer diagnosis and recovery, and purpose, hopes and future plans. Thematic Apperception Test was used to assess the purpose of the study.

The results were interpreted in terms of themes (for example, distress during treatment, post-treatment distress, renewed meaning in life, support system, faith and religiosity, hope and purpose) that were emerged on the narratives from the life experiences of the participants. Participants viewed life being predestined and guided by fate. In some cases, the realization of immortality resulted in peace and satisfaction. This renewed meaning was strongly mediated by faith in God and increased religiosity which facilitated hope and resilience. Strong support systems further enhanced meaning in their lives. However, underlying factors like fatigue, fear of recurrence of the disease and perceived burden continue to be distressing factors for them. On the other hand, some participants who experienced a preoccupation with somatic complaints and ambivalent feelings towards God, experienced a sense of meaninglessness, lack of purpose and diminished hope. The most frequently used defence mechanisms were sublimation, reaction formation, undoing, displacement and projection.

Meaning in Life and Mental Health

An enlightening study about the role of meaning in life in bullying victimization and suicidal ideation among US adolescents was done by Henry, Lovegrove, Steger, Chen, Cigularov and Tomazic (2014). They studied the two potential mechanisms, i.e. mediator and moderator by which meaning in life indicated the relationship between bullying victimization and suicidal ideation. The study reported that bullying victimization was associated with weaker meaning in life and further weaker meaning in life was associated with more frequent suicidal ideation. In this study dissimilar role of meaning in life for male and female was outlined. There was moderation role of meaning in life for males and mediation role of meaning in life for females which indicated that it served as buffering factor for males but not for females between bullying victimization and suicidal ideation. Meaning in life reduced the mental health problems as depression of adolescents (Hedayati and Khazaei, 2014).

Mascaro and Rosen (2009) examined whether the sense of existential meaning buffers against the effect of stress on depression and hope on an ethnically diverse sample (N = 143) of college undergraduates. Spiritual meaning was assessed by the Spiritual Meaning Scale and personal meaning as measured by the framework subscale from the Revised Life Regard Index. Both were found to be significantly negatively correlated with depressive symptoms and positively correlated with hope. Spiritual meaning moderated the relationship between stress and depression but not personal meaning, such that there was a strong relationship between depression and stress for individuals with low levels of spiritual meaning, but no relationship between stress and depression for individuals with high levels of spiritual meaning. Though both spiritual and personal meaning were inversely related to depression and positively related to hope, only spiritual meaning moderated the relationship between daily stress and depression.

Several studies have reported that meaning in life is negatively associated with psychological symptoms (Baiocco, Crea, Fizzotti, Gurrieri, Laghi and Paola, 2009) and mediate the relation between psychological distress and well-being (Korte, Cappeliez, Bohlmeijer and Westerhof, 2012). In a clinical psychiatric sample (N = 49, 15 male and 34 female) the role of purpose in life and satisfaction with life was assessed in protecting against suicide ideation. Purpose in life mediated the relation between satisfaction with life and suicide ideation and also moderated the relation between depression and suicide ideation (Heisel and Flett, 2004).

Sometimes, meaning in life may play role as a protective factor in adolescent development and foster psychosocial adjustment. Brassai, Piko, and Steger (2011) examined the protective role of meaning in life among Romanian adolescents (N = 2152). The result of this study reveals that meaning in life played a protective role in minimizing the health risking behaviours. Findings revealed that meaninglessness was associated with a poor psychological health (high psychosomatic symptoms, poor psychological well-being, and quality of life). A gender difference was observed, among females lower levels of meaning in life enhanced poor psychological well-being and quality of life, as well as higher levels of psychosomatic symptoms. Among males, lower levels of meaning in life increased the poor perception of quality of life and psychosomatic symptoms.

Conclusion

Researches in the field of positive psychology have highlighted the beneficial impact of meaning in life on health and well-being of people. This construct is dualistic as existential and positive psychological in nature and positively associated with different positive psychological variable such as optimism, hope, spirituality, positive emotions, feeling of fulfilment etc. Studies focusing on the concept of meaning in life have identified it as an important indicator of mental and physical health, and well-being. It acts differently among different age groups especially in the phase of crisis. Studies conducted in this area provide different mechanism through which meaning in life changes at the different life span. For obtaining the clear picture there is need to open the thread of culture in which individuals grow and acquire meaning in their life. There is also a need to reveal the family dynamics of an individual, because the characteristics and constituents of a family may also have an influence on the development of meaning in life of an individual. Studies generally indicated adolescents to be involved deeply in the search of meaning in life and elderly people reported greater importance for the presence of meaning in their life.

Findings also revealed that the sources of meaning are different for different age group of people. The studies regarding presence and search of meaning in life generally indicated higher search of meaning in life to be associated with maladaptive psychosocial functioning of individuals while higher presence of meaning in life contributed in adaptive psychosocial functioning and associated with greater sense of well-being. Studies also indicate that sometimes search is higher and it does not impact on subjective well-being of an individual, so it is a point of assessment that why it happens.

Studies focusing on chronic illness showed that meaning in life act as a buffer during stressful situation and are inversely related to psychosocial problems of illness. Studies also reported gender difference regarding meaning in life. Male experienced greater meaning in life than females. On the other hand, females reported greater search of meaning in life while males reported greater presence of meaning in life as compared to their counterparts. Review reveals that meaning in life act as a moderator between stress and coping. Meaning in life also predicted health behaviours and illness. Higher meaning in life reduced the tendency of the engagement in health risking behaviours of adolescents and also enhanced physical and mental health.

Disability studies show that meaning in life reduces the psychosocial problems of physical disability and helps in adaptation towards physical disability. In this context there is a real dearth of studies on severely disabled population.

Oncological studies reveal the meditational role of meaning in life between physical and social functioning, and distress. Meaning in life enhanced psychological health and reduced mental health problems.

In the present review, most of the studies are cross-sectional in nature that provide little direction of influence, longitudinal studies are in need to explore the role of presence and search for meaning in life for different developmental period. The findings related to meaning in life and personality of an individual may be helpful in better understanding of psychosocial adjustment of normal people. By revealing this aspect new insight can be gained. Since, meaning in life is an individual's specific belief about the significance of one's life and an individual is a cultural being, more qualitative analyses regarding this construct is needed to execute in order to understand its significance in development and maintenance of meaning in life during life-course.

References

Addad, M. and Himi, H. (2008). Meaning of life and drug use among Israeli teenagers. *International Forum of Logotherapy, 31*, 43-8.

Baiocco, R., Crea, G., Fizzotti, E., Gurrieri, G., Laghi, F., and Paola, R. (2009). Meaning in life and attachment to parents/peers among Italian high school students. In *International Forum for Logotherapy, 32*(2), 65.

Battista, J., and Almond, R. (1973). The development of meaning in life. *Psychiatry: Journal for the Study of Interpersonal Processes*.

Baumeister, R.F. (1991). *Meanings of Life.* New York: The Guilford Press.

Baumeister, R.F., and Newman, L.S. (1994). How stories make sense of personal experiences: Motives that shape autobiographical narratives. *Personality and Social Psychology Bulletin, 20*(6), 676-690.

Bhattacharya, A. (2011). Meaning in life: A qualitative inquiry into the life of young adults. *Psychological Studies, 56*(3), 280-288.

Bower, J.E., Ganz, P.A., Desmond, K.A., Bernaards, C., Rowland, J.H., Meyerowitz, B.E., and Belin, T.R. (2006). Fatigue in long-term breast carcinoma survivors. *Cancer, 106*(4), 751-758.

Brassai, L., Piko, B.F., and Steger, M.F. (2011). Meaning in life: Is it a protective factor for adolescents' psychological health? *International Journal of Behavioural Medicine, 18*, 44-51.

Bruner, J. (1990). *Acts of Meaning.* Cambridge, MA: Harvard University Press.

Cervinka, R., Roderer, K., & Hefler, E. (2012). Are nature lovers happy? On various indicators of well-being and connectedness with nature. *Journal of Health Psychology, 17*, 379-388.

Cohen and Cairns (2010). Is searching for meaning in life associated with reduced subjective psychological well-being? *International Journal of Existential Psychology and Psychotherapy, 3*, 1.

Cohen, K., and Cairns, D. (2012). Is searching for meaning in life associated with reduced subjective well-being? Confirmation and possible moderators. *Journal of Happiness Studies, 13*(2), 313-331.

Dezutter, J., Waterman, A.S., Shwartz, S.J., Luyckx, K., Beyers, W., Meca, A., Kim, S.Y., Whitbourne, S.K., Zamboanga, B.L., Lee, R.M., Hardy, S.A., Forthun, L.F., Ritchie, R.A., Weisskirch, R.S., Brown, E.J. and Caraway, S.J. (2014). Meaning in life in emerging adulthood: A person oriented approach. *Journal of Personality, 82*(1), 58-68.

Dittman-Kohli, F., and Westerhof, G.J. (2000). The personal meaning system in a life-span perspective. In G.T. Reker and K. Chamberlian (Eds.), *Exploring existential meaning: Optimizing human development across the life span* (pp. 107-122). Thousand Oaks, CA: Sage Publications.

Dogan, T., Sapmaz, F., Tel, F.D., Sapmaz, S., and Temizel, S. (2012). Meaning in life and subjective well-being among Turkish university students. *Procedia-Social and Behavioural Sciences, 55*, 612-617.

Elliott, M., and Hayward, R.D. (2007). Religion and well-being in a church without a creed. *Mental Health, Religion and Culture, 10*(2), 109-126.

Emmons, R.A. (2005). Striving for the sacred: Personal goals, life meaning, and religion. *Journal of Social Issues, 61*, 731-745.

Frankl, V.E. (1959). *Man's Search for Meaning.* Simon and Schuster, New York.

Frankl, V.E. (1967). The doctor and the soul: From Psychotherapy to Logotherapy. New York: Washington Square Press.

Frankl, V.E. (1969). *The Will to Meaning.* New York: New American Library.

Frankl, V.E. (1976). *Man's Search for Meaning.* New York: Pocket.

Frankl, V.E. (1984). *Man's Search for Meaning: An Introduction to Logotherapy* (3rd Ed). Simon and Schuster, New York.

Frankl, V.E. (1988). *The Will to Meaning: Foundations and Applications of Logotherapy.* New York: Meridian.

Frankl, V.E. (2006). *Man's Search for Meaning.* Boston Beacon Press.

Freud, S. (1991). Civilization and its discontents. In A. Dickson (Ed.), *Sigmund Freud: 12. Civilization, Society, and Religion* (pp. 245-341). New York: Penguin. (Original work published in 1930).

García-Alandete, J., Soucase, B., Sellés, P., and Rosa, E. (2013). Predictive role of meaning in life on psychological well-being and gender-specific differences. *Acta Colombiana de Psicología, 16* (1), 17-24.

Halama, P., and Bakosova, K. (2009). Meaning in life as a moderator of the relationship between perceived stress and coping. *Studia Psychologica, 51*(2-3), 143-148.

Halama, P., and Dedova, M. (2007). Meaning in life and hope as predictors of positive mental health: do they explain residual variance not predicted by personality traits? *Studia Psychologica, 49*(3), 191.

Harter, S. (1996). Scholastic motivation, self-esteem. *Social motivation: Understanding children's school adjustment*, 11.

Hedayati, M., and Khazaei, M. (2014). An Investigation of the Relationship between Depression, Meaning in Life and Adult Hope. *Procedia-Social and Behavioural Sciences, 114*, 598-601.

Heisel, M.J. and Flett, G.L. (2004). Purpose in life, satisfaction with life and suicide ideation in a clinical sample. *Journal of Psychopathology and Behavioural Assessment, 26*, 127-135.

Henry, K.L., Lovegrove, P.J., Steger, M.F., Chen, P.Y., Cigularov, K.P., and Tomazic, R.G. (2014). The potential role of meaning in life in the relationship between bullying victimization and suicidal ideation. *Journal of Youth and Adolescence, 43*(2), 221-232.

Howell, A.J., Passmore, H.A. and Buro, K. (2013). Meaning in nature: Meaning in life as a mediator of the relationship between nature connectedness and well-being. *Journal of Happiness Studies, 14*, 1681-1696.

Jim, H.S., and Andersen, B.L. (2007). Meaning in life mediates the relationship between social and physical functioning and distress in cancer survivors. *British Journal of Health Psychology, 12*(3), 363-381.

Jim, H.S., Richardson, S.A., Golden-Kreutz, D.M., and Andersen, B.L. (2006). Strategies used in coping with a cancer diagnosis predict meaning in life for survivors. *Health Psychology, 25*(6), 753.

Karoly, P. (1999). A goal system-self regulatory perspective on personality and psychopathology, and change. *Review of General Psychology*, 3, 364-391.

Kernan, W.D. and Lepore S.J. (2009). Searching for and making meaning after breast cancer: Prevalence, patterns, and negative affect. *Social Science and Medicine, 68*, 1176-1182.

Klinger, E. (1977). *Meaning and Void: Inner Experience and the Incentives in Peoples' lives*. U of Minnesota Press.

Klinger, E. (1998). The search for meaning in evolutionary perspective and its clinical implications. In P.T.P. Wong and P.S. Fry (Eds.), *The Human Quest for Meaning: A Handbook of Psychological Research and Clinical Application* (pp. 27-50), Mahwah, NJ: Erlbaum.

Korte, J., Cappeliez, P., Bohlmeijer, E.T., and Westerhof, G.J. (2012). Meaning in life and mastery mediate the relationship of negative reminiscence with psychological distress among older adults with mild to moderate depressive symptoms. *European Journal of Ageing, 9*(4), 343-351.

Koushede, V. and Holstein, B.E. (2009). Sense of coherence and medicine use for headache among adolescents. *Journal of Adolescent Health, 45*, 149-55.

Krause, N. (2003). Neighbourhoods, health, and well-being in late life. *Annual Review of Gerontology and Geriatrics, 23*, 223-249.

Krause, N. (2004). Stressors in highly valued roles, meaning in life, and the physical health status of older adults. *Journal of Gerontology: Social Sciences, 59B*, S287-S297.

Krause, N., and Hayward, R.D. (2012). Religion, meaning in life, and change in physical functioning during late adulthood. *Journal of Adult Development, 19*(3), 158-169.

Lazarus, R.S., and Folkman, S. (1987). Transactional theory and research on emotions and coping. *European Journal of Personality, 1*(3), 141-169.

Lazarus, R.S., and Folkman, S. (1984). *Stress, Appraisal and Coping*. New York: Springer.

Lee, V., Cohen, S.R., Edgar, L., Laizner, A.M., and Gagnon, A.J. (2004). Clarifying "meaning" in the context of cancer research: A systematic literature review. *Palliative and Supportive Care, 2*(3), 291-303.

Maddi, S.R. (1970). The search for meaning. In *Nebraska Symposium on Motivation* (Vol. 17, pp. 134-183). Lincoln, NE: University of Nebraska Press.

Mascaro, N., and Rosen, D.H. (2006). The role of existential meaning as a buffer against stress. *Journal of Humanistic Psychology, 46*, 168-190.

Mayer, F.S., and Frantz, C.M. (2004). The connectedness to nature scale: A measure of individuals' feeling in community with nature. *Journal of Environmental Psychology, 24*, 504-515.

Mohamad, M., Abd Razak, A., and Mutiu, S. (2011). Meaning in Life among Muslim Students. *Procedia-Social and Behavioural Sciences, 30*, 743-747.

Murphy, G.L., and Medin, D.L. (1985). The role of theories in conceptual coherence. *Psychological Review, 92*(3), 289.

Myrin, B., and Lagerström, M. (2006). Health behaviour and sense of coherence among pupils aged 14-15. *Scandinavian Journal of Caring Sciences, 20*, 339-46.

Naylor, T.H., Willimon, W.H., and Naylor, M.R. (1994). *The Search for Meaning*. Nashville, TN: Abingdon Press.

Nisbet, E.K., Zelenski, J.M., and Murphy, S.A. (2011). Happiness is in Our Nature: Exploring Nature Relatedness as a contributor to subjective well-being. *Journal of Happiness Studies, 12*, 303-322.

Öztekin, C. and Tezer, E. (2009). The role of sense of coherence and psychical activity in positive and negative affect of Turkish adolescents. *Adolescence, 44*, 421-32.

Pargament, K.I. (1997). *The Psychology of Religion and Coping: Theory, Research, Practice*. New York: The Guilford Press.

Park, C.L. (2010a). Making sense of the meaning literature: An integrative review of meaning making and its effects on adjustment to stressful life events. *Psychological Bulletin, 136*, 257-301.

Park, C.L. (2010b). Stress, coping, and meaning. In S. Folkman (Ed.), *Oxford*

Handbook of Stress, Health, and Coping (pp. 227-241). New York: Oxford University Press.

Park, C.L., and Folkman, S. (1997). The Role of Meaning in the Context of Stress and Coping. *General Review of Psychology, 1*, 115-144.

Park, C.L., Malone, M.R., Suresh, D.P., Bliss, D., and Rosen, R.I. (2008). Coping, meaning in life, and quality of life in congestive heart failure patients. *Quality of Life Research, 17*(1), 21-26.

Park, N., Park, M., and Peterson, C. (2010). When is the search for meaning related to life satisfaction? *Applied Psychology: Health and Well-Being, 2*(1), 1-13.

Psarraa, E. and Kleftaras, G. (2013). Adaptation to Physical Disabilities: The role of meaning in life and depression. *The European Journal of Counselling Psychology, 2*(1), 79-99.

Proulx, T., and Heine, S.J. (2006). Death and black diamonds: Meaning, mortality, and the meaning maintenance model. *Psychological Inquiry, 17*, 4, 309-318.

Rahe, R.H., Veach, T.L., Tolles, R.L. and Murakami, K. (2000). The Stress and Coping Inventory: An educational and Research Instrument. *Stress Medicine, 16*, 199-208.

Rahe, R.H., and Tolles, R.L. (2002). The Brief Stress and Coping Inventory: A useful stress management instrument. *International Journal of Stress Management, 9*(2), 61-70.

Rathi, N., and Rastogi, R. (2007). Meaning in Life and Psychological Well-being in Pre-adolescents and Adolescents. *Journal of the Indian Academy of Applied Psychology, 33*, 31-38.

Reker, G.T. (1992). Life Attitude Profile—Revised.

Reker, G.T. (2000). Theoretical perspective, dimensions, and measurement of existential meaning. In G.T. Reker and K. Chamberlain (Eds.), *Exploring Existential Meaning: Optimizing Human Development Across the Life Span* (pp. 39-55). Thousand Oaks, CA: Sage Publications.

Reker, G.T., and Wong, P.T.P. (1988). Ageing as an individual process: Toward a theory of personal meaning. In J.E. Birren and V.C. Bengston (Eds.), *Emergent Theories of Ageing* (pp. 214-246). New York: Springer.

Reker, G.T., and Woo, L.C. (2011). Personal Meaning Orientations and Psychosocial Adaptation in Older Adults. *SAGE Open*.

Ryff, C.D. (1989). Happiness is everything, or is it? Explorations on the Meaning of Psychological Well-being. *Journal of Personality and Social Psychology, 57*, 1069-1081.

Ryff, C.D., and Keyes, C.L.M. (1995). The Structure of Psychological Well-being Revisited. *Journal of Personality and Social Psychology, 69*(4), 719.

Ryff, C.D., and Keyes, C.L.M. (1995). The Structure of Psychological Well-being Revisited. *Journal of Personality and Social Psychology, 69*, 719-727.

Ryff, C.D., and Singer, B. (1998). The role of purpose in life and personal growth in Positive Human Health. In P.T.P. Wong and P.S. Fry (Eds.), *The Human Quest for Meaning: A Handbook of Psychological Research and Clinical Applications* (pp. 213-235). Mahwah, NJ: Lawrence Earlbaum Associates.

Santos, M.C.J., Magramo Jr., C., Oguan Jr., F., Paat, J.N., and Barnachea, E.A. (2012). Meaning in life and subjective well-being: Is a satisfying life meaningful? *Researchers World: Journal of Arts, Science and Commerce*, *3*.

Saraf, S., Singh, T.B., and Khurana, S. (2013). Cervical Cancer Survivors: Meaning in Life. *Psychological Studies*, *58*(2), 144-152.

Schnell, T., and Becker, P. (2006). Personality and Meaning in Life. *Personality and Individual Differences, 41*, 117-129.

Schwartzberg, S.S., and Janoff-Bulman, R. (1991). Grief and the search for meaning: Exploring the assumptive worlds of bereaved college students. *Journal of Social and Clinical Psychology*, *10*(3), 270-288.

Simonelli, L.E., Fowler, J., Maxwell, G.L., and Andersen, B.L. (2008). Physical Sequelae and Depressive Symptoms in Gynaecologic Cancer Survivors: Meaning in Life as a Mediator. *Annals of Behavioural Medicine*, *35*(3), 275-284.

Skrabski, Á. Kopp, M.S., Rózsa, S., Réthelyi, J. and Rahe, R.H. (2005). Life meaning: An important correlate of health in the Hungarian population. *International Journal of Behavioural Medicine, 12*, 2, 78-85.

Steger, M.F. (2009). Meaning in life. In S.J. Lopez (Ed.), *Oxford Handbook of Positive Psychology* (2nd ed.). Oxford, UK: Oxford University Press.

Steger, M.F., Fitch-Martin, A.R., Donnelly, J., and Rickard, K.M. (2014). Meaning in Life and Health: Proactive Health Orientation Links Meaning in Life to Health Variables among American Undergraduates. *Journal of Happiness Studies*, 1-15.

Steger, M.F., Frazier, P., Oishi, S., and Kaler, M. (2006). The meaning in life questionnaire: Assessing the presence of and search for meaning in life. *Journal of Counseling Psychology, 53*(1), 80-93.

Steger, M.F., Oishi, S. and Kashdan, T.B. (2009). Meaning in life across the life span: Levels and correlates of meaning in life from emerging adulthood to older adulthood. *The Journal of Positive Psychology, 4*(1), 43-52.

Stroope, S., Draper S. and Whitehead, A.L. (2013). Images of a Loving God and Sense of Meaning in Life. *Social Indicators Research, 111*, 25-44.

Taylor, S.E. (1983). Adjustment to threatening events: A theory of cognitive adaptation. *American Psychologist*, *38*, 1161-1173.

Thege, B.K., Urbán, R., and Kopp, M.S. (2013). Four-year prospective evaluation of the relationship between meaning in life and smoking status. *Substance Abuse Treatment, Prevention, and Policy, 8*(8), 1-5.

Tomasello, M., Kruger, A.C., and Ratner, H.H. (1993). Cultural learning. *Behavioural and Brain Sciences*, *16*(03), 495-511.

Walton, G.E., and Bower, T.G.R. (1993). A Modal Representation of Speech in Infants. *Infant Behaviour and Development*, *16*(2), 233-243.

Wong, P.T. (Ed.). (2013). *The Human Quest for Meaning: Theories, Research, and Applications*. Routledge.

Wong, P.T.P. (1998). Implicit theories of meaningful life and the development of the Personal Meaning Profile (PMP). In P.T.P. Wong and P.S. Fry (Eds.),

The Human Quest for Meaning: A Handbook of Psychological Research and Clinical Applications (pp. 111-140). Mahwah, NJ: Erlbaum.

Wong, P.T.P. (2010). Meaning Therapy: An Integrative and Positive Existential Psychotherapy. *Journal of Contemporary Psychotherapy, 40*, 2, 85-93.

Wrosch, C. (2010). Self-regulation of Unattainable Goals and Pathways to Quality of Life. In S. Folkman (Ed.), *Oxford Handbook of Stress, Health, and Coping* (pp. 319-333). New York: Oxford University Press.

Yalom, I. (1980). *Existential Psychotherapy.* New York: Basic Books.

Zika, S., and Chamberlain, K. (1992). On the relation between meaning in life and psychological well-being. *British Journal of Psychology, 83*, 133-145.

5

Spiritual Psychology

An Overview

Ram Kalap Tiwari

Human nature has been a matter of fascination since ancient times. We desire to understand ourselves and our place in the world and at times we also ask questions like—Why am I here? What is the meaning or purpose of my life? Why do people suffer? These questions have been attempted to answer on the basis of spirituality and psychology. Over the past century there has been interchange of ideas and views between psychologists and spiritual practitioners about these questions.

Spirituality

Spirituality is a broad term covering multiple domain of meaning that may differ among various cultural, national and spiritual/religious groups (Roeklkepartain *et al.*, 2006). Roof (1999) argues that spirituality encompasses 4 themes:

(1) a source of values and meaning or self-transcendence,
(2) method of understanding,
(3) inner awareness, and
(4) personal integration (MacInner, 2003).

Spirituality has an integrative and harmonizing function that involves (a) Person's inner unity and (b) Person's relationship and connectedness with others and to a broader reality that powers person's ability to be transcendent (McGrath, 2006).

Spirituality has a powerful quality and takes us beyond ordinary daily experience and has a transforming effect on our relationship. It is not just about being and experience, it is also about doing. It involves a search for higher values, inner freedom and things that give life meaning (Vergote, 2003).

Spirituality is an important aspect of our lives. It radiates positively and leads personal and organizational development. Spirituality in the body, mind and spirit or soul of people would change the attitude and life style of millions of people all-over the world. Spirituality offers solutions for personal and social problems and is instrumental in developing human potential and human nature.

Spirituality is the cure to all hidden wounds and it seeks to purify our true nature. It gives a new dimension to see the worldly problems as transitory in nature. Those who followed the spiritual tradition would reach the highest realm of spirituality through knowledge, piety and righteousness. Those who sought knowledge and science through education would show the exemplary life in every sphere of activity. Spirituality is a part of life.

Spirituality is reflected in everyday life as well as in disciplines ranging from philosophy and popular literature to psycho-therapy, health psychology, medicine, nursing, sociology and science (Pullen, 2001). While no one has been able to provide a universally accepted definition of spirituality, theorists and researchers agree that it is a multi-dimensional phenomenon and descriptions of its characteristics abound in the literature. In psychology, spirituality is explained as an expression of one's internal motives and desires concentrating on the self instead of God. Psychology examines one's spiritual search for meaning, purpose and guidance.

Spirituality provides higher level of intelligence and wisdom which integrates the emotional with the moral. It acts as a guide in integrating different aspects of personality and ways of being and living. It is found in the integration of several deep connections: the connection with one's true and higher self; the connection with society and especially with the poor, the deprived and underprivileged; the connection with the world of nature and other life forms; and for some, a connectedness with the transcendent.

A person's spirituality is not separate from the body, the mind or material reality, for it is their inner life. It is the practice of loving, kindness, empathy and tolerance in daily life. It is a feeling of solidarity with our fellow humans while helping to alleviate their suffering. It brings a sense of peace, harmony and conviviality with all. It is the essence and significance behind all moral values and virtues such as benevolence, compassion, honesty, sympathy, respect, forgiveness, integrity, loving, kindness towards strangers, and respect for nature. Spirituality creates and connects these virtues. This is what lies behind moral intuition. It is about knowing, and experiencing deeper meaning and connection behind apparently random events and processes such as illness and an awareness of human vulnerability.

Spirituality development is individualistic and involves a series of steps or cycles that occur in no particular order or time frame throughout the life of an individual. It is just possible as physical, intellectual, emotional or moral development. Traditional Hindu thoughts see spiritual development in the context of human life span. There are four stages or *Ashrams: Brahmacharya, Grihastha, Vanaprastha* and *Sannyasa*. Spiritual development in Buddhism happens in relation to meditation practice.

Early psychological theories of spiritual development focused on childhood and adolescence, but they have old history. Piaget (1896-1980) was interested in how we acquire knowledge or epistemology. His thinking had a strong influence on religious education. Kohlberg (1927-1987) developed a theory of justice reasoning. Fowler (1981-1996) developed a theory of faith development. Faith is based in our sense of self that develops on several level: An emergent self, embodied self, inter-subjective self (Fowler, 1989). Wilber outlined transpersonal theory of development that draws upon sources in religion, psychology and philosophy. He believed that all have a drive towards spirit. He stated that the goal of evolution is "*Atman*" or ultimate unity consciousness in only "God" and is part of the "drive of God towards God" (1996). There exists a complexity in theoretical views about spiritual development. Psychological research has tended to focus more on childhood and adolescence and neglected spiritual issues.

Spiritual process of development is an important part of the human experience. Spiritual experience has also significant effect on the physical and mental health of the individual. The relationship between spirituality and mental health has been a subject of intense interest. There is a strong connection between spiritual activities and mental health of the people. More recent research has often suggested that spiritual activities has a positive effect on mental health and that good mental health is an important prerequisite for spiritual development (Stoeber, 1994).

Another group of researchers (Welch, 1996) argues that while there is important connection between the two, they are also somewhat independent of each other so that a person might have a rich spiritual life while suffering from mental illness, or be psychologically healthy, but have deep spiritual problems. Various models have been advocated to discuss these issues. In some models of human health, spirituality is about power, and spiritual practices are tools for increasing human power and control in the search for happiness and well-being. Spirituality that leads to freedom man involve relinquishing constant needs for power and control, accepting mystery that is inherent in life and welcoming gratitude with others have to offer. Acceptance of that is key to a genuine spiritual life as well as freedom from illusion and attachments that leads to pain and suffering. Scholars who evaluate the research on spirituality and health caution against overinterpreting or underinterpreting its findings. Just because spiritual exercise is beneficial it cannot be concluded that everyone and everything will benefit from it. It effects also appear to be limited.

Science and spirituality are twin endeavours of human quest for truth and happiness. However, the two ran on parallel lines in the West. Spiritual psychology was considered as oxymoron by those with the Western mindset where psychology is considered a science and therefore, could not have a link with spirituality. While, in Indian tradition, science and spirituality are complementary and reinforcing pursuits. They have the same goal—liberation, liberation from physical world, external constraints and the inner spirit.

Spiritual Experiences

The concept of spiritual experience is relatively new. Psychologists have found the concept of religious experience to be useful way of talking about features of spirituality that are found in various religious traditions.

Expressions: Spirituality can be expressed through rituals such as praying, meditation, guided imagery, visualization, practicing gratitude, spending time in nature, viewing and engageing in art and through storytelling and questioning.

Psychology: Like the term spirituality, the meaning of the word psychology has changed over times. The term originally comes from the Greek word 'Psyche' or soul and 'Logos' or study. Historically, most definitions of psychology have labelled it as the study of mental life or mind. Prior to 1850, most works in psychology were written by philosophers, but in the latter half of the nineteenth century experimental laboratories for the study of psychology were established in Europe and north America and researchers began applying methods from the natural sciences to study of mind. After long journey psychology became seen as the scientific study of behaviour. Later on cognitive psychology came into existence, which uses scientific method to study method processes like language, reasoning and memory. The rise of biological and cognitive models has displaced behaviourism as the dominant models in psychology (Miller, 2003).

The work of William James (1842-1910) and Hall (1924) did not continue. By the 1920s, behaviourism and positivism had became the dominant paradigms in psychology. Hall advocated for the Genetic Psychology. He tried to apply psycho-analytic principles to explain Christianity as a pure psychological projection (Hall, 1924). Leuba viewed spirituality in positive light. He studied religious beliefs of scientists. He also believed that all religious experiences or needs could be explained on a purely psychological basis, with the help of biological and evolutionary theory and an understanding of normal thought processes. He believed that all behaviour is instrumental, designed to achieve gratification of needs and desires, and that religion was about how we relate to and use the power of psyche. Religion is thus a psychological phenomenon, and should be studied by psychological experts. When this happened rapid spiritual improvement would follow (Leuba, 1925).

Freud's (1856-1939) contribution of psycho-analytic psychology put strong support for researcher. In the 1960s, humanistic psychology joined psycho-analysis and behaviourism as a "third force" within the larger field of psychology. Maslow (1908-1970) advocated for transpersonal psychology. Transpersonal psychology has provided a forum for dialogue between psychology and some religious traditions. Maslow developed and produced a motivational theory of personality. He talked about self-actualization.

Social psychologists like Allport and Gorsuch have frequently pointed out positive aspects of religious behaviour on personal and social levels. Allport argued that psychology and religion were both about truth. Many different schemes for relating psychology and religion have been proposed. It can be argued that integration movement has had a significant role in changing negative views toward religion and spirituality within the profession of psychology.

Spiritual Psychology: The movement to relate psychology and spirituality together has progressing for decades. Today, more alternative beliefs are coming out of the closet and working to reconcile the spiritual and physical aspect of human self for healing the whole of a person: mind/body/spirit.

Spiritual psychology is a blend of spirituality and science. It uses elements of both traditional psychology and spirituality in order to help individuals feel better and more content with their lives. Researchers in the field of spiritual psychology understand that the body, mind and spirit all work together, therefore, they must be studied together. Each of these elements must be healthy and "in shape" to achieve optional harmony. Spiritual psychology focuses on repairing fractured soul or replacing missing pieces of the soul. Spiritual psychology has been around in some form for centuries. Spirituality counseling has also been available to everyone who needs it for century.

Spiritual psychology is based on an understanding of human being multi-layered entities with a body (Physical dimension), mind (Psychological dimension), and spirit (Spiritual dimension). Commonly known as integral, transpersonal or spiritual psychology, it is a method that seeks to explore the full range of human potential in relation with soul.

Spiritual psychology takes the step beyond scientific psychology and tries to merge the wisdom of both the physical and spiritual experiences together. Regardless of what that spiritual path is.

Spiritual psychology seeks to understand the three dimensions of human being: as a person, as having a self and the person we really are within our spiritual existence. This process of understanding helps an individual to gain insight into the trials we feel that have moved us away from our spiritual path created *Karma* and consequently caused us to feel separated from the Divine force within our life and our own higher self. Through spiritual work we gain a new insight.

Despite its popularity, spiritual psychology is still not recognized by APA. It does, however, have a division for the psychology of religion and spirituality is more focused on understanding the impact that these elements have on individual.

Spiritual psychology enables a person to better understand their own beliefs and work through confusion. Spiritual psychologists or experts can help individuals by allowing them to explore their spiritual side and work towards repairing and wounded signs of their soul. Spiritual experts can usually help people feeling disappointed and dejected with a number of problems that cannot usually be solved by traditional psychological methods. Spiritual psychologist or expert provides a counselling and help people to achieve spiritual well-being as well as mental and emotional well-being.

Spiritual psychology examines spiritual self-transcendent or transpersonal aspects of human consciousness. Spiritual psychology studies the spiritual aspect of human beings. Its premise is that we cannot really understand human being unless we also appreciate their spiritual dimension. Spiritual psychology combines scientific and spiritual understanding of people in trying to help these to cope with the exigencies of their daily living. Spiritual psychology borrows religious terminologies, it does not belong to any extant-religion; it is a spiritual science, an attempt to understand spirit through the scientific method, not through faith and belief.

Spiritual psychology attempts to understand the nature of human mind and behaviour from the perspective of spiritual growth and evolution of human conciseness. A study of spiritual psychology can be highest rewarding, at a personal level, it deepens our understanding of ourself, helping people to become more self-aware. At a larger level, it widens our perception of life in general, allowing us to view the grander scheme of things.

Indian psychology is not Hindu psychology, rather it is spiritual psychology. Its seeds are found in all the Hindu systems of thought, in Buddhism and Jainism as well as in Indian Sufism.

Another positive contribution of psychology to spirituality has been the work of psychiatrists and psychologists on the psychology of meditation. The work explicitly on the psychology of meditation has been helpful in analyzing and describing practices, structures, goals and interrelationships among a number of spiritual practices.

Transpersonal Psychology

Transpersonal psychology is an outgrowth of the humanistic psychology movement that gained momentum in the 1960s, especially in the US and Europe. Transpersonal psychology had its formal origin in 1967. It emerged as a "fourth force" in psychology with a mission to investigate human spirituality in its broadest expression. Transpersonal psychology investigates the significance and validity of spiritual experience and tries to understand its meaning and implication for our world and future.

Transpersonal psychology is a school of psychology that integrates the spiritual and transcendent aspects of the human experience with the framework of modern psychology. It is also possible to define it as a spiritual psychology. Maslow and his colleagues expected that transpersonal psychology would constitute a "Fourth force" in psychology, complementing and pulling the field beyond behaviourism, psycho-analysis and humanistic psychology—the first three major psychological systems of the twentieth century.

Transpersonal psychology is a field centred on the spiritual aspect of human life. The term transpersonal psychology was first introduced in the 1960 by Maslow and Frank. This field utilizes psychological methods and theories to examine spiritual subject matter. The *Journal of Transpersonal Psychology* began publication in 1969 and in 1971 the Association of Transpersonal Psychology was established. It has its roots in early work by psychologist James and Jung who were deeply interested in the spiritual aspects of human nature. In addition to using psychology to better understand spiritual experiences, transpersonal psychology also strives to provide a deeper and rich understanding of individuals and to help them to achieve their greatest potential.

Psychology as a Resource for Spirituality

In modern era, the discipline of psychology and of spirituality is inextricably related to each other. Researchers of spirituality take help from psychology. As an academic discipline, the study of spirituality is a recent development although the phenomena and texts which are the objectives of its study is not new. Among the behavioural science, the discipline of psychology emerged late in nineteenth century and has contributed significantly to spirituality. Psychology can and should be an important resource for spirituality. Various schools of psychology serve different functions within the study of spirituality. Developmental psychology contributed spirituality in a number of ways. Psychopathology in human behaviour serves as a critical check on theory and on practice in spirituality. Further, psychology offers a number of developmental theories which influence our knowledge of various stages of growth towards transcendent reality and the interaction of the self with superpower throughout the life-cycle. The psychology of meditation illuminates the activity of the self to its own consciousness as well as to the super power of God. These areas exemplify closeness and deep relationship between these two disciplines.

Psychology and spirituality have problematic relationships. There are differences in assumptions and methods of both fields as well as overlapping subject matter and interests. The most important issue is the difference between the way these two disciplines view transcendent reality and the nature of the relationship of the human to transcendence.

Psychology is a useful and necessary tool for spirituality. Conversely, spirituality is frequently a source for psychology, providing a number of new research area for exploration. Literature with spiritual tradition, often rooted in individual experience, describe psychological experience and offer pre-scientific theories about it.

Psychology and spirituality both have been concerned with the same phenomena which are often interpreted from quite different perspective. There is a reciprocal relationship between psychology and spirituality. Researchers in the spirituality can use developmental theory of psychology as one of understanding the psychological development.

Organizational Spirituality

Organizational spirituality can be defined as: "Enabling each employee to be able to realize their highest human potential, by embodying spiritual values and attitudes within the workplace such as meaning, love, compassion, acceptance, forgiveness, value, and integrity" (Alfred, 2002).

There are a number of benefits of a more positive workplace spirituality, where staff are valued and find meaning in their daily work:

- Enhancement of a culture of 'service' to other staff and the organization, rather than competition or undermining. This can only happen if staff personal values resonate with organization's values and culture.
- Employees find 'meaning' in the workplace situation, which leads to improved personal job satisfaction, low rates of workplace stress and absenteeism.

Signs of Flourishing Organizational Spirituality

- Policies and procedures of the organization promoting a culture of personal growth, self-knowledge and the maintenance of integrity. Employees enabled to create, achieve, and influence in their daily work.
- Organization having shared values which generate not only supportive relationship between employees, but also a sense of belonging and meaning.
- Management should encourage creativity, sensitivity, and empathy and have the ability to inspire employees to reach their full potential.

It is now accepted that those organizations which have a 'spiritually-friendly' culture, show universally lower than average rates of absenteeism, workplace stress and employee turnover. Spiritual culture also provide opportunities for transcendence and interconnectedness through the work processes which, within the moral framework, results in increased and better output. Thus, workplace spirituality is not only just good for the 'soul', but is also good for the workplace itself.

According to Karakas, Fahri (2010), incorporating spirituality at work: (a) increases employees well-being by increasing their morale, commitment and productivity; (b) decreases employees' stress, burnout, and workholism in the workplace. A 'spiritually-friendly' workplace will have greater staff-retention rates, so lowering recruitment costs. It will see an increase in innovation, better cooperation and team work and superior interface between organization and its customers. It is a source of inexhaustible faith and will power. It covers a broad range of phenomena, pertains employees' hopes and dreams, their patterns of thoughts, emotions, feelings and behaviours.

Organizational spirituality include: meditation time at the beginning of meetings, retreat or spiritual training time set aside for employees' appropriate accommodation of employee prayer practices and openly as King questions to test of company actions are aligned with higher meaning and purpose (Srishti, 2010)

Role of spirituality in an Organizational set-up goes a long way in correcting prevailing conditions so as to inculcate the values into the employees with a viewpoint to serve better in a society, country and in the world. Spiritual values promote economic efficiency and cause equality improvements in productivity. It promotes an understanding amongst employees and smoothen employee and employer relationship. Every organization strives to strengthen this relationship with sole motto of creating a conducive environment to develop mutual trust, understanding, cooperation and coordination.

Organization based on modern management system looks for dynamism, openness, enthusiasm, sustainability in the procedure and action. In addition more kindness, fairness, democratic principles and power sharing can be attributed to spirituality in the workplace. Employees are empowered and they thus contribute to the strength of the organization and a renewed competitive energy. If employees are encouraged to become more conscious of their 'highest' selves and are made aware that the purpose of life and work is both material and spiritual, organizational effectiveness is enhanced.

References

Alfred, R. (2002). *Spirituality at Work.* First International Conference on Organizational Spirituality, University of Surrey.

Fowler, J.W. (2001). Faith development theory and post-modern challenges. *The International Journal for the Psychology of Religion, 11*, 159-172.

Frank, A.W. (2004). Narratives of spirituality and religion in end-of-life. In B. Hurwitz, T. Green Halgh and V. Skultans (Eds.) *Narrative Research in Health and Illness* (pp. 132-145) Maldeen, M.A: Blackwell.

Freud, S. (1961 a). *Civilization and its Discontent.* NY. W.W. Nton.

Hall, G.S. (1924). *Life and Confusions of a Psychologist.* New York: D. Appleton.

James, W. (1961). *The Varieties of Religious Experiences*, New York: Collier.

Karakas, Fahri (2010) Spirituality and performance in organizations: A literature review. *Journal of Business Ethics, 94* (1), 89-106.

Kohlbeg, I. (1984). *The Psychology of Moral Development: The Nature and Validity of Moral Stages, Essays on Moral Development*, Vol. 2nd. San Francisco: Harper and Row.

Leuba, J.H. (1925). *The Psychology of Religions Mysticism.* NY: Harcourt, Brace.

Mac Innes, E. (2003). *Zen Contemplation for Christian.* Lanham, M.D.: Shed & Ward.

Maslow, A.H. (1990). *Toward a Psychology of Being* (3rd Edition), New York, John Willey & Sons.

Mc Grath, P. (2006). Defining Spirituality: From meaning making to connection. In S. Ambrose (Ed.) *Religion and Psychology: New Research* (pp. 223-239) NY: Nova Science.

Miller, G.A. (2003). The cognitive revaluation: A historical perspective. *Trends in Cognitive Science, 7*, 141-144.

Piaget, J. (1954). *The Construction of Reality in the Child.* NY: Basic Books.

Puffer, K.A. (2001). The church as an agent of help in the battle against late life depression. *Pastoral Psychology, 50*, 125-136.

Roehlkepartain, E., Benson, P., King, P. and Wagener, I. (2006). Spiritual development in childhood and adolescents: Moving to the scientific mainstream. In E. Roehlkepartain, P. King, I. Wagener, and P. Benson (Eds.) *The Handbook of Spiritual Development in Childhood and Adolescence,* (pp. 1-15). Thousand Oaks, C.A. Sage.

Roof, W.C. (1999). *Spiritual Market Place. Baby Boomers and the Remaking of American Religion.* Princeton, NJ: Princeton University Press.

Srishti, J. (2010). Impact of workplace spirituality on organizational culture through improved employee productivity. *AIMS International Conference on Value-Based Management,* August 11-13, 2010.

Stoeber, M. (1994). *Theo-monistic Mysticism: A Hindu Christian Comparison.* New York: St. Martin's Press.

Vergote, A. (2003). Playing between psychology and mysticism. In J. Belzen and A. Geels (Eds.) *Mysticism: A Variety of Psychological Perspectives* (pp. 81-107), Amsterdam: Rodopi.

Welch, J. (1996). *The Carmelite Way: An Ancient Path for Today's Pilgrim*. NY: Paulist Press.

Wilber, K. (1996). *The Atman Project: The Transpersonal View of Human Development* (2nd ed.). Wheaton, 11: Guest Books.

6

Mindfulness

Structure, Function and Consequences

Aradhana Shukla

In these days researchers and health care professionals are paying their attention on positive topics and mindfulness as a source of increasing personals strength is becoming more attractive (Aspinwell and Staudinger, 2003; Peterson and Selligman, 2004). Researches on positive psychotherapy and general use of mental strength suggest that it cannot be possible without having mindfulness. Fluckiger and Perks (2006) have suggested that nurturing strength in clients may be injected through therapeutic bonding, mastery experience and declined in the symptoms of disorder. Researches done on educational setting suggest strength base curriculum as a means of fostering intrinsic motivation and strength (Hayes, 2002; Louis, 2009; Bowers and Lopez, 2010). All these things are possible by the existence and development of mindfulness.

Mindfulness—A Mental State

Although mindfulness is a new age and recently emerged concept it can be comparable with the traditional concept of Buddhism (*cultivating awareness of everybody happening and psycho-physical sensation*) and modern therapeutic devices of increasing attention in order to identify distortion in thinking (Miller, 1995). Longer (2002) presided a very extensive definition of mindfulness.

"It is important to take at least a brief look at what mindfulness is and is not: It is a flexible state of mind, an openness to novelty, a process of actively drawing novel distinctions. When we are mindful, we become sensitive to context and perspective; we are trapped in rigid mind-sets, oblivious to contest or perspective. When we are mindless our behaviour is rule and routine governed. In contrast, when mindful, our behaviour may be guided rather than governed by rules and routine. Mindfulness is not vigilance or attention when what is meant by those concepts is a stable focus on an object or idea. When mindful, we are actively varying the stimulus field. It is not controlled processing (e.g. 31*267), in that mindfulness requires or generates novelty."

Thus, it is surely fair to say that mindfulness is active research of novelty in everybody life (as the situation be).

Being mindfulness requires us to (1) Overcome the desire to reduce uncertainty in daily life, (2) Override a tendency to encourage in automatic behaviour, and (3) Engage less frequently in the evaluation of self, others and situations.

Bishop *et al.* (2004) have produced an operational definition of mindfulness, but they have stressed more on cognitive and emotional components of mindful engagement. They have focused on self-regulated attention (*based on current personal experiences*) and emotional openness (*appreciations and acceptance of all internal experiences*). Thus, mindful is emerged by own personal experiences and it is incorporated with meta-cognition and emotional awareness.

Shapiro (2002) suggested some qualities of mindfulness and they are directly related to the qualities of a person having positive orientation towards life. They are:

- *Non-judgemental:* Impartial, observation of any event without any categorization or judgement.
- *Non-striving:* No attachment on goals, no outcome orientedness.
- *Acceptance*: Observing things and events in present base.
- *Patience*: Patience to ownself, others and the present moment.
- *Trust*: Trust on ownself, others, emotions, intuition and situations and overall life.
- *Openness*: Observation of anything as presented in first time.
- *Letting go*: Less attachment on thoughts, feeling, experiences and the people.
- *Gentleness*: Characterized as soft and tender personally, but not passive.
- *Generosity*: No attachment of gaining or any positive work to be returned.
- *Empathy:* The quality of feeling the thoughts and/or emotions of the other person as he thinks or feels and show it by their action.

- *Gratitude*: The quality of reverence, appreciating and being thankful for the present moment.
- *Loving-kindness:* Benevolent, compassionate and cherish a quality of giving unconditional love.
- *Meditation and mindfulness*: Origin from Buddhism.

It can be said that mindfulness is said to have emerged in the East and is growing popular in West due to the widespread implication of mindfulness-based intervention (MBI), which integrates traditional mindfulness practice with contemporary psychological practice in order to improve well-being. Originally, the concept of mindfulness has been associated with spiritual movements rather than mainstream psychology (Cardaciotto *et al.*, 2006). Mindfulness as such refers to a way of orienting one's self to the present moment (Thompson and Waltz, 2007). It is believed to promote well-being of human since Buddhism teaches Western psychologists as to how they can relate to their own experiences. The trending research on mindfulness looks at how the brain responds to mindful practices, how relationship benefit, and how physical and mental health improves, in addition to similar other topics. It should also be kept in mind that howsoever novel the construct of mindfulness looks like, the body of research on mindfulness has also been criticized because of the scarcity of rigorous empirical research on mindfulness.

Mindfulness Research at a Global Level

Researcher's interest in mindfulness practice has steadily increased as studies continue to reveal its beneficial effects. For instance, Singla (2011) in her study reflects on how theoretical knowledge can be applied to meditation practices and how to relate East and West psychology. She further advocates that with mindfulness, one can learn to experience difficult thoughts, emotion and pains in a less judgemental manner. She considered it to be beneficial for modern world which is under the clutches of social fragmentation.

Thompson and Waltz (2007) examined the relationship between measures of everyday mindfulness, mindfulness during meditation, and the effect of sitting meditation on mood. The aim of mindfulness meditation is the development of deep insight into conscious cognitive processes and development of optimal states of psychological well-being and consciousness (Wallsh, 1983). The scales used were: Mindful Attention Awareness Scale (MAAS: Brown and Ryan, 2003), Cognitive and Affective Mindfulness Scale-Revised (CAMS-R: Feldman, Hayes, Kumar, Greeson and Laurenceau, 2007), the Toronto Mindfulness Scale (TMS: Lau *et al.*, 2006) and Positive and Negative Affect Schedule (PANAS, Watson, Clark and Tellegen, 1998). They found that everyday mindfulness correlated positively with agreeableness and conscientiousness, and correlated negatively with neuroticism. Little to no relationship was found between mindfulness during meditation and everyday mindfulness. Also, experienced meditation practitioners exhibited stable mood compared to non-practitioners.

Brown and Ryan (2003) developed Mindful Attention Awareness Scale (MAAS) to examine the role of mindfulness on psychological well-being. They examined relationship between MAAS and well-being indicators. MAAS was found to be positively related with openness to Experienced, Feelings, Actions, Ideas and Values; and inversely with Depression, Angry Hostility, Self-consciousness, Impulsiveness and Vulnerability. The result also suggested that MAAS well-being relations cannot be explained by Social Desirability. It was observed that people who consciously practice this skill have higher MAAS and show closer relations between implicit and explicit affective states than those scoring low. The scale is also used to study the well-being in cancer patients.

Schreiner and Malcolm (2008) investigated how mindfulness meditation affects the emotional states of depression, anxiety, and stress. They conducted tests using depression, anxiety, and stress scale, before and after a 10 week mindfulness meditation programme and found a decrease in above mentioned symptoms after the programme. Meditation reduces ruminative tendencies and simultaneously increases intentional control. It works on two levels: one, by increasing awareness about the present; and two, by accepting emotions non-judgementally (Baer, 2003). They also predicted that individuals with higher levels of depression, Anxiety, and Stress benefits more from mindfulness training. Cardaciotto, Herbert, Furmam, Moitra and Farrow (2006) developed a two dimensional measure of mindfulness to evaluate present-moment awareness and acceptance with Philadelphia Mindfulness Scale (PHLMS). This measure of mindfulness can be applied in populations without meditation experienced and assesses acceptance distinctly from ongoing awareness. Cardaciotto *et al.,* (2006) theorized mindfulness as "*tendency to be highly aware of one's internal and external experiences in the context of an accepting, non-judgemental stance toward those experienced*". A clear two factor solution and good internal consistency was demonstrated in both non-clinical and clinical samples. The PHLMS Awareness sub-scale was found to be positively related to measures of acceptance, happiness and quality of life. It was negatively related to rumination, thought suppression and anxiety.

Clinical and non-clinical groups showed significantly lower score of awareness and acceptance in the general psychiatric sample and significantly less acceptance in the eating disorders sample. Also, from correlation test, it was found that two sub-scales were not related which suggests that awareness can be disambiguated from acceptance.

In one intervention study, Kabat-Zinn and Skillings (1989) examined the effects of an 8 week, Mindfulness Based Stress Reduction (MBSR) programme on stress hardiness and sense of coherence in hospital patients. MBSR programme are designed to treat chronic stress and there happens to be blending discussion about stress reactions and active mediation skills training. MBSR also teaches individuals how to direct attention to their body parts and observe the sensation in each area (Segal, Williams and Teasdale, 2002). Stanley and Jha (2010) studied how mindfulness training effect working memory capacity and affective experience in military service members preparing for deployment. They found participants practicing meditation at home have increased working memories and higher level of positive affect. Likewise, Key and Wang (2008) examined the relationship between mindfulness, flow dispositions and mental skills adoption in athletes using cluster analytic approach. Participants were tested using Mindfulness/Mindfulness Scale (MMS: Bonder and Langer, 2001) and Dispositional Flow Scale (DFS: Jackson and Eklund, 2004). Moderate high correlation was found between flow dispositions and attentional control and goal setting. A four-point cluster was found to be optimal and no gender difference was observed in clusters. The finding suggested that more mindful, experienced more flow states.

Cullen (2011) discussed the contemplative practices that are integral to MBSR and examined how they have developed over the years. Participants in MBI report a deeper connection to their own faith tradition. The two most comprehensively used MBIs are mindfulness-based stress reduction (MBSR: Kabat-Zinn, 1994) and mindfulness-based cognitive therapy (MBCT; Segal, Williams and Teasdale, 2002; 2013). These teach mindfulness skills through range of formal and informal mindfulness practices. Both MBSR and MBI has revolutionized the understanding and delivery of health care. To cohort groups such as people with depression, cancer patients, overweight women, medical students etc. specific modules are added according to difficulties faced by that group. Mindfulness tendency is linked to the flow dispositions of clear goals, concentration with a sense of control and loss of self-consciousness (Key & Wang, 2008). Mindfulness is positively correlated with openness to experience, but no relationship is found between mindfulness and neuroticism. Increased mindfulness facilitates the positive effects of mindfulness-based stress reduction intervention.

Above all, Nyklicek and Kujipers (2008) examined meditating effects of mindfulness in a randomized controlled trial. Participants were randomly assigned into a group receiving MBSR or a waiting list control group. They were given questionnaires on psychological well-being, quality of life, and mindfulness. MBSR group showed stronger reductions of perceived stress and vital exhaustion and stronger elevations of positive affect, quality of life and mindfulness. Gu, Strauss, Bond and Cavanagh (2015) in their latest meta-analysis defines Mindfulness Based Cognitive Therapy (MBCT) as a psychotherapeutic treatment with *"established efficacy in preventing relapse of depression for individuals in complete remission."* They conducted Two Stage-Structural Equation Modelling (TS-SEM) meta-analyses by choosing mental health outcomes such as global psychopathological, depressive and anxiety symptoms, stress, and negative affectivity as the target psychological outcomes. SEM analyses and sobel tests found strong, consistent evidence for cognitive and emotional reactivity, moderate, consistent evidence for mindfulness and RNT, and preliminary but insufficient evidence for self-compassion and psychological flexibility as mechanisms. Furthermore, the study demonstrated proof for mindfulness and RNT as significant of the impact of MBIs on clinical outcomes.

The above mentioned review of the research conducted on mindfulness and mindfulness-based techniques the richness and depth of studies conducted and made available on the construct. And, at the same time it points to the overall significance of a purportedly meaningful construct having foundation in Eastern Worldview with more or less no empirical documentation in the eastern cultural context. This gap makes the topic worthy of investigation and appealing to researches interested in the construct and is taken up for further exploration from an Indian perspective.

According to Indian Ethos

> "Mindfulness is seeing yourself by SELF in simple terminology,
> 'Mindfulness is the practice of loosening the ties that bind our Spirit with the body, senses, mind, and intellect; and thereby a

> person realizing his true nature which is pure, illuminating, and ever-shining free from all mental impurities."

In Sanskrit the definition of mind is '*sankalpa vikalpatmako mannhe*'. Our mind vacillates between past and future hardly comes to present moment ....where life is. It will either agree or disagree with the situation, but we are not aware of it. We have to learn how to manage our own mind. The rapport between us and the world is through our mind and spirit. The mind is like mudded water. When the mind is disturbed simply observe what is happening and give it a little time. It will settle down without any effort on our part. Don't accept when mind is in pieces, accept when mind is at peace because only then the clarity comes and mind becomes as sharp and powerful as a laser beam. The mind has the capacity to heal and elevate itself. It is full of joy, ease and love and true knowledge depends upon calmness of mind (Talwar, 2013).

In *Kathopanishad (1.3.4)*, an ancient Indian sacred text, it is mentioned:

> *Aatmanam rathinam viddhi, shariram rathameva tu,*
> *Buddhim tu sarathim viddhi manah pragrahmeva cha.*
> *Indriyani hayanahuh, vishayamsteshu gocharan,*
> *Aatmendriya manoyuktam, bhoktertyahurmanishinah.*
>
> "Wise people know that body is the chariot, senses are the horses, objects of the senses are the paths, intellect is the charioteer, mind is the rein of the horse lying in the hands of intellect, and Spirit is the Lord of the chariot enjoying the ride."

The underlying message for Mindfulness in the above text is:

> "Be the knower and be the enjoyer. Know the causal process of our sufferings. It starts when senses aimlessly draws towards sense objects. These senses have to be controlled through mind. But mind is in the hand of intellect which is knowledge developed through past experiences. Intellect is required to be under the command of Spirit. Otherwise, the chariot will move aimlessly from one path to another reaching nowhere. Those people enjoy who know this truth and follow inside-out approach of Spirit controlling the intellect, intellect controlling the mind, mind controlling the senses, and senses no more move aimlessly. Person sees himself (body, senses, mind, and intellect) with SELF

(Spirit or *Atman* or Individual Consciousness). Serenity prevails. Remove the cause of suffering and effect goes automatically is the *mantra*. This is Mindfulness."

Breath is the first act in our present life. When we are born first we take a long deep breath and cry and our last act is we breathe out. In between we always breathe in and out but we are not aware about it. There are many secrets that can be revealed by the breath and we can access a vast mind and intellect through breath. This along with cosmology can make a big difference (Talwar, 2013). Observing the breath for few minutes brings relaxation to the body and mind and energizes our whole system. These days in Mindfulness meditation for stress reduction most of the training programmes across the world make the practitioner concentrate on the breath to live in the present moment.

In Indian ethos meditation is concentration. Concentration on the breath is one way of meditation. In *Katha Upanishad*, the utility of concentration on breath is explained. It says, by concentrating on breath that flows in and out make a person realize that the source of life is not breath. Instead, the source is somewhere else and is the cause of the breath. Mindfulness takes the person to that cause which is the Spirit and the realization makes the person enlightened as now he knows the source of his life which is no different than the source of any other life. Fire in coal looks different than fire in jungle, but fire is same so is the wind, though one, takes different form. Similarly, Spirit though one, takes different form. Our illusion, called as *avidya* or *maya* (ignorance) is a result of perceptions and inferences drawn through senses, mind, and intellect. Mindfulness makes us realize the oneness of omnipresent Spirit in all. He who see many and not the ONE wanders. This truth could be learned even by the mind through practice by surrendering senses to mind and surrendering mind to know Thyself. Indian ethos calls for overcoming two mental sufferings for Mindfulness and they are:

- Attachment (*Raaga*)
- Aversion (*Dvesha*)

Attachment for something that is transitory like wealth and fame and aversion toward any object makes the mind wander. Aversion arises out of our ignorance of 'I' and 'Others'. It burns the person in hatred. Mindfulness prescribes search for Eternal. Attachment and Aversion makes the mind wandering for transient. Calmness of mind is lost. Calmness makes the mind attentive and receptive to present moment. Attachment and Aversion make the mind dwell in the past. Attachment to transitory things and aversion are evils. Most learned person could be its victim. Evil of mind has to be removed only then there will be rest in senses, concentration in mind, peace in heart and Mindfulness achieved.

Gautama Buddha in his Doctrine of Origination (*Pratityasamutpada*) explains the foundation of Mindfulness. This Doctrine explains the cause of human sufferings (2nd Noble Truth) and the way to cessation of these sufferings (3rd Noble Truth). Uncontrolled mind works in relative way through its interaction with the *Samsara* (world). Controlled mind is an enabler in realizing the reality the Absolute (*nirvana*). *Pratityasamutpada* as told by Buddha so explicitly explains that the world perceived through gross (senses, mind, intellect) results in skewed definition of all creations and destruction arising out of empirical analysis, conditionality, relativity, and dependence. Fixing the mind to transient (impermanent and neither real nor unreal) is the cause. Mind becomes shuttlecock moving from one side to another.

Chandradhar Sharma (1970) explains the Doctrine of Gautama Buddha in following words: "*The causal formula is: 'This being, that arises', i.e., 'depending on the cause, the effect arises.' Thus, every object of thought is necessarily relative. And because it is relative, it is neither absolutely real (for it is subject to death) nor absolutely unreal (for it appears to arise).*"

The remedy for this is prescribed by Gautama Buddha in Eight Noble paths out of which two paths given below are presently linked with Mindfulness:

- Right Thoughts (*smriti*)
- Right Concentration (*samadhi*)

But one thing should be remembered that there are prerequisites for right thoughts and right concentration. As in *Astanga Yoga; yamas* (don'ts of life), *niyama* (discipline), *asana* (postures for making body fit for deep meditation), *pranayama* (practice of breath control for deep meditation) and *pratyahara* (control of senses) are described as prerequisites for deep meditation; similarly, Gautama Buddha has prescribed right living (*ajiva*), right action (*karmanta*), right effort (*vyayama*) and right speech (*vak*) as noble paths making a person fit for right concentration (*samadhi*). Before starting concentration or deep meditation, preparedness of mind is a pre-requisite. Mind is prepared by deciding the object on which mind has to be fixed for meditation. This process is *dharana* in *Astanaga Yoga*. In eight noble paths of Gautama Buddha, this process could be related to right thoughts, so that, mind does not waver and fix itself to the *shreya* (good) and not *preya* (pleasure). In current Mindfulness Based Training Programmes world-wide, mind is made to fix on the breath so that mind does not wander in bad thoughts.

Point here is that for Mindfulness there is a complete and holistic process in Indian ethos and teachings of Gautama Buddha. Simply jumping to meditation in Mindfulness based training programmes of few hours, days or week is a gross injustice to the practitioners. Mindfulness is a sacred way of life embracing withinn itself the material values also resulting in proper synthesis of spiritual values (*Shreya* or *Dharma* and *Moksha*) and material values (*Preya* or *Artha* and *Kama*).

There are five levels of mental life which are given below:

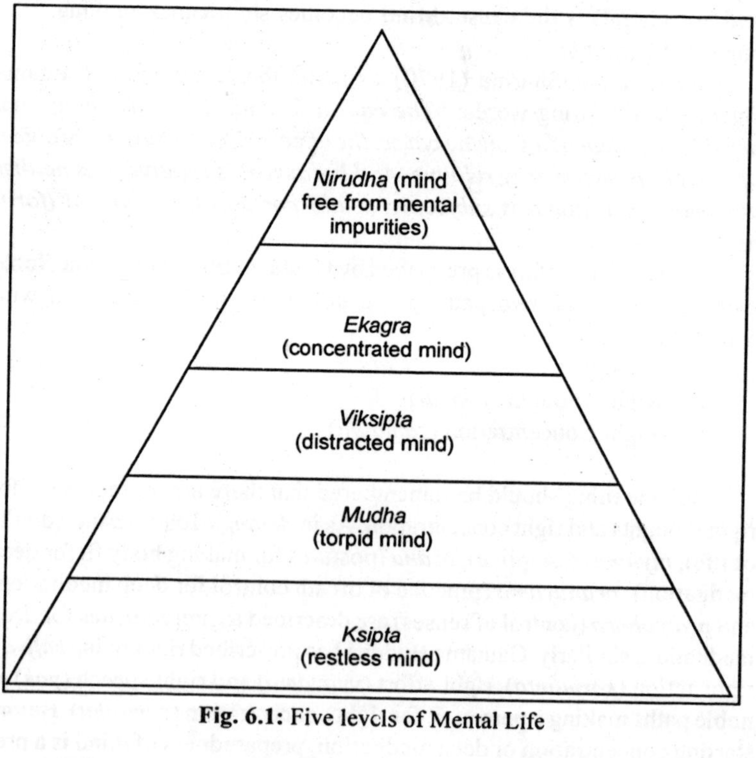

Fig. 6.1: Five levcls of Mental Life

The purpose of Mindfulness is to reach to the highest level of *nirudha* where the mind is in pure and calm state free from all the modifications from the lowest level of *ksipta* where the mind is restless. Initially, any practitioner of Mindfulness need to practice *Ekagra* (concentration) taking care of the prerequisites mentioned earlier. Normally, *Ekagra* is sufficient for Mindfulness.

According to Sharma (1970) difference in *Ekagra* and *Nirudha* meditation is that *Ekagra* is conscious meditation (*samprajnata*) in which the end state is that mind is fully concentrated on the object of meditation and *Nirudha* is supra-conscious meditation in which the object of meditation is transcended. Further, *Ekagra* meditation could be done in four ways (Sharma, 1970):

Table 6.1: Four ways of Meditation for Concentrated Mind

Four ways of Meditation for Concentrated Mind	
1. *Savitarka*	Concentrating mind on gross objects like the tip of the nose or the mid-point of the eyebrows or the image of the deity.
2. *Savichara*	Concentrating mind on a subtler object of meditation like the sound.
3. *Sananda*	Concentrating mind on a still subtler object of meditation like senses which produce joy.
4. *Sasmita*	Concentrating on the ego-substance with which the self is generally identified. Here, we have conscious ecstasy where individuality persists.

Benefits of Mindfulness

Affective Benefits

Emotion Regulation: There is evidence that mindfulness helps to effective emotion regulation in the brain (Corcoran, Fasb, Anderson and Segal, 2010; Siegel, 2007), in term of proposed mechanism of change. Corcoran *et al.* (2010) have emphasized that mindfulness meditation promotes meta-cognitive awareness, and develops intentional capacities, cognitive gains which, in term, contribute to effective emotion regulation strategies, i.e. directly associated with effective emotional regulation (Chambers, Lo and Allen, 2008). Chambers and associates have found that mindfulness training decreased rumination is consistent with research with participants having chronic mood disorders. In other study efficacy of mindfulness based therapy for reducing anxiety and depression symptom was also noticed (Halfman, Sawyer, Witt and Oh, 2010).

Thus, it is sure that meditation may *elicit* positive emotion, minimize negative effect and enable emotion regulation.

Interpersonal benefits: There are so many evidences indicating the fact that mindfulness trait predicts satisfaction ability to maintain positive and constructive relation skill in identifying and communicating the relation, reducing relational stress (Barnes, Brown, Krusemark Campbell and Rogge, 2007). Barns *et al.* (2007) have also noticed that people having higher trait mindfulness show less emotional stress, anger and anxiety. Thus, it is surely fair to say that mindfulness protects against stressful conditions and promotes ability to deal the environment with positive orientation, other benefits of mindfulness meditation practice include increased information processing speed (Moore and Melinowski, 2009), decreased task effort (Lutz *et al.*, 2009) and having fewer thought that are unrelated to the task at hand.

Enhancing mindfulness: There are so many strategies and discipline that are found useful in enhancing mindfulness (Siegel, 2007b), but many writings of ancient and modern time have shown that mindfulness can be increased through meditation. In Buddhism, mindful practice and its significance has also been stated and used synonymously as *Vipassana.* This is a Pali word and derived from *Theravada Buddhism* (Gunaratana, 2002, Young, 2007). The term *vipassana* deals with the insight or awareness (Gunaratana, 2002), moreover, mindfulness, can systematically be cultivated by *vipassana* practice emotion, thoughts and especially on the surrounding (Bodhi, 2002; Germer, 2005; Wallace, 2001; Young, 1997).

Although, it is true that all meditational practices enhance mindfulness yet different types and styles of meditational activities stimulate different types of brain activity (Cohn and Polich, 2006; Lut, Dunne and Davidson, 2007). For example mindful meditation focusing on *mantras* stimulate prefrontal brain including self-observation and meta-cognition (Cohn and Polich, 2006) and faster specific attentional mechanism (Valentine and Sweet, 1999). With the advent of new thoughts and vision in the mindful investigation, many other areas life focused attention, open monitoring (non-judgemental and moment to moment observation of one's experience) and loving endless compassion practice and their specific physiological outcomes are also being examined (Lutz, Slagter, Dunne and Davidson, 2008; Lutz *et al.*, 2009).

Being benefited by mindfulness: As it is appeared that mindfulness research reveal a sense of positivism, that is so many benefits of mindfulness.

Intervention: Mindfulness meditation noticed can successfully use in the promotion of therapist client relations.

Empathy: There are numerous evidences related to empathy (Anderson, 2005; Shapiro and Izett, 2008; Walsh and Shapiro, 2006) therapist track their internal response to client and make them feel more and less empathetic towards client. Wang (2007) found that therapist who were experienced mindfulness meditators scored higher as measure of self-reported empathy than therapists who did not meditate.

Compassion: Next to empathy, the second attribute that a client should have is compassion. Shapiro *et al.* (2005) have stressed the need and importance of MBSR training for professionals. Kingsbury (2009) found that non-judgementatism and non-creationism (important components of mindfulness) are associated with compassion.

Counselling Skill: We have so many evidences which suggest that mindfulness inventions in psychotherapy can become so helpful for the skill development and client counsellor in training. Who have participated in similar mindfulness based intervention have reported significant increase in self-awareness and insights about their professional identity (Birn Baum, 2008) and overall wellness (Rybak and Russell-Chopin, 1998).

Decrease in Stress and Anxiety: Evidences suggest that mindfulness based interventions can bring faster emotional intelligence and social connectedness and reduce stress and anxiety (Cohen and Iniller, 2000), depression, fatigue and anger (Tang *et al.*, 2007) and promotion of greater attention, self-regulation and immunoreactivity was also visited (Waelde, 2008).

So far as, the matter of other benefits is concerned, it can be said that relationship between mindfulness and counselling self-efficacy was predicted by self-reported mindfulness technique. Dreifuss (1990) interviewed six therapists who practiced one of these mindfulness meditation style (*Vipassiana, Zename Vajrayana*) for more than five years to examine the influence of their meditation practice on their work as therapists. Findings suggested that long-term mindfulness meditation practice can positively impact therapists' ability to distinguish their own experience from their client experience, can enrich therapists clarity in their work with clients, and may help therapists' self-insight. Other potential benefits of mindfulness include increase in the magnitude of patients, intentionality, gratitude and body awareness (Rolhaupt and Morgan, 2007).

In conclusion, it is surely to say that mindful in practice has a potential transformation in ways to facilitate therapist insight as well as total humanity development. Not only in the field of therapy but also general human life can also be nourished by mindfulness meditation practice.

References

Anderson, D.T. (2005). Empathy, psychotherapy integration, and meditation: A Buddhist contribution to the common factors movement. *Journal of Humanistic Psychology, 45*, 483-502. doi:10.1177.

Baer, R.A. (2003). Mindfulness training as a clinical intervention: A conceptual and empirical review. *Clinical Psychology: Science and Practice, 10*(2), 125-143.

Barnes, S., Brown, K.W., Krusemark, E., Campbell, W.K., and Rogge, R.D. (2007). The role of mindfulness in romantic relationship satisfaction and responses to relationship stress. *Journal of Marital and Family Therapy, 33*, 482-500. doi:10.1111/j.1752–0606.2007.00033.x

Bishop, S.R., Lau, Shapiro, S., Carlson. L., Anderson, N.D., Carmody, T., *et al.* (2004). Mindfullness: A Proposed operational definition. *Clinical Psychology: Science and Practice, 11*, 230-241.

Birnbaum, L. (2008). The use of mindfulness training to create an "Accompanying Place" for social work students. *Social Work Education, 27*, 837-852. doi:10.1080/02615470701538330

Bodner, T., and Langer, E. (2001). Individual differences in mindfulness: The Langer Mindfulness Scale. *Post-session presented at the annual meeting of the American Psychological Society*, Toronto, Ont., Canada.

Bodhi, B. (2000). *A Comprehensive Manual of Adhidhamma*. Seattle: BPS Pariyatti.

Brown, W.K., Ryan, R.M. (2003). The benefits of being present: mindfulness and its role in psychological well-being. *Journal of Personality and Social Psychology. 84*(4), 822-848.

Cahn, B.R., and Polich, J. (2006). Meditation states and traits: Eeg, erp, and neuroimageing studies. *Psychological Bulletin, 132*, 180-211. doi: 10.1037/0033-2909.132.2.180

Cardaciotto, L.A., Herbert, J.D., Forman, E.M., Moitra, E. and Farrow, V. (2006). The Assessment of Present-Moment Awareness and Acceptance: The Philadelphia Mindfulness Scale.

Chambers, R., Lo, B.C.Y., and Allen, N.B. (2008). The impact of intensive mindfulness training on attentional control, cognitive style, and affect. *Cognitive Therapy and Research, 32*, 303-322. doi:10.1007/s10608-007-9119-0

Cohen, J.S., and Miller, L. (2009). Interpersonal mindfulness training for well-being: A pilot study with psychology graduate students. *Teachers College Record, 111*, 2760-2774. Retrieved from http://www.tcrecord.org

Corcoran, K.M., Farb, N., Anderson, A., and Segal, Z.V. (2010). Mindfulness and emotion regulation: Outcomes and possible meditating mechanisms. In A.M. Kring and D.M. Sloan (Eds.), *Emotion Regulation and Psychopathology: A Trans-diagnostic Approach to Etiology and Treatment* (pp. 339-355). New York: Guilford Press.

Cullen M. (2011). Mindfulness-Based Interventions: An Emerging Phenomenon. Springer Science Business Media.

Dreifuss, A. (1990). A phenomenological inquiry of six psychotherapists who practice Buddhist meditation. *Dissertation Abstracts International: Section B: Science and Engineering, 51*, 2617.

Feldman, G.C., Hayes, A.M., Kumar, S.M., and Greeson, J.M., and Laurenceau, J.P. (2007). Development, factor structure, and initial validation of the Cognitive and Affective Mindfulness Scale. *Journal of Psychopathology and Behavioural Assessment, 29*, 177-190.

Germer, C.K. (2005). Mindfulness: What is it? What does it matter? In C.K. Germer, R.D. Siegel, and P.R. Fulton (Eds.), *Mindfulness and Psychotherapy* (pp. 3-27). New York: Guilford Press.

Gu, J., Strauss, C., Bond, R. and Cavanagh, K. (2015). How do Mindfulness-Based Cognitive Therapy and Mindfulness-Based Stress Reduction Improve Mental Health and Well-being? A Systematic Review and Meta-Analysis of Meditation Studies, *Clinical Psychology Review, 37*, 1-12.

Gunaratana, H. (2002). *Mindfulness in Plain English.* Somerville, MA: Wisdom Publications.

Hoffman, S.G., Sawyer, A.T., Witt, A.A., and Oh, D. (2010). The effect of mindfulness-based therapy on anxiety and depression: A meta-analytic review. *Journal of Consulting and Clinical Psychology, 78*, 169-183. doi: 10.1037/a0018555

Jackson, S.A., and Eklund, R.C. (2004). The flow scale manual. Morgantown, WV: Fitness Information Technology.

Kabat-Zinn, J. and Skillings, A. (1989). Sense of coherence and stress hardiness as predictors and measure of outcome of stress reduction programmes. *Poster presented at the Society of Behavioural Medicine Conference*, San Francisco, USA.

Kabat-Zinn, J. (1994). *Wherever you go, there you are: Mindfulness meditation in everyday life*. New York: Hyperion Books.

Kee, Y.H. and Wang, C.K.J. (2008). Relationships between mindfulness, flow dispositions and mental skills adoption: A cluster analytic approach. *Psychology of Sport and Exercise, 9*, 393-411.

Kingsbury, E. (2009). The relationship between empathy and mindfulness: Understanding the role of self-compassion. *Dissertation Abstracts International: Section B: Science and Engineering, 70*, 3175.

Lau, M.A., Bishop, S.R., Segal, Z.V., Buis, T., Anderson, N.D., Carlson, L., *et al.* (2006). The Toronto Mindfulness Scale: Development and validation. *Journal of Clinical Psychology, 62*, 1445-1467.

Langer, E. (2002). Well-being: Mindfulness *versus* positive evaluation. In C.R. Snyder and S.J. Lopez (Eds). *The Handbook of Positive Psychology*. New York: Oxford University Press.

Lutz, A., Slagter, H.A., Rawlings, N.B., Francis, A.D., Greischar, L.L., and Davidson, R.J. (2009). Mental training enhances attentional stability: Neural and behavioural evidence. *The Journal of Neuroscience, 29*, 13418-13427. doi:10.1523/JNEUROSCI.1614-09.2009.

Olendzki, A. (2008). The real practice of mindfulness. *Buddhadharma, The Practitioner's Quarterly*. 37-44.

Miller, J. (1995). *How to want about you have: Discovering the magic and grandeur of ordinary existence*. New York: Avon Books.

Moore, A., and Malinowski, P. (2009). Meditation, mindfulness and cognitive flexibility. Consciousness and Cognition, *18*, 176-186. doi: 10.1016/ j.concog. 2008. 12.008

Nyklíček I. and Kujipers, K.F. (2008). Effects of Mindfulness-Based Stress Reduction Intervention on Psychological Well-being and Quality of Life: Is Increased Mindfulness Indeed the Mechanism? Springer Science Business Media.

Rothaupt, J.W., and Morgan, M.M. (2007). Counselors' and counselor educators' practice of mindfulness: A qualitative inquiry. *Counselling and Values*, 52, 40-54.

Rybak, C.J., and Russell-Chapin, L.A. (1998). The teaching well: Experience, education and counselling. *International Journal for the Advancement of Counselling, 20*, 131-139.

Shapiro, S.L., and Izett, C.D. (2008). Meditation: A universal tool for cultivating empathy. In S.F. Hick and T. Bien (Eds.), *Mindfulness and the therapeutic relationship* (pp. 161-175). New York: Guilford Press.

Shapiro, S.L., Astin, J.A., Bishop, S.R., and Cordova, M. (2005). Mindfulness-based stress reduction for health care professionals: Results from a randomized trial. *International Journal of Stress Management, 12*, 164-176. doi: 10.1037/1072–5245.12.2.164

Shapiro, S.L., Schwartz, G.E.R. and Santerre, L. (2002). Meditation and Positive Psychology. In C.R. Snyder and S.J. Lopez (Eds.) *The Handbook of Positive Psychology.* New York: Oxford University Press. 0022167805280264

Sharma, C. (1970). *A Critical Survey of Indian Philosophy*. Delhi: Motilal Banarasidass.

Schreiner, I., and Malcolm, J.P. (2008). The Benefits of Mindfulness Meditation: Changes in Emotional States of Depression, Anxiety, and Stress. *Behaviour Change. 25* (3), 156-168.

Schui, G. and Krumpen, G. (2010). Bibliometric Analyses on the Emergence and Present Growth of Positive Psychology. *Applied Psychology: Health and Well-Being, 2* (1), 52-64.

Segal, Z.V., Williams, J.M.G., and Teasdale, J.D. (2002). *Mindfulness-based cognitive therapy for depression: A new approach to preventing relapse.* New York: Guilford.

Singla, R. (2011). *Origins of Mindfulness and Meditation Interplay of Eastern and Western Psychology*. Psyke & Logos, *32*, 220-239.

Siegel, D.J. (2007b). *The mindful brain: Reflection and attunement in the cultivation of well-being*. New York: Norton.

Stanley, E., and Jha, A. (2010). Examining the protective effects of mindfulness training on working memory capacity and affective experience. *Emotion, 10*, 54-64.

Tang, Y., Ma, Y., Wang, J., Fan, Y., Feng, S., Lu, Q., Posner, M.I. (2007). Short-term meditation training improves attention and self-regulation. *PNAS Proceedings of the National Academy of Sciences,* USA of the United States of America, *104*, 17152-17156. doi:10.1073/ pnas.0707678104

Talwar, R. (2013). Role of Spirituality in Human Decision Making. In Singh, S. (Ed.), *Spiritual Paradigm for Management.* New Delhi: Excel India Publishers, p. 44.

Thompson, B.L. and Waltz, J. (2007). Everyday mindfulness and mindfulness meditation: Overlapping constructs or not? *Personality and Individual Differences*, *43*, 1875-1885.

Walsh, R.N. (1983). Meditation Practice and Research. *Journal of Humanistic Psychology, 26*, 113-121.

Watson, D., Clark, L.A., Tellegen, A. (1988). Development and validation of brief measures of positive and negative aspect: The PANAS scales. *Journal of Personality and Social Psychology. 54*(6), 1063-1070.

Valentine, E.R., and Sweet, P.L.G (1999). Meditation and attention: A comparison of the effects of concentrative and mindfulness meditation on sustained attention. *Mental Health Religion and Culture*, *2*, 59-70. doi:10.1080/ 13674679908406332

Waelde, L.C., Uddo, M., Marquett, R., Ropelato, M., Freightman, S., Pardo, A., and Salazar, J. (2008). A pilot study of meditation for mental health workers following hurricane Katrina. *Journal of Traumatic Stress*, *21*, 497-500. doi:10.1002/jts.20365

Walsh, R., and Shapiro, S.L. (2006). The meeting of meditative disciplines and Western psychology: A mutually enriching dialogue. *American Psychologist*, *61*, 227-239. doi:10.1037/0003-066X.61.3.227

Wang, S.J. (2007). Mindfulness meditation: Its personal and professional impact on psychotherapists. *Dissertation Abstracts International: Section B: Science and Engineering, 67*, 4122.

Young, S. (1997). *The Science of enlightenment.* Boulder, CO: Sounds True.

7

Understanding Positivism in Westo-Eastern Perspective

A Comparative Vision

Anubhuti Dubey

Similar to other cultures, the traditional Indian (Hindu) culture, embraces numerous values, placed in the context of philosophy, religion and spiritualism, generally regarded as both Indian philosophy and Indian psychology. With the aim to comprehend the core Indian culture, it is imperative to understand that....the moral and social qualities that are valued in a society have their roots in religion, philosophy and tradition (D. Sinha, 1972: 153). By Hindu tradition we refer to the world-view that has emerged from Vedic texts in the Indian subcontinent.

There is an immense call for understanding human behaviour and psychological processes in specific cultural context and through culturally-appropriate research approaches. To facilitate better appreciation to positive psychology, it is fine to value the interaction between culture and positive psychology because it will explain how positive psychology varies across culture. Cultural psychologist Shweder (1984) maintains that cultural factors help out to form what people reckon is good, moral, and virtuous. Outside the United States, Shweder's main fieldwork had been in the temple town of Bhubaneswar in the State of Odisha, India. His fieldwork in India has looked at cross-cultural concepts of the person, self, emotions, and moral reasoning.

Azuma (1984) remarked on the diverse world-views of Western and Non-Western researchers that "*When a psychologist looks at a non-Western culture through Western glasses, he may fail to notice important aspects of the non-Western culture since the schemata for recognizing them are not provided by his science.*"

In support of culturally-embedded psychological inquiry, Misra (2011: xv-xvi), commented, "*Since culture is a process involving engagement and participation of people, psyche and culture are intricately linked and influence each other. This motivates researchers in the direction of extending, elaborating and refining theories and appreciating linkages between socio-cultural and psychological processes. The culturally informed inquiry is becoming indispensible in all traditions of psychological research.*"

Cross-cultural psychologists (e.g. Markus and Kottayam, 1991; Smith and Bond, 1994; Triandis, 1989) have stressed that in collective cultures there are strict social norms governing people's appropriate behaviours, whereas in individualistic cultures people's behaviours are governed by their own internal attributes, such as their personal beliefs or attitudes.

Western literature generally stresses autonomy, individuality, and personal satisfaction, their Eastern counterparts generally believe in harmony, collective cooperation, and group satisfaction. In this chapter firstly, I will discuss the Eastern and Western perspectives of positive psychology in short, then particularly emphasize on the Hindu philosophy of life and its application in the present-day positive psychology.

Western Perspective

The thousands years of Western ideology and traditions were—Athenian, and Judaeo-Christian. Ancient Greek philosophers Aristotle and Plato focused on human strengths and stated about 11 moral virtues: courage, moderation, generosity, munificence, magnificence, even temper, friendliness, truthfulness, wit, justice, and friendship (Solomon, 2006). The main religious book of Judaism and Christianity "The Holy Bible" delineate the human virtues like faith, hope, and charity in Old Testament. Scholars also cite the Ten Commandments given by Moses in the Old Testament as directives towards cultivating certain strengths. The New Testament also illustrates the virtues that are valued by God are leadership, faith, mercy, love, joy, hope, patience, and hospitality (12:3-21).

Eastern Perspective

Four eastern philosophies, namely Confucians, Taoism, Buddhism and Hinduism have a great impact on the way of life of people in Asia as well as many parts of world. The Chinese homeland sage Confucius emphasized on five virtues which are deemed central to living a moral existence are *jen* (humanity), *yi* (duty to treat others well), *li* (etiquette and sensitivity for others' feelings), *zhi* (wisdom) and *xin* (truthfulness). Another Eastern perspective on life is explained in Taoism. Achieving naturalness and spontaneity in life is the most important goal in Taoist philosophy. One more Eastern philosophy Buddhism refers to the teachings of the "Enlightened One" which state that life is full of suffering brought on by human desire and attachment. There is, however, a possible end to the suffering through transcendence and ultimate understanding. Virtues are of utmost importance, and include love, joy, compassion, and composure. One of the main Eastern philosophy, i.e. Hinduism emphasizes the interconnectedness of all things. It advocates for the harmonious union among all individuals. Individuals are to strive for ultimate self-betterment and also encouraged to be good to others. Good deeds are motivated by the process of *karma.* In the religious-spiritual sphere of Indian thought, every human enterprise displays a striving towards the attainment of one of four fundamental goals, namely, *dharma* (duty), *artha* (economic welfare), *kaama* (enjoyment of life), and *moksha* (salvation). In most of Asian cultures (Hindu, Muslims, Sikh, Buddhists, even Christians living in various Asian countries) religious philosophies play important role in leading human beings towards attainment of positive goals of life; whereas Western 'secular' approach always attempt to separate religion from spirituality and humanity, individuals from society and community, state from citizen and so on (Laungani, 2007; Husain, 2011).

Western and Eastern Approaches to Positive Psychology

Indeed there are factors common to both the indigenous and Western cultures. There are also, however, factors unique to indigenous cultures. For example, cross-cultural researches conducted on the meaning of life with Koreans (Kim, Lee & Wong, 2005), Japanese (Takano & Wong, 2004) and Chinese (Lin & Wong, 2006); the results support both the culture free and culture specific positions.

Western approaches have faith in linear notion of positive-negative (two extreme ends of the line); whereas Eastern (Asian) approach spots mutuality of positive-negative (i.e. two sides of the same coin). A great deal of widely researched positive psychology concepts, e.g. happiness, optimism, self-efficacy, hope, life satisfaction which are defined and measured from 'Western American Individualistic' model; are not understood in the same way in other cultures (Indian, Chinese, Arabic, African and many others).

Virtues and strengths are esteemed in different ways across cultures. Hence, efforts to construct strengths related concepts using positive psychology can only be successful if they embrace significant cultural contemplations. The code of righteous living as stated in Hindu philosophy is—

> *Dhritih kshama damo'steyam shauchmindriyanigrahah,*
> *Dhirvidya satyamakrodho dashakam dhramalakshanam.*
> (Resolve, forgiveness, controlled mind, never stealing, cleanliness, control over senses, intellect, education, honesty and never getting angry are the ten facets of *Dharma*).
>
> (*Manu*.VI.92)
>
> *Ashtaugunapurusham dipayanti pragya sushilatvadamau shrutam cha,*
> *Prakram ashchbehubhashita chadanam yathashakti kritagyata cha.*
> (Eight qualities adorn a man—intellect, good character, self-control, study of scriptures, valour, less talking, charity as per capability and gratitude).
> *Dhairya yasya pita kshma cha janani shantih chiram gehini,*
> *Satyam soonuh aayam daya cha bhagini bhrata manah sanymah;*
> *Shayya bhumitalam dishah aapi vasanam gyanamtram bhojanam,*
> *Aite yasya kutumbinah vada sakhai kasmad bhayam yoginah.*
> (To a *yogi*, courage is his/her father, forgiveness mother, calm mind wife, truth son, compassion sister, control of mind brother, earth bed, directions (*disha*) garment, and knowledge is food. With the foregoing as one's family members, why would be one afraid of anything?).

Manu Samhita, one of the manual of the Hindu code of conduct, initially listed ten virtues necessary for a human being to live a *dharmic* (moral) life: *Dhriti* (courage), *Kshama* (forgiveness), *Dama* (temperance), *Asteya* (Non-covetousness/Non-stealing), *Saucha* (purity), *Indriyani-graha* (control of senses), *dhi* (reflective prudence), *vidya* (wisdom), *satyam* (truthfulness), *akrodha* (free from anger). In later verses this list was reduced to five virtues by the same scholar, by merging and creating a more broader concept. The shorter list of virtues became: *Ahimsa* (Non-violence), *Dama* (temperance), *Asteya* (Non-covetousness/Non-stealing), *Saucha* (purity), *Satyam* (truthfulness) (Gupta, 2006).

In the following part of this chapter, I will discuss only those above-mentioned virtues as pointed out in different Hindu treatise which are also well researched in contemporary positive psychology.

Happiness and Well-being

In Western society, Happiness is defined as gaining self-esteem, self-confidence, being materially and financially comfortable, being successful, being attractive, being equal, being treated with respect, being able to one's rights and enjoy pleasures and comforts of life (Laungani, 2007: 199). In Eastern cultures, in the *Bhagavad Gita* (5.21), it is said: "He who is unattached to the external world and its objects, and is attached to the inner Self, will attain supreme happiness, which is everlasting." Upanishads declared that the true nature of self is blissful (*Ananda*) (Paranjpe, 1998). Ordinarily what we call happiness (*sukha*) and misery (*duhkha*) are relâtive experiences. They are termed *dvandvas*—dualities.) Real happiness, called *ānanda* in Sanskrit, is the goal of all beings. All are seeking that goal only—some ignorantly, some with knowledge. Therefore, according to all the different philosophies of Hinduism—*Yoga*, *Vedanta*, *Samkhya*, dualists, non-dualists—our goal is to transcend dualities like happiness and misery and reach the state of supreme Bliss. Self-realization is the highest quality of life. The ideal of *Jivamukta* (Self-realization in this life) is achievable by transcending dualism in life (e.g. happiness-sorrow, pleasure-pain, love-hate) (Misra, 2013). Thus, happiness is defined as an internal state of mind; being in peace; doing one's duties; keeping others happy; being responsible and respectful to oneself, family and society; and enjoying life as it goes with oneself, family and others (Laungani, 2007 : 199). For Hindus, happiness comes from following one's *dharma* (duties); for Muslims, it comes from obeying to wish of *Allah* (God); for Chinese, it comes from balancing *Yin* and *Yang* (opposite life forces). In other communities (e.g. tribal communities), these positive psychology concepts may not be understood at all. Taken together, eastern traditions generally emphasize balance in life as the key to happiness.

As far as the conceptualization of well-being is concerned, the Hindu philosophy see wellness for all. By cultivating the capacity to remain unaffected by dualities one lives in a steady state of mind (*sthitapragya*) and person remains self-satisfied (Kiran Kumar, 2006). This view recognizes the significance of collective well-being, the complementary nature of pleasure and pain and pursuit of desirables (*shreyes*) (Misra, 2013).

> *Sarve bhavantu sukhinah, sarve santu niramayah,*
> *Sarve bhadrani pashyantu, ma kashchit duhkha bhag bhavet.*
> (May All become Happy, May All be Free from Illness, May All See what is Auspicious, May no one Suffer.)

In a study by Fazal and Young (Tibetan refugees) (Mahayana Buddhists, N = 59) and native Hindus (N = 66) residing in Himachal Pradesh in India were administered the Life Quality Scale. The Tibetan refugees displayed greater life satisfaction than Hindu natives despite language problems and fewer financial resources for the Tibetan participants. The high life quality reported by the Tibetan sample is interpreted in terms of their religious beliefs which stress self-contentment and the pleasure of existing in the presence of the living God, the Dalai Lama. While both Hindus and Tibetans subscribe to the fatalistic attitude of *Karma*, the Tibetans report greater life satisfaction. If one looks beyond the superficial similarities in the concept of *Karma*, however, it becomes clear that Tibetans adopt a "proactive" posture as opposed to the "reactive" fatalism of the Hindus (Fazal and Young, 1988).

Glimpses of Future through Positive Psychology: Hope, and Optimism

Fatalistic belief systems allow people to deem that life outcomes can be interpreted and managed by means of these forces. The Hindu concept of *karma* is merit accumulated in past lifetimes. Through the system of *samsara*, or the cycle of rebirth, each person is born with head writing—an invisible inscription on the forehead that commands when and where they will encounter good and bad fortune, based on their *karma*. As the fixed, mechanistic nature of this system through which fortunes are assigned means that the forms of Fatalism cannot be altered, it also means that they are potentially discoverable in advance. One can try to find control through the strategy of hearing one's fortune and then adapting one's actions to minimize its consequences. In harmony with this, Hindus offer conviction to the conception that seers or psychics can determine a person's fortune from signs, such as the astrological conditions of the person's birth (Young, Morris, Krishnan and Regmi, 2005). Both Hindus and Christians hold divergence conceptions of fate that produce diverse precedents of fatalistic thinking (Young *et al.*, 2005).

A well researched concept in positive psychology is hope, which is defined as "Hope is a goal directed thinking in which a person has the perceived capacity to find routes to desired goals (pathway thinking) and the requisite motivations to use those routes (agency thinking) (Snyder, 1994). Snyder believes that hope is not genetically based but an entirely learned and deliberate way of thinking. In Hinduism, hope is referred to with *Pratidhi* (Sanskrit: प्रतिधी), or *Apêkshā* (Sanskrit: अपेक्षा). It is discussed with the concepts of desire and wish.

> *Ashanam nadi manorathjala krishnatarangakula, raag grahwati vitrak vihada dhairaya drum dhvansini.*
> *Mohavartsudurahratigahana prottungachintatati, tasyah paragat vishuddhmanaso nandanti yogishwarah.*
>
> (Bhartrihari's *Vairagya Shataka*, 43)
>
> (Hope, like a river, with fantasies as water, agitated by waves of desires; attachments to various objects serving as prey; abounding in thoughts of greed, like birds; destroying the foes of courage; surrounded by eddies of ignorance deep and difficult to cross; with precipitous banks of anxiety—such a river the perfected *yogis* of pure minds, cross to enjoy beatitude.)

In Vedic Philosophy, *karma* was linked to ritual sacrifices (*yajna*), hope and success linked to correct performance of these rituals. In *Vishnu Smriti*, the image of hope, morals and work is represented as the virtuous man who rides in a chariot directed by his hopeful mind to his desired wishes, drawn by his five senses, who keeps the chariot on the path of the virtuous, and thus is not distracted by the wrongs such as wrath, greed, and other vices. In the *Bhagavad Gita,* Hope is a long-term *karmic* concept in the structure of beliefs and motivations. In Hindu belief, actions have consequences, and while one's effort and work may or may not bear near term fruits, it will serve the good, that the journey of one's diligent efforts (*karma*) and how one pursues the journey, sooner or later leads to bliss and *moksha* (De John Romus, 1995; Krieger, 1989).

Chang (1996) found that Asian Americans reported higher levels of pessimism than Caucasians, however, within that population pessimism was not found to contribute to depression and was associated with positive problem-solving strategies. This suggests that while pessimism is considered a weakness in some cultures, it might actually serve as strength in others. Defensive pessimism, for example, leads people to set lower expectations for themselves. This supports the idea that applications of positive psychology to cultivate strengths need to be altered to fit the clients' cultural backgrounds.

In their study Young, and associates (2005) reported that Christians were more likely to attribute misfortune to supernatural punishment for a target person who had behaved badly earlier in life, while Hindus call upon supernatural force without needing confirmation that the victim had misbehaved earlier in life. In addition, Christians in general preferred petition, but Hindus by and large favoured divination strategies. It should be mentioned that some petition and divination practices subsist in both cultural settings. For instance, in parts of India people look for intervention of deities by carrying out a *vrat*—a vow—"to influence some deity to come to one's aid," even though the aid may not be expected until one's next lifetime (Wadley, 1993). Similarly, Americans take up a great number of psychics, astrologers, and other experts with mystical testimonials who pronounce to predict people's futures. In spite of the availability of these strategies in both cultural settings, there was a clear difference in which practices participants endorsed (Young, Morris, Krishnan, & Regmi, 2005).

Hindu perceivers hold a person responsible for misfortunes that are judged to be their *karmic* rewards. These results do not support the view that Hindu fatalism engrosses a passive outlook of persons and corresponding reluctance to allocate responsibility.

Pro-social Behaviour: Altrusim, Gratitude and Forgiveness

Altrusim: *Dānam* apparently resembles what is called prosocial behaviour in contemporary social psychology, but an analysis based on major traditional Indian texts reveals several crucial divergences between the two concepts (Krishnan, 2005). *Dānam* in Sanskrit (*dāna* in Hindi) literally means "giving". In the context of contemporary psychology, *dānam* would bet spontaneously included under charity, altruism, generosity, benevolence, or what social psychologists would collectively call helping and pro-social behaviour. A more careful examination indicates that *dānam* as a traditional Indian concept goes beyond the commonly understood meaning of helping/pro-social behaviour (Krishnan, 2005). *Dānam* is one of the prescribed actions. Actually, certain transcripts (for example, the *Dharma-shastras*) have been dedicated to the inventory of prescribed actions and practices in different conditions, and for different social roles (for example, for the householder, the lady of the household, the husband, the wife, and so on). Specification of these practices are introduced in the *Grihya-sūtram* and *Dharma-sūtram*, two divisions of the *Kalpa-sūtras.* Virtualy, these texts function as rule-books or manuals, and also be full of descriptions of the outcomes of performance (or non-performance) of these actions. Some of the recommended actions are said to be part of daily behaviour (*vyavahāra*), and others, part of moral conduct (*āchāra and nīti*). *Dānam* appears to have elements of both *vyavahāra* and *āchāra. Dānam* is said to be a considered necessary action as well, since, it is an excellent mode of using one's assets. It is said that wealth should be either consumed by oneself, or given away as *dānam*. If one does neither and merely store it, then it will only be destroyed (Bhartrihari's *Nīti-shatakam).*

> *Ātmartharam jivalokea'smin ko na jivati manavah,*
> *Paramparopakarartham yo jivati sajivati.*
> (In this world who doesn't live for oneself? but one lives for others is true living) (*Nīti Shatakam*)
> OR
> *Paropakaraya satam vibhutayah*
> (The life of good people is for others) (*Nīti Shatakam*)

***Gratitude*:** The construct of Gratitude has received attention of positive psychologists in recent times in field of psychology. Gratitude is an emotional state and an attitude towards life that is a source of human strength in enhancing one's personal and relational well-being. The experience of gratitude has historically been a focus of several world religions. As far as the theological origins of gratitude is concerned, it is a virtue which is advocated to be cultivated in the major monotheistic traditions of Judaism, Christianity, Islam, Buddhism and Hinduism. Each tradition emphasizes the development of gratitude as a path to a good life, and prescribes approaches for practicing (Emmons, and Crumpler, 2000). Cicero (Pro Plancio) held that "gratitude is not only the greatest of virtues, but the parent of all others".

The experience of gratitude has historically been a focus of several world religions. Grateful people are happier, less depressed, less stressed, and more satisfied with their lives and social relationships (McCullough, Emmons, and Tsang, 2002; Wood *et al.*, 2007, 2008). Gratitude may also serve to reinforce future prosocial behaviour in benefactors. Every Hindu festival is about counting one's blessings and thanking God for them.

Indeed, buying a new car or new home entails special *puja* or prayer ceremonies to bless the new item and to offer thanks. Gratitude is exalted as one of the most important virtues (*dharma*) in many Hindu texts. Gratitude, thankfulness, gratefulness, or appreciation is a feeling or attitude in acknowledgement of a benefit that one has received or will receive.

Forgiveness: The concept of Forgiveness as understood through the Western approach of positive psychology as "Forgiveness is a suite of prosocial motivational changes that occurs after a person has incurred a transgression" (McCullough, 2001). Forgiveness is distinct from pardon (which is more apposite to the legal realm), condonation (which implies justifying the transgression), and excusing (which implies recognition that the transgressor had a good reason for committing the transgression) (Enright, Gassin, and Wu, 1992). In their study of 'Indigenous forgiveness' in Hmong culture, Sandage, Hill and Vang (2003) discovered that there is no term comparable to 'forgiveness' in native Hmong language and they came across a great deal of difficulties in obtaining suitable equivalent concepts to explain 'forgiving behaviour' in Hmong culture. Similarly, in Hinduism Forgiveness is explained as—

> *Kshama balam ashaktanam shaktanam bhushanam kshama,*
> *Kshama vashikarate loke kshamah kim na sidhayat.*
> (Forgiveness is the power of powerless. Forgiveness adorns the powerful. Forgiveness has controlled this entire world. What cannot be achieved by forgiveness!).

The conceptualizations about forgiveness of Indians from the Hindu community were explored by Tripathi and Mullet (2010). The four-factor structure of conceptualizations found among Western Europeans from Christian backgrounds (Encourages Repentance, Immoral Behaviour, Broad Process, and Change of Heart) fit the data collected among the Hindus, and the three-factor structure of forgivingness found among Europeans (Lasting Resentment, Sensitivity to Circumstances, and Unconditional Forgiveness) fit the data collected among the Hindus. It was found that, among Hindus, the relationships between conceptualizations about forgiveness and propensity to forgive were basically the same as the ones found among Western Europeans.

Resilience: Resilience is the process of adapting well in the face of adversity, trauma, tragedy, threats, or even significant sources of stress — such as family and relationship problems, serious health problems, or workplace and financial stressors. It means "bouncing back" from difficult experiences (Masten, Cutuli, Herbers and Reed, 2009). It is one of the important features of Hinduism which distinguishes it from other religions. The Sanskrit word for resilience is आततिशक्ति (*ātishakti*) means an occurrence of rebounding or springing back. Many researchers also differentiate resilience from the following terms: competence, hardiness, optimal functioning, and thriving. The distinction they draw between resilience and these is twofold: first, they see resilience as requiring the presence of substantial risk, while optimal functioning and thriving do not; and second, resilience may include optimal functioning and thriving, but it is more often understood as "normal" (Fonagy *et al.*, 1994) or "ordinary" (Masten, 2001) development. Hardiness carries the connotation of a "hardy constitution", while most researchers view resilience, as we have seen, not as an intrinsic trait but a dynamic process occurring under specific circumstances.

In Norway, individualism is a central value for many, and the emphasis in childrearing is more on the parents supporting the child making his/her own choices and standing on its own feet, while in Southern Africa the advice and opinion of parents and the rest of the extended family are more important even for young people, e.g. in choice of education, work etc. Even in Latino culture and Indian First Nation culture it seems that the unity and fellowship in the family is playing a more vital role (Gunnestad, 2004).

Conclusion

On emergence of global psychology of future, Tripathi (2011) commented, "*the usefulness of indigenous and cultural psychologies is going to come in handy to understand the variability of people not only within their own cultures but also those who migrate to other cultures taking with them memories of their cultures which shaped their minds*". Nandy (2011) argued for a '*more plural culture of world psychology*' which should work like a confederation of mutually tolerant and mutually critical cultures of understanding the human mind. On developing a multicultural positive psychology perspective, Sandage *et al.* (2003) commented, "A *multicultural* positive psychology will require that researchers and clinicians explore the roles of cultural and contextual factors in the diverse expressions of virtues such as forgiveness."

In her ethnographic study of Tibetan refugees in India, Vahali (2009) explored psychologically devastating consequences of refugeehood and torture and how Tibetan refugees have developed resilience through Dalai Lama's teachings and philosophy of Buddhism. Similarly, in another ethnographic study on survivors of Kachchh earthquake in 2001, Priya (2007) reported on how survivors regained their self-confidence and healing through their belief and faith in their *Karma* (internalized duty towards family, community and nature). For discovering such social phenomena, researchers need to go for alternative approaches.

References

Azuma, H. (1984). Psychology in a Non-Western Country, *International Journal of Psychology, 19*, 45-55.

Chang, E.C. (1996). Cultural differences in optimism, pessimism, and coping: Predictors of subsequent adjustment in Asian, American and Caucasian American College Students. *Journal of Counselling Psychology, 43*(1), 113.

Cheng, D.H. (2000). *On Lao Tzu*. Belmont, CA: Wadsworth.

Ching, C.C. (1984). Psychology and the Four Modernizations in China. *International Journal of Psychology, 19*, 57-63.

De John Romus (1995). *Karma* and *Bhakti* ways of Salvation: A Christological Perspective. *Indian Journal of Theology, 37* (1), 1-14.

Emmons, R.A., and Cheryl, A.C. (2000). Gratitude as a Human Strength: Appraising the Evidence. *Journal of Social and Clinical Psychology, 19* (1), 56-69.

Emmons, R.A., and Crumpler, C.A. (2000). Gratitude as a Human Strength: Appraising the Evidence. *Journal of Social and Clinical Psychology, 19*(1), 56-69.

Enright, R.D., Gassin, E.A., and Wu, C.R. (1992). *Forgiveness: A Developmental View*. Vol. *21* (1), 99-114.

Fazel, M.K., and Young, D.M. (1988). Life Quality of Tibetans and Hindus: A function of religion. *Journal for the Scientific Study of Religion*, 229-242.

Fonagy, P., Steele, M., Steele, H., Higgitt, A., and Target, M. (1994). The Emmanuel Memorial Lecture 1992, The Theory and Practice of Resilience. *Journal of Psychology and Psychiatry, 35* (2), 231-257.

Gunnestad, Arve (2004). *The Role of Culture in Early Childhood Education.* Report from the 6th Network Conference in Gantsi, Botswana. Trondheim: Queen Maud's College.

Gupta, B. (2006). *Bhagavad Gītā* as duty and virtue ethics. *Journal of Religious Ethics, 34*(3), 373-395.

Hussain, D. (2011). Spirituality, Religion, and Health: Reflections and Issues. *Europe's Journal of Psychology, 7*(1), 187-197.

Karsaz, A. and Singelis, T. (2009). Qualitative and Mixed Methods Research in Cross-Cultural Psychology. *Journal of Cross-Cultural Psychology, 40*, 6, 909-916.

Kim, M., Lee, H.S., and Wong, P.T.P. (2005). *Meaning of life according to Koreans: The Korean personal meaning profile*. Poster presented at the Annual Convention of the American Psychological Association, Washington, DC.

Kiran Kumar, S.K. (2006). Happiness and well-being in Indian tradition. *Psychological Studies, 51*, 105-112.

Krieger, D. (1989). Salvation in the World—A Hindu-Christian Dialogue on Hope and Liberation. In Jerald Gort (Eds.), *Dialogue and Syncretism: An Interdisciplinary Approach*, ISBN 0-8028-0501-9.

Krishnan, L. (2005). Concepts of social behaviour in India: *Daana* and distributive justice. *Psychological Studies, 50*(1), 21.

Laungani, P.D. (2007). *Understanding Cross-Cultural Psychology*. New Delhi: Sage.

Lin, A., and Wong, P.T.P. (2006). *The Meaning of Life: According to a Chinese Sample*. Paper presented at the Annual Convention of the American Psychological Association, New Orleans.

McCullough, M.E., Emmons, R.A., and Tsang, J.A. (2002). The grateful disposition: A conceptual and empirical topography. *Journal of Personality and Social Psychology, 82*(1), 112.

Markus, H.R., and Kitayama, S. (1991). Culture and the self: Implications for cognition, emotion, and motivation. *Psychological Review, 98*, 224-253.

Masten, A.S. (2001). Ordinary magic: Resilience processes in development. *American Psychologists, 56* (3), 227-238.

Masten, A.S., Cutuli, J.J., Herbers, J.E., and Reed, M.J. (2009). Resilience in Development. In S.J. Lopez and C.R. Snyder (eds.) *Oxford Handbook of Positive Psychology* (pp. 117-131). New York: Oxford University Press.

McCullough, M.E., Kilpatrick, S.D., Emmons, R.A., and Larson, D.B. (2001). Is gratitude a moral affect? *Psychological Bulletin, 127*(2), 249.

McCullough, M.E., Emmons, R.A., and Tsang, J. (2002). The grateful disposition: A conceptual and empirical topography. *Journal of Personality and Social Psychology, 82*, 112-127.

Misra, G. (2011). Preface. In *Handbook of Psychology in India*, (Ed.) Girishwar Misra, Oxford University Press, New Delhi, pp. xv-xvi.

Misra, G. (2013). Happiness. In Kenneth D. Keith (eds.) *The Encyclopaedia of Cross-Cultural Psychology*, John Wiley & Sons, Inc.

Nandy, A. (2011). Towards an Alternative Politics of Psychology. In G. Misra (Eds.) *Handbook of Psychology in India*, (Chapter 24, pp. 358-369), New Delhi: Oxford University Press.

Paranjpe, A.C. (1998). *Self and Identity in Modern Psychology and Indian Thought*. New York: Plenum Press.

Priya, K.R. and Misra, G. (2011). Ethnographic Inquiry in Psychology. In G. Misra (Eds.) *Handbook of Psychology in India*, (Chapter 6, pp. 99-110), New Delhi: Oxford University Press.

Sandage, S.J., Hill, P.C., and Vang, H.C. (2003). Towards a multicultural positive psychology: Indigenous forgiveness and Hmong culture. *The Counselling Psychologist, 31*(5), 564-592.

Shweder, R.A., and Levine, R.A. (Eds.) (1984). *Culture Theory: Essays on Mind, Self and Emotion*. New York: Cambridge University Press.

Sinha, D. (1972). *Industrial Psychology: A Survey of Research in Psychology*, 175-237.

Smith, P.B., and Bond, M.H. (1994). *Social Psychology Across Cultures: Analysis and Perspectives*. Needham Heights, MA: Allyn & Bacon.

Snyder, C.R. (1994). *The Psychology of Hope: You can get therefrom here*. Simon & Schuster.

Solomon, L.D. (2006). *From Athens to America: Virtues and Formulation of Public Policy*. New York: Lexington.

Takano, Y., and Wong, P.T.P. (2004, July). Meaning of life according to a Japanese sample. In *Annual Convention of the America Psychological Association*, Honolulu, Hawaii.

Tripathi, A., and Mullet, E. (2010). Conceptualizations of forgiveness and forgivingness among Hindus. *The International Journal for the Psychology of Religion, 20*(4), 255-266.

Tripathi, R.C. (2011). In Search of a 'Global Psychology'. In G. Misra (Eds.) *Handbook of Psychology in India*, (Chapter 25, pp. 370-373), New Delhi: Oxford University Press.

Triandis, H.C. (1989). The self and social behaviour in differing cultural contexts. *Psychological Review, 96*, 506-520.

Vahali, H.O. (2009). *Lives in Exile: Exploring the World of Tibetan Refugees*. New Delhi: Routledge, India.

Wadley, S.S. (1993). *Struggling with Destiny in Karimpur, 1925-1984*. Berkeley, University of California Press.

Wood, A.M., Joseph, S., and Linley, P.A. (2007). Gratitude: The parent of all virtues. *The Psychologist, 20*, 18-21.

Wood, A.M., Maltby, J., Stewart, N., and Joseph, S. (2008). Conceptualizing gratitude and appreciation as a unitary personality trait. *Personality and Individual Differences, 44*, 619-630.

Young, M.J., Morris, M.W., Krishnan, L., and Regmi, M.P. (2005). *Forms of Fatalism: Christian and Hindu approaches to attributing misfortune and coping with risks*. Working paper, Anderson School, University of California, Los Angeles, Westwood, CA 90024.

8

Optimism and Pessimism in Positive Psychology

Contemporary View

Shaimaa E. Basha

Introduction

People's behaviour is sometimes controlled by a tendency for expecting good and happiness, while at other times they are overcome by the tendency to expect evil and misfortune. The first state is described as optimism, while the second is described as pessimism. This state tends to recur in different situations until it becomes a trait that a person is often described with (Badr El Ansari, 1998:8).

Despite the importance of both the optimism and pessimism concepts in the human life in general, and in the psychological studies in particular, the interest in those concepts is relatively new. Notice was given to their study in the seventies of the last century, where those concepts attracted the attention of several scholars in the field of personality study, social psychology, medical psychology, and clinical psychology (Badr El Ansari, 1998: 19; Ahmed Abdel Khalek, 1998; Hassan Abdel Latif and Louloua Hamada, 1998; Scheier & Carver, 1998; Chang, 1998).

Studying optimism and pessimism acquire great attention from researchers due to the association of those two traits to the psychological health of the individual. Various theories link optimism with happiness, health, perseverance, achievement, and positive outlook of life; while pessimism is linked with despair, failure, sickness, and negative outlook of life (Ahmed Abdel Khalek, 2000; Badr El Ansari, 2003; Peterson, 2000).

The use of the words "optimism" and "pessimism" by non-specialists is longstanding where they refer to a general life orientation, a characteristic describing individuals or a psychological state affected by internal or external circumstances. Despite this old usage of the two words by non-specialists, the interest in both concepts and their detailed study in the framework of psychology have only started to take place regularly by the end of the seventies. A specialized book on this subject was issued by Tiger in 1979, called: *Optimism—The Biology of Hope.* Another book written by Badr El Ansari was issued in 1998, considered the first of its kind in Arabic, about optimism and pessimism, presenting the concept, measurement, and relationships in detail (Badr El Ansari, 2003; Badr El Ansari, 1998).

Definition of Optimism/Pessimism

Optimism (*el tafa'ol* in Arabic) is linguistically derived from the word "*fa'l*" meaning omen, and contrary to "*tira*", meaning superstition. According to El Gohary, people consider some situations to be good omens, as for example, a sick person hearing a man calling another by his name "Salem", meaning "well-being", or a person who has lost an object hearing a man calling another by his name "Wagid", meaning "finder". In those cases, they consider it a good omen, where the sick person believes he is going to be cured, or the person searching for a lost object believes he will find it. The Hadith specifies that the Prophet, peace and blessings be upon him, loved good omens and hated superstition. Superstition is contrary to good omens, where omens are related to the good while superstition is related to the bad (Ibn Manzour, 1978:1042). Thus, the "*fa'l*" or omen is a saying or an action that gives a person hope for a good situation. It is common to facilitate its pronunciation in Arabic by removing the "*Hamza*" to become "*fal*" instead of "*fa'l*"; where the saying goes "there is no fal on you" meaning, no harm will befall you (Arabic Language Academy, 1962:677; Soad El Sweed, 2003:232).

Optimism is defined with multiple definitions. Linguistically, Merriam Webster Dictionary defines it in 1991 as the inclination to anticipate the best possible outcomes (by Badr Al Ansari, 1998:14).

Scheier and Carver (1985) defined optimism as the positive outlook to life, belief in the possibility of achieving future desires, in addition to believing the likelihood of good occurrences instead of the bad. In a later text (1987), Scheier and Carver added that optimism is a personal disposition inside an individual that reflects the extent to which they hold a general favourable or positive expectation for the future, meaning expecting positive outcomes for future situations.

Marshal defines optimism as a personal inclination towards a positive expectation of events (Marshal *et al.*, 1992). Ahmed Abdel Khalek and Badr Al Ansari (1995) define optimism as a cheerful view of the future which makes an individual expect the best, anticipate good occurrences, yearn for success, and exclude all contrary to the above.

The concept of optimism is associated with unrealistic optimism, which is not justified by logic or prior experience. This optimism could prevent its holders from perceiving probable risks, leading them for example to ignore health problems and causing complications for lack of early treatment, or leading them to believe in their ability for performing difficult tasks or dangerous stunts, or dreaming of getting rich quickly pushing them to gambling addiction (Weinstein, 1980, 1983).

Taylor and Brown (1988) define unrealistic optimism as the person's feelings of optimism towards certain events without logical justifications, events, or facts that lead to this feeling. This can sometimes cause unexpected results, leaving the person highly frustrated and at risk of certain diseases like AIDS.

Unrealistic optimism could lead to biased thinking, which might result in biased decisions with realistic bases. It leads most individuals to underestimate the likelihood of their exposure to disease, accidents, familial separation, or unwanted pregnancy, in comparison to other persons. Consequently, those individuals become less inclined to take the needed precautions against risks and probable disease. Unrealistic optimism also leads individuals to have higher expectations than others for good future events. However, the feedback a person receives on his/her academic performance or the accumulated experience in performing certain tasks, can contribute to modifying the degree of optimism to a more realistic level (Othman El Khedr, 1999).

We conclude from the above that optimism is a personality trait existing with different levels in individuals, rather than a state. Although this trait is usually related to the future, it affects the human behaviour in the present. It is also believed that optimism as a trait is related to the positive aspects of the human behaviour and personality, positively affecting the individual's physical and psychological health (Badr El Ansary, 1998:22; 2003).

Pessimism (*el tasha'om* in Arabic) is linguistically derived from the source "*sha'am*" meaning bringer of bad luck. "*Al Sho'm*" is contrary to "*al yumn*", meaning blessings. Also, a man who is "*mash'oum*" to his people, "*masha'eem*" in plural, means that the man brings bad luck to his people, he became their bad luck. A man "*tasha'am*", affiliated to "*sha'am*", means that a man became associated with bad luck (Ibn Manzour, 1978:257-258). In addition, "*Sha'm bihi*" means drove him to bad luck, and "*tasha'am*" means "becoming superstitious". The saying goes "*Ash'am kol Emreen bayna lehyeyho*" means person's bad luck lies in his tongue (Magd El Din El Fayruz Abady, 1986:1453).

Pessimism is a personality trait. Individuals with high abundance of this trait often have a tendency for sadness and melancholy. Such an individual is more inclined to predict failure and has negative expectations for future events, leading him/her to expect the worst, including failure and disappointment (Hanaa Showeikh, 2007:124).

Scheier and Carver (1985) define pessimism as the general negative expectations of outcomes, and the presumption of inability for effective response. Marshal (Marshal *et al.*, 1992) finds that pessimism is a personal readiness or a latent trait inside the individual, which leads a person towards negative expectation of events.

Ahmed Abdel Khalek (1998) defines pessimism as the negative expectation of future events, leading a person to anticipate the worst and to expect failure and disappointment, excluding the contrary. Pessimism, in Showers' (1992) view, is when an individual focuses his/her attention on the negative possibilities of future events, while only imagining the adverse side. However, pessimism or the negative expectation of events motivates the individuals' objectives and efforts towards preventing the occurrence of bad events resulting in the preparedness for responding to such events.

Showers and Ruben (1995) noted that pessimism has the following functions: prepares the individual to face negative events. It thus represents a strategy for protecting oneself and increasing efforts to support good performance, and to avoid such events. Therefore, it is called Defensive Pessimism.

The concepts of defensive pessimism and unrealistic pessimism are linked with the concept of pessimism. Defensive pessimism refers to the tendency for negative expectation of future events regardless of the actual level of performance of the individuals (Showers, 1992).

Norem and Cantor distinguished between optimism and defensive pessimism. Defensive pessimists are those individuals that possess a good level of previous success in a certain situation, but they often go through similar new situations expecting bad outcomes. Defensive pessimism involves setting lower expectations for an individual's future performance, leading him/her to feel anxiety and lack of control, despite the previous good performance in the same situation. Norem and Cantor found that the optimists feel a lesser amount of anxiety and a higher level of performance in comparison to defensive pessimists. The latter often expect a bad scenario of failure or frustrating events although the level of academic performance is similar to optimists. This scary scenario increases the level of anxiety among defensive pessimists and pushes them to exert more effort. While Norem and Cantor did not find fundamental differences in performance between the two groups, Showers found that the individual's focus on the negative probabilities of future events contributes to the increase in the level of performance among pessimists more than their focus on good future probabilities would (Othman El Khedr, 1999).

Defensive Pessimism prepares a person for the probability of failure and increases the level of the person's motivation to overcoming the difficulties. Persons relying on the optimism strategy in facing the future often depend on denial, misinterpretation of unpleasant information, running from facing failure probability, and ignore thinking of probable negative outcomes, because it increases their concerns. Optimists always have unrealistic and limited alternatives for facing problems when exposed to hypothetical situations that require solutions, in comparison to defensive pessimists (Othman El Khedr, 1999).

The concept of unrealistic pessimism is referred to as the tendency for negative expectations of future events though there exists a general belief that exposure to such events is difficult. The individual is convinced he/she is more susceptible than others to be exposed to mishaps such as becoming the victim of an accident or an incurable illness, flood, earthquake, or theft. While people believe that such unfortunate incidents may occur, they have the tendency to believe that they are protected against them and that others become the victims of those incidents (Badr El Ansari, 1998:30-31).

There is also what is called oral optimism/pessimism, which is based on the Freud's division of the psychosexual development stages in childhood: oral, anal, and phallic. Psychoanalysts assume that depression is due to fixations during the oral stage, where a person who was frustrated or lacked fulfilment at that stage become pessimistic in his view of the world, and acquires a sad, depressed, and withdrawn mood, along with a feeling of insecurity and the constant need to self-assertiveness (Badr El Ansari, 1998:22; Ludwing and Idelberg, 1968).

Abraham, in 1924, indicated that an optimistic person is one who acquired his experiences during the oral stage, which forms his personality.

That person could be a normal person facing life with expectations of success, and expecting others to take care of him at work. In other cases, a person's personality might be influenced completely by the oral stage. This could be clearly defined through a comprehensive analysis performed by the individual. Anny Angel, in 1934, described three cases of optimistic behaviour. The first is where the patient possessing the attributes of optimism use them to deny any cognition of emotion of anxiety. The second case is where the patient uses optimism as a preventive rather than a denial factor to decrease the effect of external. The third type is that of normal persons (through: Ludwing and Idelberg, 1968:283-284).

We can conclude from the above that pessimism is a personality trait that exists in moderate levels among the sample population, rather than it being a state. We can assume that pessimism may negatively affect human behaviour and humans' physical and mental health. It may also hold a positive and fundamental correlation to psychological disturbances or susceptibility (Badr Al-Ansari, 2003:17-18; 1998:22).

Importance of Optimism and Pessimism

The significance of studying optimism and pessimism lies in their association to the various aspects of the personality. Optimism is a key factor for human survival. The desire to have children, ideas for social and economic development, as well as religious and political concepts can all be predictable through the optimistic attitude towards the future. Optimism enables individuals and communities to set specific targets and to overcome difficulties and adversities that may afflict society (Ahmed Abdel Khalek, 2000).

Studies have demonstrated the existence of a high positive correlation between optimistic view of the future and current happiness. Optimism is associated with the perception of control over and response to pressures, using effective confrontation and positive reinterpretation of situations, solving problems successfully, seeking social support, positive outlook of stressful situations, academic achievement, job performance, self-control, self-esteem, quick recovery from illness, happiness, compatibility, physical health, healthy behaviour, and the quick resumption of normal activities after surgeries. On the other hand, studies revealed that pessimism associated with high rates of depression, despair, suicide, anxiety, OCD, neuroticism, hostility, feeling of loneliness, decreased morale, and reduced motivation for work and accomplishment, feelings of sadness, desolation, social withdrawal, failure to solve problems, and the negative view of life adversities (Ahmed Abdel Khalek, 2000; Bader Al-Ansari, 1998; Taylor *et al.*, 1992; Atienza *et al.*, 2002; Lobel *et al.*, 2000; Marshall *et al.*, 1992).

Optimism, Pessimism, and Stress

Stress causes a mixture of emotions that are affected by optimism. Optimists expect positive outcomes even in complicated situation, while pessimists expect the worst of outcomes. That is why they possess strong negative emotions like anxiety, sadness, and despair. Studies examined the correlation between optimism and response to stressful events like exams, intense business competition, earthquakes, and other disasters. Other studies focused on the role of optimism among caregivers of cancer patients, Alzheimer patients, bone marrow transplant cases, and cases of repeated miscarriages. Studies found that optimism has a role in modifying the emotional responses to severe stress (Mamdouha Salama, 2009:281).

Scheier and Carver (1985) found that optimists suffer less symptoms physically in response to stress as they use a "problem focus" strategy once they realize that the situation could be controlled. On the other hand, pessimists use an "emotional focus" strategy represented in denial, behavioural withdrawal, and avoiding stress inducing objectives (Hoda Hassan, 2006).

One of the personality dimensions associated with experience of stress and risk of disease is the feeling of either optimism or pessimism (Wortman *et al.*, 1992:474). In a study, Sheier and Carver (1985) asked the students at the beginning of the academic year to fill in a survey designed for measuring their tendency towards optimism and pessimism. At the end of the term, the study found that students who had acquired high scores in optimism suffer less physical symptoms (headache, stomach disorders) than those who scored lower on the scale.

This was supported by empirical studies, which findings indicated that persons having pessimistic explanations for life events suffer from weaker physical health, are more susceptible to depression, and possess lower levels of attainment and achievement (Malin Choc *et al.*, 1996).

Some studies have also found that the personality dimensions of optimism and pessimism play an important role in the psychological and behavioural reactions of individuals when faced by crises or distress. Optimists are better in those situations than pessimists because they are capable of responding more effectively. A strong evidence of the difference in response between both groups exists. Both groups differ in their methods of response, attitudes, tendencies, reactions to certain situations, ability to deal with a past stressful experience, dealing with serious problems, overcoming the vicissitudes of life, and confronting serious diseases and threats to health (Carver *et al.*, 1993). People with an optimistic view experience less physical symptoms than those with a pessimistic view, for they suffer less from fatigue, cramps, dizziness, and blurred vision, in comparison to pessimists who experience more pain and are often more upset (Ali Askar, 2000:135).

Optimism/Pessimism, Self-Esteem, and Locus of Control

Some studies indicate the existence of positive correlation between optimism and high self-esteem, while it is negatively correlated to external locus of control. This means that the higher the score is on the optimism scale, the higher the individuals' confidence in the existence of an internal locus of control on his/her actions. On the other hand, the higher the score is on the pessimism scale, the higher the individual's confidence in the existence of an external locus of control on his/her actions, where there is a negative correlation with internal locus of control (Badr El Ansari, 2003:22; Badr El Ansari, 1998; Ahmed Abdel Khaled, 1999; Chang *et al.*, 1994; Carver *et al.*, 1993).

Optimism/Pessimism and the Academic and Professional Performance

The results of some studies indicate the existence of a positive relationship between optimism and work knowledge, work quality, production rate, discipline, tact, motivation, planning, direction and general performance, in addition to initiative, cooperation, and capability for planning. On the other hand, a negative relationship exists between all the mentioned performance variables and pessimism.

One other study also found that optimists are more compatible with the new university life in comparison to pessimists. Another study indicated that the academic results of pessimistic children in the third primary grade were lower than the grades of optimistic children (Badr El Ansari, 2003:23).

Optimism/Pessimism in Different Theoretical Approaches

The use of the words "optimism" and "pessimism" by non-specialists is too old, where they refer to at least three meanings including a general life orientation, a characterization describing individuals, or a psychological state affected by internal or external circumstances. Despite this old usage of the two words by non-specialists, the interest in both concepts and their detailed study in the framework of psychology have only started to take place regularly by the end of the seventies (Ahmed Abdel Khalek, 2008:189).

Thus, the concepts of optimism and pessimism are considered relatively modern concepts. Therefore, the theoretical frameworks behind them seem fairly low, presented below:

Social and Psychological Development Theory

If optimism means expecting positive outcomes, it is due to the internal certainty and absolute confidence that were formed in the early stages of life that started with the first interactions with others. Eric Erikson refers to eight stages of personality development characterizing human growth. However, he believes that there are cultural differences that govern the method by which individuals handle the problems of each stage and the appropriate solutions for those problems. In every culture, there is a synergy between the individual in the different stages of development and the social environment. The first stage (Hope: Trust *versus* Mistrust) of the psychological and social development is formed during infancy. It results from the ease of feeding, depth or sleep, ease of excretion, as well as the presence of caregivers and their continued presence to ensure satisfaction and fullness, which in turn is psychologically translated to feelings of safety and reassurance, feelings that everything is alright, and that the world as a whole is safe and can be trusted. In this stage, the general sense of absolute confidence, which Erikson considers the cornerstone of a normal personality, is formed. Based on such absolute confidence, the infant derives an internal feeling of safety, and sees the world as a place that radiates security and satiability, full of trustworthy and dependable caregivers. As for inadequate and undependable care which cannot be trusted as an external reality, it leads to the development of a social and psychological trend of fear, mistrust, and suspicion towards the world in general and people in particular (Mamdouha Salama, 1997: 123-125).

Based on the above, as a result, the individual either becomes an optimist, expecting good and feeling safety and stability, or becomes a pessimist, feeling fear and suspicion towards the world and people.

Expectancy and Value Theory

The theory is based on the idea that behaviour aims to achieve a desired goal, and without this goal with its importance and value, there would be no motivation for behaviour or action. The second component, the expectancy, is the confidence or doubt concerning achieving the goal. If a person lacks the confidence, there will be no action or behaviour. Adequate confidence is what drives people to take action or continue their efforts for achieving goals of value. The same concepts apply to optimism and pessimism. Optimists, when faced with obstacles or problems and challenges, continue to exert effort even if the progress towards the goal is difficult or slow. Pessimists on the other hand are more hesitant and doubtful. The same happens in response to adversity or bad events, where optimists feel that however difficult the adversity is, it can be overcome successfully, while pessimists expect future disasters (Mamdouha Salama, 2009:280).

The third assumption in this theory is about the self-regulation behaviour, which assumes that internal values are the goals providing feedback for the individual and governing his or her behaviour through self-regulation. Those goals become active in directing action, providing a positive meaning for life, which in turn provides a person with the ability to give and to rise over the self, thus affecting the whole humanity (Badr El Ansari, 2002).

Based on the above, Scheier and Carver (1985) assumed that optimism and pessimism include future expectations of objectives that individuals seek to achieve, and which they might consider as more valuable than their own lives. Motivation for life is also affected by the cognitions that an individual has acquired regarding the future, in addition to the value related emotional components associated with such cognitions.

Theory of Social Learning

Theorists of social learning believe that building an individual's personality consists of expectations, objectives, ambitions, and personal activities, all of which work interactively through learning by observation. This learning occurs in light of response and support. Consequently, the behaviour of the individual is associated with the history of support in a certain amount of time. As a result, some individuals might succeed in performing certain tasks in certain situations, while fail in others. They thus build negative expectations towards some of the situations causing pessimism to prevail on their behaviour. In light of those two criteria, expectation for future success and failure differ between individuals (Badr El Ansari, 11: 1998; Aweed El Meshaan, 2002).

Learned Helplessness Theory

Theorists of Learned Helplessness believe that a person recognizes his inability to respond when exposed to stressful events. This leads to a feeling of helplessness and hopelessness as well as decreased self-esteem, lack of efficacy depression and sadness. Finally, recognizing failure and helplessness leads to building expectation of future failures based on the failed experiences. Despair prevails as the person believes that there is no hope in the future and trying is futile as long as any attempts are doomed to failure (Abramson *et al.*, 1978).

Seligman presented the Optimistic Explanatory Style and the Pessimistic Explanatory Style. The Pessimistic Explanatory Style may cause the risk of helplessness and depression when a person faces events that are beyond his control, causing him to amplify psychological states, and thus increasing the risk for disease and early death. Studies confirmed that the Pessimistic Explanatory Style in adults is associated with somatic diseases and low academic and professional performance (Peterson *et al.*, 1988).

Seligman also conducted a series of longitudinal studies that revolve around one axis, which is the relation of pessimism to an individual's general health. Seligman found that individuals interpreting bad events occurring to them as a general and constant state that is caused by them (internal) were less healthy than those individuals who believed that the bad events they faced were caused by temporary and external factors (Aweed El Meshaan, 2000).

Individuals acquiring learned helplessness because of the repeated and unavoidable occurrences of bad events in their lives strongly believe that external factors are responsible for those events. Experiments show that two-thirds of the sample succumbs to the bad circumstances they are exposed to during the experiment due to their inability to overcome them. The other third of the sample, however, refuse to succumb and continue trying to get out of the situation. Seligman found that the difference between those two groups lies in the level of optimism/pessimism they possess, for the sample individuals that continued trying were more optimistic than the rest of them. A study implemented by Roden on seniors receiving in home support from nurses revealed that 93 per cent of the sample individuals who exert some effort for affecting the surrounding environment (self care, changing furniture, garden care, washing dishes) were more active, happier, and more attentive (Othman El Khedr, 1999).

Seligman has noted in his book "Learned or Acquired Optimism" in 1988 that optimism can be learned, for we are not optimistic or pessimistic by nature. Contrary to a pessimist, an optimist believes that disappointment and frustration are temporary challenges or disabilities that will not defeat them. Seligman used a method called Cognitive Restructuring, which includes identifying negative thoughts and beliefs and substituting them with more positive and optimistic thoughts that help replace the individuals' negative mood with positive mood (Aweed El Meshaan, 2002; Ahmed Ismail, 2001).

Seligman presented the Optimistic Explanatory Style and the Pessimistic Explanatory Style. The Pessimistic Explanatory Style may cause the risk of helplessness and depression when a person faces events that are beyond his control, causing him to amplify psychological states, and thus increasing the risk for disease and early death. Studies confirmed that the Pessimistic Explanatory Style in adults is associated with somatic diseases and low academic and professional performance (Aweed El Meshaan, 1999).

Cognitive Appraisal Theory

Lazarus and Folkman (1984) present a different theory. They consider that cognitive appraisal, personal efficacy, and outcome expectation represent responses to specific situations rather than tendencies or personality traits. Therefore, a person could feel optimistic towards some situations or issues in his/her life and pessimistic towards others (by Nagwa El Yahouft and Bad Al Ansary, 2005).

Adler's Theory of Individual Psychology

Alfred Alder stressed that people are motivated by objectives formed through their own views and their interpretations of current and future events. Such objectives organize their behaviour, or an individual behaves according to his own beliefs whether those beliefs represent an objective reality or not. The result is the same in both cases, meaning that, according to Adler, behaviour is a reflection of the individual's personal view of reality (by Mamdouha Salama, 1997:47).

Adler focused on cultural influences on behaviour, assuming that a personality is innately social, and that the sense of inferiority is the core of human motivation. Adler's words read: "I began to see clearly a drive for excellence in every psychological phenomenon, and that the driving force from the negative to the positive never ends, as is the push from the low to the high." Adler believed that the sense of inferiority highly increases in cases of failure to achieve life objectives, where it forms a unique lifestyle for each individual (by Roh El Fouad Ibrahim, 2002).

References

Abeer, Anwar and Faten Sadek (2009). *Role of Tolerance and Optimism in Predicting the Quality of Life among a Sample of University Students*, First Regional Conference of the Psychology Department, Faculty of Arts, Cairo University.

Ahmed Abdel Khalek (1996). *Instruction Manual for the Arab List of Optimism and Pessimism*, Alexandria: University Dar El Maarefa.

Ahmed Abel Khalek (1998). Optimism and a Healthy Body: A Practical Study, *Journal of Social Sciences*, Kuwait, *26* (2), 45-62.

Ahmed Abdel Khalek (2000). Optimism and Pessimism, a Presentation of Arab Studies, *Psychology Journal*, (56), 6-27.

Ahmed Abdel Khalek (2005). Arab Scale for Optimism and Pessimism: Results for Egypt, *Journal for Psychological Studies*, *15* (2), 307-318.

Ahmed Abdel Khalek (2008). *Personality Psychology Laboratory,* Alexandria, University, Dar El Maarefa.

Ahmed Abdel Khalek and Badr El Ansari (1995). *Optimism and Pessimism: An Arab Study of the Personality*, Second International Conference of the Psychological Counselling Center, Ain Shams University, 25-27.

Ahmed El Kandary (1992). *Family Psychology*, Kuwait, El Falah Bookshop for Publishing and Distribution.

Ahmed Ismail (2001). *Optimism and Pessimism and Some Psychological Variables among a Sample of Om El Qora University Students*, Education Magazine, Kuwait, *15* (60), 51-81.

Arabic Language Academy (1962). *El Waseet Lexicon*, Cairo, Dar El Maaref.

Arabic Language Academy (1985). *El Waseet Lexicon*, Cairo, Dar El Maaref.

Aweed El Meshaan (1999). *Optimism and Pessimism in Relation to Physical and Psychological Disorders*, The Sixth Conference of the Psychological Counselling Center, Ain Shams University, 949-969.

Aweed El Meshaan (2002). The Relation Between Job Satisfaction, Optimism and Pessimism, and Psychosomatic Disorders among Employees of the Public Sector in Kuwait, *Social and Humanitarian Sciences Journal*, Kuwait, *18* (1), 1-38.

Aweed El Meshaan, Optimism and Pessimism in Relation to Physical and

Psychological Disorders and Stressful Life Events among University Students, *Psychological Studies Journal, 10* (4), 505-532.

Badr El Ansari (2001). Preparing Unrealistic Optimism Scale among a Sample of Male and Female Students, Kuwait, *Psychological Studies Journal, 11* (2), 194-243.

Badr El Ansari (2002). Preparing an Arabic Version of Life Direction Assessment as an Optimism Scale, *Social Sciences Journal,* Kuwait, *30* (4), 775-812.

Badr El Ansary (1997). Gender Differences in Personality Traits, *Arabic Journal of Humanities*, Kuwait, *59* (16), 52-88.

Badr El Ansary (1998). *Optimism and Pessimism, the Concept, Measurement, and Related Matters*, Kuwait, Scientific Publishing Council of Kuwait University.

Badr El Ansary (2000). *Measuring Personality*, Kuwait: Dar El Kitab El Hadith.

Badr El Ansary (2003). Optimism and Pessimism: Measurement and Relation to Personal Variables among Kuwait University Students, *Annals of Arts and Social Sciences*, Annal 192, Kuwait, Scientific Publishing Council, Kuwait University.

Blankstein, K., Flett, G., and Koldin, S. (1991). The brief college student hassles scale: development, validation and relation with pessimism, *Journal of College Student Development*, *32*(2), 258-264.

Carver, C. (1989). How should multifaceted personality constructs be tested?—Issues illustrated by self-monitoring, attribution style, and hardiness. *Journal of Personality and Social Psychology*, *56*(4), 577-585.

Carver, C., and Pozo, C., Harris, S., Noriega, V., Scheier, F., Robinson, D., Ketcham, A., Moffat, F., and Clark, K. (1993). How coping mediates the effect of optimism on distress: A study of women with early stage breast cancer. *Journal of Personality and Social Psychology*, *56*(2), 375-390.

Chang, E. (1988). Dispositional optimism and primary and secondary appraisal of a stressor: controlling for confounding influences and relations to Coping and psychological and physical adjustment. *Journal of Personality and Social Psychology, 74*(4), 1109-1120.

Colligan, R., Offord, K., Malnchoc, M., Schulman, P., and Seligman, M. (1994). Caveing the MMPI for an Optimism—Pessimism Scale: Seligman's attributional model and the assessment of explanatory style. *Journal of Clinical Psychology*, *50*(1), 71- 95.

Fereih El Anzy and Aweed El Meshaan (1998). The Relation between the Schizophrenic Personality and Optimism and Pessimism, *Psychological Studies Journal*, *18* (2), 128-156.

Hassan Abdel Latif and Louloua Hamada (1998). Optimism and Pessimism and their Relation to Personality Dimensions: Diastolic and Neuroticism, *Social Sciences Journal*, Kuwait, *26* (1), 83-104.

Hoda Hassan (2006). Optimism and Pessimism and their Relation to Job Stress and Satisfaction, *Psychological Studies Journal*, *16* (1), 83-111.

Ibn Manzour (1978). *Lissan El Arab El Moheet* (Lexicon), Volume 2, Beirut, Lissan El Arab.

Ibn Manzour (1979). *Lissan El Arab El Moheet* (Lexicon), Volume 3, Cairo, Dar El Maaref.

Kivimaki, M., Vahtera, J., Elovainio, M., Heleius, H., Singh—Manoux, A., and Pentti, J. (2005). Optimism and pessimism as predictors of change in health after death or onset of severe illness in family. *Health Psychology, 24*(4), 413-421.

Malinchoc, M., Colligan, R., and Offord, K. (1996). Assessing explanatory style in teenagers: adolescent norms for the MMPI Optimism-Pessimism Scale, *Journal of Clinical Psychology. 52*(3), 285-295.

Marshal, G., Wortman, C., Kusulas., J., Herring, L., and Vickers, R. (1992). Distinguishing optimism from pessimism: Relations to fundamental Dimensions of mood and personality. *Journal of Personality and Social Psychology, 62*(2), 1067-1074.

Martin Seligman (2005). *Authentic Happiness: Using the New Positive Psychology to Realize Your Potential for Lasting Fulfilment,* Translated by Safaa El Assar, Alaa Kafafy, Aziz El Sayed, Faisal Younis, Fadya Elwan, and Soheir Ghobashy, Cairo, Dar El Ein for Publishing.

Maysa Shoukry (1999). Optimism and Pessimism and the Relation to Methods of Facing Hardships, *Psychological Studies Journal, 9* (2), 378-416.

Nagwa El Yahfoufy (2002). Optimism and Pessimism and Their Relation to Social Demographic Variables among University Students, *Psychology Journal*, Issue (62), 132-151.

Nagwa El Yahfoufy and Bade Al Ansary (2005). Optimism and Pessimism: A Comparative Cultural Study between the Lebanese and Kuwaitis, *Social Sciences Journal*, Kuwait, *33* (2), 313-336.

Othman El Khedr (1999). *Optimism and Pessimism and Job Performance,* Arab Magazine of Humanitarian Sciences, Kuwait, *17* (67), 214-242.

Peterson, C., Seligman, M., and Vaillant, G. (1988). Pessimistic explanatory style is a risk factor for physical illness: A thirty five year longitudinal study. *Journal of Personality and Social Psychology, 55*(1), 13-27.

Peterson, C. (2000). The future of optimism. *American Psychologist, 55*(1), 44-55.

Samer Radwan (2001). Depression and Pessimism, Comparative Correlative Study, *Psychological and Education Studies Journal*, Faculty of Education, Bahrain University, *2*, 14-48.

Sarmany, I. (1996). Optimism and Cognitive Style. *Studio Psychologia, 34*(3), 261-267.

Scheier, M., and Carver, C. (1985). Optimism, Coping, and Health: Assessment and implications of generalized outcome expectancies. *Health Psychology. 4*(3), 219-247.

Scheier, M., and Carver, C. (1987). Dispositional optimism and physical well-being: The influence generalized outcome expectation on health. *Journal of Personality, 55*(1), 169-210.

Scheier, M., and Carver, C. (1992). Effects of optimism on psychological and physical well-being: Theoretical overview and empirical update. *Cognitive Therapy and Research, 16*(2), 201-228.

Srivastava, S., Mcgonigal, K., Richards, J., Butler, E., and Gross, J. (2006). Optimism, in close relationship: How seeing things in a positive light Makes them so. *Journal of Personality and Social Psychology, 91*(1), 143-153.

Taylor, S., Keneny, M., Aspinwall, L., Schneider, S., Rodriguez, R., and Herbert, M. (1992). Optimism, coping, psychological distress, and high-risk sexual behaviour among men at risk for acquired immune deficiency syndrome (AIDS). *Journal of Personality and Social Psychology, 63*(3), 460-473.

Turkum, A. (2005). Do optimism, social network richness, and submissive behaviours predict well-being? Study with a Turkish sample. *Social Behaviour and Personality, 33*(6), 619-628.

Weiner, B. (1980). *Human Motivation*, New York: Springer Verlag.

Weinstin, N. (1980). Unrealistic optimism about future life events. *Journal of Personality and Social Psychology, 39*(5), 806-820.

Weinstin, N. (1983). Reducing unrealistic optimism about illness susceptibility. *Health Psychology, 2*(1), 11-20.

Wong, S., and Lim, T. (2009). Hope versus optimism in Singaporean adolescents: Contributions to depression and life satisfaction. *Personality and Individual Differences, 46*(5-6), 648-652.

9
Promoting Positive Mental Health

V. Smitha Ruckmani, A. Shanmugiah and *R. Jeyaprakash*

Mental health is an important agenda in today's life. As there is an increase in the rates of homicide, suicide, rape, violence and assault across different age groups in society has led the society to brainstorm about mental health at large.

Promotion of Mental Health refers to the positive mental health. Mental health promotion or Positive Mental Health is defined as the creation of individual, social and environmental conditions that help optimal psychological and psycho-physiological development. Prevention of mental disorders is the aim and outcome of a broader mental health promotion strategy (Hosman & Janellopis, 1999).

Mental ill-health refers to signs and symptoms leading to distress and disability. The strategies to improve or promote mental health towards positive side or focusing on reducing risk factors and enhancing protective factors that lead to mental ill-health. In the context of public health, positive mental health aims at reducing the magnitude of mental disorders and identifying and reducing the risk factors. Mental health promotion in turn reduces the incidence and prevalence of mental disorders. Positive mental health serves as a powerful protective factor against mental illness. Mental disorders and positive mental health cannot be described as the different ends of a linear scale, but rather as two overlapping and interrelated components of a single concept of mental health (Detels *et al.*, 2002).

Through negative attitudes about mental illness that pervade in public thinking, young people learn from very early age view that psychiatric problems are personal failures. The sense of embarrassment around the concept of mental health difficulty contributes to the fact that such problems are often unrecognized or even denied. Young people often deal with personal mental health problems in an unsophisticated ways such as bottling them up, sleeping, drinking alcohol, simply hoping that they would go away.

We need to define mental health, and understand various concepts like risk factors, protective factors, vulnerability and resilience. This will help to classify risk factors into modifiable risk factor and non-modifiable risk factors. Risk factors which cannot be changed is called non-modifiable like family history of mental illness, gender, age and life events. Modifiable risk factors are those which can be changed like social isolation, unhealthy lifestyle, coping mechanism, emotional reactions and motivation. Factors that protect young people with mental health difficulties work in complex ways. We need to identify factors that are amenable for intervention and in the promotion for building positive mental health.

WHO (2007) defines that mental health is not just the absence of mental illness. It is defined as a state of well-being in which every individual realizes his or her own potential, can cope with the normal stresses of life, can work productively and fruitful, and is able to make a contribution to his or her community.

Mental health is about three aspects:

1. how we feel about ourselves;
2. how we feel about others; and
3. how we deal with demands of life.

Poor mental health does not mean that one is suffering from mental illness or disorder. It is a kind of general mental health difficulty that all of us experience in specific stressful circumstance, for example not able to balance between home life and work pressure, academic pressure, uncertain situations. Everyone of us faces pressures, everyday tensions and problems and challenging life situations. Problems are classified into the following—certain problem has immediate solutions, one has to think different ways of dealing with the problems successfully. Few problems do not have immediate solutions, but it takes time to solve for example debts, financial crisis, and physical health problems. During these periods one has to keep his mental status at peace and continue to function at optimal level without getting affected emotionally and impair the function and have a realistic and optimistic attitude to keep him going with life.

Few problems do not have solutions, which is not in their hands; for example alcoholic spouse, handicapped children, poverty which is a limitation. One has to learn to get adapted to situations and change the reactions and thoughts towards experiencing the situations without getting affected psychologically. They should be able to change their attitude, approach and reactions which help in strengthening their psychological immunization.

Determinants of Mental Health

Multiple biological, psychological and social factors determine the mental health of the person at any point of time. Poor mental health is associated with specific temperamental personality factors, stressful work pressure, conditions, unhealthy lifestyle and physical ill-health, exposure to violent environment, social exclusion, gender discrimination and rapid social change. Few biological causes are of genetic factors and biochemical changes in the brain which lead to the development of mental disorder. These factors predispose the individual and environmental factors act as precipitating factor and make people vulnerable to mental illness.

Characteristics of Individual with Good Mental Health

- Individual with value based mental set.
- Individual with cordial and harmonious relationship in the family.
- Persons, who are able to take appropriate, right decisions in life.
- Persons who are responsible in their life (Internally driven).
- Person's having good interpersonal relationship.
- Attitude of flexibility and adaptability to face demands in life and occupation.
- Frustration tolerance and patience.
- Engageing oneself in healthy lifestyle practice.

Characteristics of Individual with Poor Mental Health

- Family history of mental illness, suicide, alcohol.
- Impaired emotional and social development in childhood is precursor for poor mental health in adulthood.
- An individual who is externally driven.
- An attitude of rigidity and uncaring.
- Ruminating on past bad experiences and unwilling to accept the negative aspects.
- Sensitive and touchy nature.

- Engageing in impulsive and self-harm behaviour.
- Impatience and a strong desire for immediate gratification.

Resilience and Protective Mechanism

Resilience is a critical skill where an individual bounce back when there is a life adversity. It is like try, try, and try again. People differ in the presence of severity of risk factors. Many individuals exposed to risk factors, everyone are not vulnerable to develop mental health problems. Few individuals engage in high risk behaviours and some do not. What makes the difference in the two groups. The term resilience is used, despite the severity of risk factors the individual do well and maintain optimal functioning. Resilience is determined by the following aspects:

- A sense of self-esteem and self-confidence.
- A belief in one's own self-efficacy and ability to deal with change and adaptation.
- Social Problem Solving Skills.
- Enhance tolerance and understanding in general.

Research suggests that as children and young people are surrounded by risk factors, protective factors help in developing resilience trait in the individual. This in turn counterbalance and reduces the impact of risk factors. Characteristics related to resilience lie within the individual, family, community and society. The following illustration about two children who are facing a parental conflict may clear the issue. Two children who were from the same family, who had alcoholic father. One grew up and became responsible, affectionate and a successful person. Another grew up and became an irresponsible, unemployed and alcoholic. When they were asked about what made them. For both father was the role model as to how to choose their life. First person told I didn't want to become like my father. Second person told life is easy, free like my father. In both of them father was the role model for choosing how their lives had to be.

Individual Protective Factors

Self-esteem, Emotional resilience, Positive thinking, Problem solving skill, Social skill, Coping strategy, Familial protective factors, Good parenting, Attachment and Positive parent-child interaction.

Social Protective Factors

Empowerment, Social participation, Social support, and Community networks.

Through the understanding of factors related to resilience which lies within the individual, family, community and society, we need to look at how to develop qualities related to resilience. Few factors are discussed below.

Temperament: Easy temperament, flexible trait will make an individual to adapt to changes and cope with stressful events. Individual capacity to adapt in a healthy manner is referred to as tolerance trait. Youth who, when exposed to multiple risk factors, shows successful responses and looks at the situation as challenging and tries to get adapted without getting affected and gets back to the routine life as early as possible. Williams *et al.* (2000) noted that temperament in early infancy and early childhood was an important aspect in protecting young people from substance abuse by 15 years of age.

Intelligence: When a person has high I.Q. which helps him to negotiate with high risk environments. High on emotional quotient help the individual to cope with negativity, unpleasant feelings and emotions when faced with adverse life situation as they will be able to regulate and modulate negative emotions in a healthy and adaptive manner.

Social competence: Interpersonal skills which help an individual to integrate feelings, thoughts, and actions in a meaningful way to achieve goals in specific are referred to as social competence. These skills help an individual to pick up relevant social cues, generate a range of effective solutions, take appropriate social decisions, and translate decisions into behavioural terms/actions when faced with obstacles and frustrations. Studies have shown that enhancement of competence is a preventive measure.

Pro-social behaviour: Research studies have shown that pro-social behaviour is negatively correlated with mental health problems and hence pro-social behaviour is a promotive factor. Research evidence suggests that role of pro-social behaviour; pro-social peers can mitigate and have a buffer impact on anti-social peer influence of drug use behaviours (Kaufmann *et al.*, 2007).

Family Environment: Family has vital effects on the development of the child. According to Morris *et al.* (2007) children learn emotions by observing the people around them. Their experiences and behaviours related to parent's emotion help children to understand what is appropriate behaviour expected in society. The qualities of emotional attachment between parents and children, attitudes of parents, marital relationships between the parents are some of the factors related to the family which have an impact on emotional skills.

Positive opportunities to develop key interpersonal skills in early development should be made available. Interactions with good peer group, involvement in roles which contribute to their group, family and friends or larger community are important (Dryfoos, 1990) which works as a protective mechanism during adolescence, where substance abuse is a proximal behaviour.

Bonding: The other important protective and promotive factor is bonding. Individuals who have developed healthy positive bonds from early years to their family, peer, schools are less likely to develop high risk behaviour. Young Individuals aged 10 years, 14 years, 16 years who have positive bonds to school and have educational aspirations predicted lower alcohol abuse at age 21 years (Guo *et al.,* 2001). Alcoholics in the age of thirties were found to have poorer educational achievement during elementary school, not completing high school.

Schooling: Students come from different family background, family types. School is a common platform and is one of the important sources for socialization process. Students spent more time in school. School has a great impact on the personality development of an individual. Students should develop a positive bond to the school. He/She should be able to develop a commitment for studies. A school which encourages extracurricular activities has an impact on emotional and social development in the individuals. For students who come from unhealthy, pathological families which pose as a risk factor. School environment can act as a catalyst which can bring down the negative effects of family on the individual. Teacher can play a positive role model in such students, instead of developing a negative and neglect attitude towards students with problem behaviour.

Care, trust, commitment and respect for diversity are some of the qualities which are developed in school environment. Philosophers such as Benjamin Franklin, John Stuartmill, Herbert Spencer and John Dewey had emphasized on talents of students. Simon and Binet who are known for their work on mental age, also emphasized on enhancement of students' academic and non-academic skills rather than remediation and weakness.

Quality and attitude of the teachers act as positive role models. Such teachers provide positive emotional development, a secure environment for young people to explore and find way to achieve their own academic and life goals.

Trust has received less attention among educators. It has effects on both Psychological and Performance. Development of trusting relationship is crucial from elementary grades. Learning to trust help in the classroom management of thorny problem with the most difficult students and this in turn has a ripple effects that spread to the rest of the class.

Based on attachment theory Watson and Ecken (2003) developed the concept of developmental discipline. This advocates helping students who have insecure attachment to caregivers. According to them, building caring and trusting relationship will be the important goal for the socialization process in these students. Non-punitive methods should be used as disciplinary modes in the management of aggressive students. For withdrawn and dependent students self-reliance and confidence should be the goal for the development. They should avoid judgemental and cynical attitude about students which will undermine trust which is crucial for learning. Unless students sense the teachers respect for them they will not give full cooperation. When the mentor is not sure about the student, silence is the best approach. Observation with a non-judgemental attitude will help in understanding the student. The importance of diversity encourages students to become sensitive to the ideas and opinions of other persons.

Culture, Society and Religion: Insight into culture shows how people of varied background generate psychological well-being. In examining how adverse experiences could promote psychological well-being, adaptive psychological functioning gives us an understanding/clues on optimal human function.

Cultural values provide the basis in which behaviour, thoughts, and feeling are deemed as normal/abnormal. These values influence, experience/meaning.

There is a national difference with related to homicide across different nations and laws related to control of guns also differ. Studies have shown that suicidal rates are less in religious countries compared to non-religious countries.

Risk Factors: Risk factors are those factors that increase the susceptibility of an individual to develop mental health problems. One becomes vulnerable when faced with a risk factor. Risk factors are negative life events, negative life experiences which affect the individual negatively. It brings in negative emotions like shock, fear, anxiety and depression.

Risk factors are accumulative in nature. When the individual is faced with risk factor his chance of developing poor mental is 1-2 per cent chances. However, with 3 risk factors it is thought to be increased by 8 per cent and with more than 4 risk factors in the individual life the likelihood of increase is 20 per cent. Risk factors are those predictors associated with the likelihood of development of drug abuse and other behavioural disorders (Hawkins *et al.*, 1992). Risk factors predict future problem behaviours, those risk factors which are amenable to change are targets for preventive measures.

Patterns of Risk Exposure: Two types of patterns appear one in which a risk factor get accumulated from early experiences even before the protective factors gets available in the child's life. For instance, smoking in mother during pregnancy might impact foetus and infancy development, leads to cognitive impairment, and the foetus is at risk to develop other health problems, and is at greater vulnerability. And secondly, children who are not exposed to early risk factors and only during adolescence and youth exposed to risk factors, they are likely to develop mental health problems in absence of protective factors (for example greater availability of drugs, peer influence, weak ties with protective factors like decrease in family ties, increase independence lead the youth towards participating and engageing in high risk behaviour). Risk factors have been found in individual level (e.g. genetic predisposition) and in environments in which young people are socialized family, school, peer group, community, culture and society.

National surveys show that approximately 85 per cent of adolescents experiment with drugs before completing high school and individuals who begin drug use during adolescence have an increased risk of progression to addiction leading to make a diagnose of substance abuse disorder, compared to individuals who delay the use of drug until adulthood (Winters *et al.,* 2008). Most young people who initiated or experimented with drugs do not end up as dependence or develop chronic problem but one-third of such young people's journey end to the road of abuse and dependence. Alcohol substance abuse, reckless driving, aggression, suicidal behaviour, irresponsible sexual behaviour is little high risk behaviour in youth. The behaviours that are impulsive, disinhibited not driven by consequences and not able to effectively use executive functions lead to high risk behaviours.

Individual Risk Factors: Behaviour patterns in the form of anti-social behaviour, rebellious attitude, poor emotional modulation skills, and external locus of control, poor/unhealthy coping pattern, low self-esteem, low self-efficacy and negative belief systems are the factors at individual level which puts a person to participate in high risk behaviour.

Personality as a Predictor: Research has examined various variables of personality traits/temperamental traits, which pose a adolescent vulnerable to participate in risky behaviour.

Based on five factor model of personality, extroversion (activity level, sociability and dominance) has been associated with externalizing behaviours. Agreeableness (kindness, likeability, trustworthiness) appears to be negatively associated with risky behaviour and delinquency among youths. Conscientiousness (organization, reliability, impulse control) was related negatively with risky behaviours and youth deviance. Openness to experience (originality, intellect and creativity) has been related positively to risky behaviour in early maturing adolescent girls. Neuroticism (emotional instability, anxiety and sadness) has been related to poor mental health positively. Though there was a relation with the risky behaviour, but has not emerged as a consistent predictor.

Charlotte (2006) in his study found that girls who expressed behaviours like neuroticism, introversion, disagreeableness and low conscientiousness are the one who engage in risky behaviours. Boys who participate in risk behaviours were related to behaviour expressions associated with extroversion and disagreeableness.

Research has come out with a consistent finding that conscientious individuals have been found to take care with their health, avoid participate in health compromising behaviours and live longer than their unconscientiously peers.

Another consistent finding raised from past research was that youths who are sociable, outgoing and dominant are susceptible to risk behaviour. Girls who behaved introvert (passive, quiet and shy) are vulnerable to risk behaviours to receive peer approval, acceptance and cope with their negative moods.

Another consistent finding is children and adolescent who have difficulties in regulating negative emotions lead a person to participate in risk behaviour and pose risk for later mental health problem like personality disorder (Mark *et al.,* 2003).

Low in emotional intelligence, perceiving the family environment as critical, low pro-social behaviour contributes to mental health problems in adolescents and youth (Ruckmani & Balachandran, 2010). Emotional intelligence, pro-social behaviour and critical family environment are the promotive factors for mental health problems. Individual perception of the environment may show a significant relationship to absence of sickness behaviour. Henderson and colleagues used longitudinal data to show that children whose teachers described them as having frequent aches and pains, appearing miserable and being off school for trivial reasons were more likely to be permanently work sick and disabled. They suggest that how temperament interacts with individual perceptions of the workplace requires a life course approach to clarify the mechanisms by which these variables contribute to long-term sickness behaviour.

***Parental/Family Characteristics*:** Parent-child relationships are well recognized cause of behavioural problems in childhood. Behavioural problems are a predictor of depression in later life. Mental illness of parents interferes with parenting mediated through maltreatment, neglect, emotional deprivation and other relationship problems, further exposure to trauma and abuse lead to later psychiatric disorders. Prospective long-term cohort studies over periods ranging from 10-37 years support the view that abuse in childhood is inextricably linked with common psychiatric disorders in later life.

Family relationship measures in the form of abuse (physical, emotional and sexual) and neglect, lack of parent-child affection, parent-child discord, affectionless control, harsh discipline, perceived negative role in the family and poor care and mothering are risk factors at family level in a person's life.

The analysis of cohort studies showed those children with conduct problems at the age of 7-9 years likely to experience depression, die by suicide, have drug problem or to be involved in crime in later life. This brought out the importance of child development for later adult life.

***School Factors*:** Poor commitment to school, academic failures, school refusal and school truancy, victim of bullying, and other negative school experience place an individual at risk for associated emotional, behavioural and addiction problems.

***Community and Cultural Factors*:** Easy accessibility and availability of drugs in community, media portrayals, technological changes, where child and adolescents are exposed to lot of entertainments in the form of internet, highly sophisticated mobiles pose a risk factor. The individual himself not aware of its ill effects become a victim for abuse and addiction without their knowledge. Less neighbourhood attachment and extreme economic deprivation, high rate of transitions and mobility, prejudice ideas, cultural and racial discrimination, ethnicity emphasizes the culture bound syndrome, social distance among members of the culture are a few community factors which breeds poor mental health. Individuals who have multiple cultural identities, cultural changes when they travel for studies and employment have difficulties to adapt to cultural transitions might have adjustment problems and experience cultural shock.

Few studies have shown that religious countries have low rates of suicide compared to non-religious countries.

Society: Mental health and mental illness are profoundly affected by the social determinants of health. Psychosocial processes are important pathways by which social environment has an impact on both physical and mental health. Discrimination in the society is a social cause for mental illness, community clashes, and war in society where everyday life is affected badly. People are living with fears related to uncertainty as what will happen to whom and when. Natural disasters like earthquake, tsunami risks the community as a whole. Manmade disasters like bomb blast, aircrash, nuclear disaster affects the groups in large community. This is one important causative factor for development of post-traumatic stress disorder. Once mental disorder has risen it leads to range of inequalities like increased health risk behaviour, reduced educational and employment outcomes. Populations living in poor socio-economic circumstances are at high risk to develop mental health problems (Jane-Llopis, 2005).

Macro factors such as urbanization, war, displacement, racial discrimination and economic instability leads to increased psychiatric morbidity. The social risk factor for the development of poor mental health are found as low socio-economic, low education, unemployment and underemployment, food insecurity, gender inequality, discrimination, prejudice etc.

Vulnerability: 'Vulnerability' is derived from the Latin word 'vulnerary' (to be wounded) and it describes the potential to be harmed physically and psychologically and suggests the opposite for the term resilience. The concept of vulnerability was introduced in 1970s by O'Keefe, Westgate and Wisner in relation to natural hazards and disasters. Vulnerability has an external and internal side. People are exposed to specific natural and social risk. At the same time people vary in capacity, strength and potentiality to deal with the exposure to abuse, hazards and disasters in life. When individuals face life events some of them develop depression and few of them do not. Concept of vulnerability and protective factors makes an attempt to explain why some individuals develop depression and some do not. Individuals differ in the extent to which they are vulnerable to depression. Blaikie *et al.* (1994) define vulnerability as the "Set of characteristics of a group or individual in terms of their capacity to anticipate, cope with, resist and recover from the impact of a natural hazard. It involves a combination of factors that determine the degree to which someone's life and livelihood is at risk by a discrete and identifiable event in nature or society."

Within the natural hazards and disasters, the concept of social vulnerability emerged. One of the dimensions of vulnerability is social vulnerability to multiple stressors and shock. Research on social vulnerability makes an attempt to understand how social conditions transform a natural hazard (e.g. flood, earthquake, mass movements) into disasters. Social processes and structures define the causes and the phenomenon of disasters. However, exposure to the event (natural hazard) is constant, but individuals and groups in society vary in their capacities to deal with the impact of hazard and its consequences.

Biological Perspectives: Biological vulnerabilities are endogenous (e.g. genetic makeup) or they arise from environmental adversity which has an effect on early brain development. The organization and maturation of central nervous system during foetal and early post-natal life are governed by genetic factors and further modulated by the environmental inputs which are experienced by developing brain. An association between birth complications and emotional dysfunction was found in a study (Fowler, Langley, Frances Rice *et al.*, 2009). Birth complications are simply an index for biological and genetic vulnerability rather than a risk factor. The susceptibility of the person is thus altered by these biological moderators. This process is called diathesis-stress model.

Diathesis is a Greek term for disposition. People differ in their vulnerability to develop disorder. The diathesis, i.e. predisposition interacts with stress response of the individual. Person's psychological equilibrium is disrupted by the life events and this serves as catalyst in disorder development. Thus, this model explores how genetic traits and non-biological factors interact with environmental factors (stress) to produce disorders like depression, anxiety and schizophrenia. When the combination of predisposition and stress exceeds a threshold the individual will have a break down. Individuals differ in their thresholds.

Diathesis stress model is used in various fields of medicine like psychiatry, cardiology and psychology in studying illness behaviour. It helps in understanding the interplay of nature and nurture in the individual susceptibility for development of disorder. It also explains why some individuals are more at risk. This model also attempts in explaining other poor developmental outcomes.

Psychological Perspectives: Bowlby's works have shown strong influence of quality of infant and caregiver relationship and its profound and lasting consequences associated with a wide range of developmental outcomes. He proposed that "the extent to which an individual makes trusting, affectionate and cooperative relations with others depends to a high degree of relationship he had with his parents especially with the mother in early years."

When there are traumatic life experiences during the developmental period which disrupts in achieving normal development tasks. A child at the age of 8 years who had a history of kidnap and sexual trauma who had to attend legal proceedings had interfered in her daily functioning, frequently absenting from school had left her not able to achieve the developmental tasks expected during that period.

Cognitive and perceptual style is referred to as vulnerable factor. Depressed individuals attribute their failures to self. They feel responsible for their failures. They attribute failures to internal factors (i.e. self-blame, negative body image, guilt, intrapunitiveness, use of introjections etc.), whereas success they attribute to external factors (luck, simplicity of task, other's support).

Weiner (1972) proposed that individuals tend to attribute their success and failures mainly to the four causes, i.e. Ability, Effort, Task difficulty and Luck.

The above mentioned causes are called locus of control and stability. Ability and task difficulty are considered as stable as this does not change across the time. Effort and luck are considered as unstable as this changes/fluctuates time to time. Ability and effort are considered as internal dimension of locus of control. Luck is considered as external dimension of locus of control. These two dimensions, i.e. Internal *versus* External and stability *versus* instability are important determinants of affective reactions to life events/experience. Individual differ in the above aspects.

Choice Theory: Choice theory is developed by Dr. William Glasser (1999). Choice theory is based on the assumption that individual's behaviour is a way to satisfy the basic five needs. The five needs are as follows:

1. Need to survive,
2. Need to belong,
3. Need to gain power,
4. Need to be free, and
5. Need to have fun.

One behaves in a particular way to satisfy the basic needs. Each one differs in their perception of world which is specific to them. When there is a discrepancy between what they have and what they want it can lead to dysfunction. This theory explains that behaviour is made of three components—what we think, what we feel and what we do. Total behaviour is the sum of feeling, thought, doing/acting and physiology. Regardless of the circumstances, the individual faces, it is this three components which makes the individual's different in their vulnerabilities. This leads one to engage in effective and ineffective behaviour. Sometimes, the ineffective behaviour persists even after the choice of effective behaviour option is available. When a person recognizes feeling is one component of behaviour then he will be more in control.

According to Glasser, feelings are expressed as verbs such as depressing anxious and head aching. The importance of this sort of language pulls down the man. By using right language we may be able to control our everyday situation.

Glasser explains further, "I do not have the ability to change how I feel, but I have the ability to change what I do, and some ability to change how I think, regardless of how I choose to feel.

Behaviours and value that satisfy needs are stored as a picture album in the brain. When we want to satisfy our needs we turn to our picture album pages. Sometimes, we do not have picture which satisfy our real life needs. Few times how we had dealt in earlier times will not be right for the present scenario. Our relentless effort to satisfy our pictures might become self-destructive and socially unacceptable. No two people share the personal album.

Societal Perspective: The major social constructs (ethnicity, gender, disability, age and sexual orientation are documented to be potential reasons for perceived discriminations. When we make choices based on ethnic background, gender, disability, age and sexual orientation, religion are few reasons leading to humiliation of humanity. Lack of participation in society; lack of social relations; social isolation and poor social support; living in violent environment war zone areas where everyday life itself is uncertain lead to anxiety; depression and poor mental health putting the individual at risk mental state.

Strategies Towards Building Positive Mental Health: Preventive science has developed over last two decades. Contribution from social, biological and neurological sciences have made insight into the role of risk and protective factors in the developmental pathway to mental health. National mental health policies should not only focus on mental disorders, but also should address broader horizons in promoting positive mental health as a preventive measure. Strategies to promote positive mental health aims to reinforce protective factors along the life span. A collective approach focusing the entire population and wide range of activities targeting positive mental health is mental health intervention spectrum. Spectrums of interventions are—

(a) Prevention,
(b) Early intervention,
(c) Treatment, and
(d) Continuing care (Mrazek and Haggerty, 1994).

Principles of Strategic Approaches in Positive Mental Health

Mental health promotion interventions have been targeted either within defined settings such as (school, work places and cities) or with identified population groups such as (older group and younger group).

The five main strategies for mental health promotion for action are:

1. Building public health policy,
2. Creating supportive environments,
3. Strengthening community action,
4. Developing personal skills, and
5. Expanding the orientation of health services (WHO, 1986).

Building Public Health Policy

Policy and funding decisions in the mainstream health, welfare, education and judiciary are important to promote positive mental health.

For example universal antenatal screening.

Follow-up of mothers at risk of postnatal depression.

Creating Supportive Environments

Supportive social, economic, cultural and physical environments provide a basic framework for and developing and maintaining mental health. Absence of war and conflict are fundamental to emotional and social well-being.

The strategies at micro levels to implement in the society (schools, work places) are:

(a) Anti-bullying schemes,
(b) To reduce the rate of physical abuse, and
(c) To reduce the rate of verbal abuse.

Improving the physical environments through infrastructure promote mental health, e.g. Good public transport.

Strengthening Community Action

Affordable and accessible leisure activities, social support, strong social networks and a sense of integration and inclusion are key predictors of positive mental health. It is important to be supportive of parents and families, as early childhood experiences within the family form a platform for later mental health.

Supportive environment at workplaces can promote positive mental health. Communities with high levels of social capital are characterized by trust, tolerance and reciprocity. They offer a wide range of networks that provide many opportunities for mutual support and participation at all levels along with exchange of skills and information. This type of community may be called as empowered community.

Media promotes mental health literacy in the community, reduces stigma and discrimination to promote recovery and understanding of mental illnesses and increase appropriate early help seeking behaviour. The media also influence attitudes on a range of everyday life issues that affect mental health.

Developing Personal Skills

Mental health promotion acknowledges the importance of psychological process, how people think, feel, interpret the world at all levels. Mental health, therefore, incorporates the development of personal skills to enhance emotional and social well-being (Health Education Authority, 1998).

Personal skills include the ability to manage change, and to recognize, acknowledge and communicate thoughts and feelings, most importantly, the ability to make and maintain relationship.

Skills are necessary to cope with stress and adversity. Every individual needs to have feelings of self-worth and empowerment, the belief that they can control and influence the environment. Personal skills can be addressed at various levels; major achievements in mental health can be attained by improving the environments that affect the development of resilience in children.

For Example—

(a) Parenting skills programme,
(b) Quality child care,
(c) Life skills training at school level, and
(d) Expanding the orientation of health services.

The component of incorporating promotion, prevention and early intervention within health services will address the positive mental health.

The objectives of these strategies are:

(a) Reducing the risk factors,
(b) Strengthen the protective factors,
(c) Decrease psychiatric morbidity,
(d) To reduce the rate of disability, and
(e) To reduce the onset of psychiatric disorders.

The prevention of mental health problem depends on identifying and modifying the determinants of mental health. Effective prevention requires an understanding of the risk and protective factors for mental health. Identification of the potential groups and individuals is very important who can benefit from interventions and the development, dissemination and implementation of effective interventions.

Principles of Early Intervention Strategy

Early intervention focuses on people with early signs and symptoms of a mental health problem or disorder or developing or experiencing a first episode of mental illness.

Identification: Early signs and symptom of developing mental disorders are:

(a) Fewer symptoms than those require for syndrome diagnosis,
(b) Present for shorter period of time, and
(c) Less intense and disruptive than those of a diagnosable disorder.

There are many diagnostic instruments for first episode of mental disorder based on the Diagnostic and statistical manual of mental disorder, fourth edition (DSM-IV) (APA1994) and the international classification of diseases, tenth edition (ICD-10) (WHO, 1992) these instruments detect only fully developed disorders.

Fully developed disorders (diagnosable) should have specific symptoms for a designated length of time and a particular intensity.

Table 9.1: Potential early signs and symptoms

Signs	*Symptoms*
Tension	Substance use
Irritability	Poor concentration
Intrusive worrying thoughts	Mood swings
Depressed mood	Appetite changes
Loss of energy/motivation	Suspiciousness

Source: Adapted from NSW Health, 1999.

The focus on early intervention will be on reducing risk factors and enhancing protective factors rather than providing treatment.

Mental Health Promotion Across Life Span Strategy

Many developmental tasks and life changes are important factors for mental health promotion. A successful negotiation of these life changes and developmental tasks enhances mental health.

Developmental Tasks and Sectors Across the Life Span

Sectors Across Life Span

(1) Community,
(2) Health care,
(3) Workforce,
(4) Social relationship,
(5) Education, and
(6) Family.

Developmental Tasks and Life Changes

1. Birth and development—marriage
2. Developing social skills—parenting

3. Academic performance—vocational
4. Psycho-social development—caregiver
5. Coping with loss—being grandparent

Life Stages (*Source*: adapted from Mrazek & Haggerty, 1994)

Mental health promotion is essential across the entire life span, regardless of current health status.

Strategies for Special Population

1. *Women:* Prevention and early intervention for post-natal depression have valuable multigenerational effects. Post-natal depression influences the women's health, development of the child, relationship with other children and the marital relationship (Boyle and Stubbs, 1994).
2. *Prevention and Early Intervention of Psychosis:* At present no known prevention for psychotic disorders such as schizophrenia and bipolar disorder, but research shows the positive effects of early intervention. The duration of untreated psychosis was associated with more complications including severe behavioural disturbances and family difficulty (Johnstone *et al.*, 1986). The time to remit and level of remission was related to duration of untreated psychosis.
3. *Substance Use Disorder:* Genetic, environmental and learned behaviours interact to determine substance misuse. Parental drug or alcohol abuse is established as a major risk factor. Emotional and behavioural problems along with peer and family influences are associated with substance misuse.
   Preventive programmes have focused on controlling access to substances, and educating people as to these harmful effects. Studies have shown that just a few minutes of structured advice is an effective and efficient intervention for harmful and hazardous drinking (Saunders and Lee, 1999).
4. *Suicide Prevention Strategy:* Individuals with mental health problem and mental disorders are at markedly increased risk of suicide. The most common mental disorder associated with suicide is depression. Suicide among younger adults is prominently associated with use of harmful drug and psychotic disorder. Therefore, early intervention of mental health problem and mental disorders has the potential to reduce the incidence

of associated suicides. Suicide is the final outcome of what is usually a complex, cumulative and interacting set of risk factors. Personal and environmental factors that place people at increased risk for suicide including hopelessness, recent loss, a previous attempt and active suicidal ideation (APS, 1999). Suicide prevention is approached indirectly through risk and protective factors.

Conclusion

Mental Health is often neglected. Due to shortage of mental health professionals preventive aspects are not targeted. Mental health policies should also focus in increasing training programmes to improve the human resources of mental health professionals in the country at various levels. Grassroots training for *anganwadi* and *balwadi* workers, caretakers, workers at rehabilitation centres is essential. Sensitization, awareness, exhibitions on mental health and screening programmes to be conducted at educational set-up, various industries for employees, military and paramilitary. Mental health education should be integrated with physical health education. Aspects of mental health could be introduced in curriculum development in educational setups. Research is another area which needs to be focused.

Acknowledgements: I thank Dr. S. Raja Rathinam, Professor of Psychiatry, Kilpauk Medical College and Hospital and Dr. Aruna, Reader in Psychology (Retd.) for their interview.

References

American Psychiatric Association (2000). *Diagnostic and Statistical Manual of Mental Disorders* (DSM-IV) 4th Ed. Washington, American Psychiatric Association.

Anderson, P., Biglen, A., and Holder. H., (2005). Preventing the Harm done by Substances. In C. Hosman, E. Jane Llopis, S. Saxena (Eds.) *Prevention of Mental Disorders, Effective Interventions and Policy Options*, Oxford Press, Oxford.

Baram, T.Z., Davis, E.P., Obenaus, A., Sandman, C.A., Small, S.L., Solodkin, A., and Stern, H. (2012). Fragmentation and unpredictability of early-life experience in mental disorders. *The American Journal of Psychiatry, 169*, 907-915.

Beardslee, W. *et al.* (1998). Psychiatric disorder in adolescent offspring of parents with Affective disorder in a non-referred sample. *Journal of Affective Disorder*, *15*(3), 313-322.

Beautrais, A.L. (1998). *Risk Factors for Suicide and Attempted Suicide amongst Young People*, NHMRC, and Canberra.

Berry, H.L. and Rickwood, D.J. (2000), Measuring Social Capital at the Individual Level: Personal Social Capital, Values and Psychological Distresses. *International Journal of Mental Health Promotion*, Vol. 2(3), 35-44.

Bhojak, M.M., Vyas, J.N., Nathawat, S.S., and Vijayvergia, D. (1989). A study of attributional style in depression compared with schizophrenic and normal patients. *Indian Journal of Psychiatry*, *31*(2), 116-121.

Birchwood, M., McGorry, P., and Jackson, H. (1997). Early intervention in schizophrenia. *British Journal of Psychiatry*, *170*(1), 2-11.

Blaikie, P., T. Cannon, I. Davis and B. Wisner. (1994). *At Risk: Natural Hazards, People's Vulnerability, and Disasters.* London, Routledge.

Boyce, P. and Stubbs, J. (1994). The Importance of Post-natal Depression. *Medical Journal of Australia*, Vol. 161, 471-472.

Brown, C. and Schulberg, H.C. (1998). Diagnosis and Treatment of Depression in Primary Medical Care Practice: The Application of Research Findings to Clinical Practice. *Journal of Clinical Psychology*, Vol. 54, 303-314.

Brown, G.W. and Harris, T.O. (1978), *Social Origins of Depression.* Tavistock, London.

Caplan, R.D. *et al.* (1998). Job Seeking, Reemployment and Mental Health. A randomized field experiment in coping with job loss. *Journal of Applied Psychology*, *74*(5), 759-769.

Catalano, R.F., Haggerty, K.P., Hawkins, J.D., and Elgin, J. (2011). Prevention of Substance Use and Substance Use Disorders: The role of risk and protective factors. *Clinical Manual of Adolescent Substance Abuse Treatment*, 25-63.

Charlotte, N., Markey, A., Patrick, M., Markey, B., Andrea, J., *et al.* (2006). Children's Behavioural Patterns, the Five-factor Model of Personality, and Risk Behaviours. *Personality and Individual Differences*, 41, 1503-1513.

Chatterjee, A. and Lieberman, J.A. (1999). Studies of Biological Variables in First episode Schizophrenia: A Comprehensive Review. In P.D. McGorry and H.J. Jackson (Eds.) *The Recognition and Management of Early Psychosis. A Preventive Approach*, (pp. 115-152). University Press, Cambridge.

Cohen, A. and Saxena, B. (2002). Ourlives were covered in darkness. The work of the national literary mission in northern India. In Social and mental health programme in low income countries (pp. 153-190). *World Mental Health Case Book*, Kluwer Academic/Plenum Publishers, London.

Cole, J.D., Watt, N.F., West, S.G. *et al.* (1993). The Science of Prevention: A Conceptual framework and some directions for a National Research Programme. *American Psychologist*, Vol. 48, 509-527.

Cotton, P. and Jackson, H. (1996). Early Intervention and Prevention in Mental Health. *Australian Psychological Society*, Melbourne.

Cowling, V.R., McGorry, P.D. and Hay, D.A. (1995). Children of Parents with Psychotic Disorders. *Medical Journal of Australia*, Vol. 163, 119-120.

Detels, *et al.* (2002). *Oxford Textbook of Public Health*, 3rd edition, Oxford University Press, Oxford.

DryFoos, J.G. (1990). *Adolescents at Risk: Prevalence and Prevention*. Oxford University Press, Oxford.

Falloon, B.J. and Bowles, T. (1999). Adolescent Help-Seeking for Major and Minor Problems. *Australian Journal of Psychology*, Vol. 51(1), 12-18.

Fowler, T., Langley, K.F., Rice, N., Whittinger, K., Ross, S., *et al.* (2009). Psychopath Traits in Adolescents with Childhood Attention—Deficit Hyperactivity Disorder. *British Journal of Psychiatry, 194*, 62-67.

Gedds, J.R., and Lawrie, S.M. (1995). Obstetric Complications and Schizophrenia: A Meta-analysis. *British Journal of Psychiatry, 167*(6), 786-793.

Glasser, W. (1999). *Choice Theory: A New Psychology of Personal Freedom*. New York: Harper Collins.

Gorden, R. (1983). An Operational Classification of Disease Prevention. *Public Health Reports, 98*, 107-109.

Gorden, R.C. (1987). An Operational Classification of Disease Prevention. In J.A. Steinberg, and M.M. Silverman (eds.) *Preventing Mental disorders: A Research Perspective*. Department of Health and Human Services, 20-26.

Guo, J., Hawkins, J.D., Hill, K.G., Abbott, R.D. (2001). Childhood and Adolescent Predictors of Alcohol Abuse and Dependence in Young Adulthood. *Journal of Studies on Alcohol, 62*, 754-762.

Hawkins, J.D., Catalano, R.F., and Miller, J.Y. (1992). Risk and Protective Factors for Alcohol and other Drug Problems in Adolescence and Early Adulthood: Implications for Substance Abuse Prevention. *Psychological Bulletin, 112*, 64-105.

Herrman, H., Saxena, S. and Moodie, R. (2004). *Promoting Mental Health: Concepts, Emerging Evidence, Practice*, WHO Report.

Hosman, C. and Jane-Llopis, E. (1999). Political Challenges 2: Mental Health. In the Evidence of Health Promotion Effectiveness: Shaping Public Health in a New Europe, *Chapter 3, 29-41. International Union for Health Promotion and Education*, IUHPE, Paris: Jouve Composition & Impression.

Hosman, C., Jane-Llopis, E. and Saxena, S. (2004). *Prevention of Mental Disorders: Effective Interventions and Policy Options:* Summary report/a report of the World Health Organization Dept. of Mental Health and Substance Abuse; In Collaboration with the Prevention Research Centre of the Universities of Nijmegen and Maastricht.

Ingram, R.E. and Porce, J.M., (2000). *Handbook of Vulnerability to Psychopathology: Risk Across the Life Span*. Guilford, New York.

Jablensky, A., *et al.* (2000). Psychotic Disorders in Urban Area: An Overview of the study on low prevalence disorders. *Australian and New Zealand Journal of Psychiatry, 34*, 221-236.

Jablensky, A.V., and Kalaydjieva, L.V. (2003). Genetic Epidemiology of Schizophrenia: Phenotypes, Risk Factors, and Reproductive Behaviour. *American Journal of Psychiatry, 160*(3), 425-429.

Jenkins, J. (2011). Psycho-social Adversity and Resilience. Rutter, M., Bishop, D., Pine, D., Scott, S., Stevenson, J.S., Taylor, E.A., and Thapar, A. (2011). *Rutter's Child and Adolescent Psychiatry*, John Wiley & Sons.

Johnstone, E.C., Crow, T.J., Johnson, A.L., *et al.* (1986). The Northwick Park Study of First episodes of Schizophrenia: Presentation of the Illness and Problems relating to admission. *British Journal of Psychiatry, 148*, 115-120.

Kaufmann, D.R., Wyman, P.A., Forbes-Jones, E.L., and Barry, J. (2007). Pro-social involvement and anti-social peer affiliations as predictors of behaviour problems in urban adolescents: Main effects and moderating effects. *Journal of Community Psychology, 35*(4), 417-434.

Lieberman, J., Jody, D., Geisler, S. *et al.* (1993). Time Course and Biological Correlates of Treatment Response in First-episode Schizophrenia. *Archives of General Psychiatry*, Vol. 50, 369-376.

Mark, T.L., Buck, J.A., Dilonard, J.D., Coffey, R.M. and Chalk, M. (2003). Medicaid expenditures on Behavioural Health Care. *Psychiatric Services, 54*, 188-194.

Morris, A.S., Silk, J.S., Morris, M.D., Steinberg, L., Aucoin, K.J., and Keyes, A.W. (2011). The influence of mother-child emotion regulation strategies on children's expression of anger and sadness. *Developmental Psychology, 47*(1), 213-225.

Mrazek, P.J., and Haggerty, R.J. (Eds.). (1994). *Reducing Risks for Mental Disorders: Frontiers for Preventive Intervention Research*. National Academies Press.

Naylor, P.B., Cowie, H.A., Walters, S.J., Talamelli, L., and Dawkins, J. (2009). Impact of a mental health teaching programme on adolescents. *The British Journal of Psychiatry, 194*(4), 365-370.

NHS Advisory Service (1995). *Together We Stand. The Commissioning Role and Management of Child and Adolescent Mental Health Services. HMSO,* London.

O'Keefe, P., Westgate, K., and Wisner, B. (1976). Taking the naturalness out of natural disasters. *Nature, 260*, 566-567.

Prevention Action. Diathesis-stress models. Retrived from http://WWW.Prevention action.org/reference/diathesis-stress models.

Ruckmani, S.R., and Balachandran, A. (2009). *School Based Behavioural Training for Adolescents with Mental Health Problems*. Unpublished doctoral dissertation. University of Madras, Chennai.

Sarah Wamala, Gunnel Bostron and Karin Nyqvist. (2007). Perceived discrimination and Psychological distress in Swedan. *British Journal of Psychiatry, 190*, 75-76.

Saunders, J.B. and Lee, N.K. (1999). Opportunistic brief Interventions. *Medicine, 27*, 22-23.

Saxena, S., Jané-Llopis, E., and Hosman, C. (2006). Prevention of mental and behavioural disorders: Implications for policy and practice. *World Psychiatry, 5*(1), 5.

Snyder, C.R. and Lopez, S. (2007). *Positive Psychology: The Scientific and Practical Explorations of Human Strengths*. Sage Publications, New Delhi, India.

Torrey, E.F., Bowler, A.E., and Clark, K. (1997). Urban birth and residence as risk factors for psychosis: an analysis of 1880 data. *Schizophrenia Research, 25* (3), 169-176.

Vanos, J., and Mcguffin, P. (2003). Can the Social Environment cause Schizophrenia? *British Journal of Psychiatry, 182*(4), 291-292.

Watson, M. and Ecken, L. (2003). *Learning to Trust: Transforming Difficult Elementary through Developmental Discipline*. Jossey Bass, San Francisco.

Weich, S., Patterson, J., Shaw, R., and Stewart-Brown, S. (2009). Family relationships in childhood and common psychiatric disorders in later life: systematic review of prospective studies. *The British Journal of Psychiatry, 194*(5), 392-398.

Weiner, B. (1972). *Theories of Motivation: From Mechanism to Cognition*. Markham Publishing Company, Chicago.

WHO (1998). *Primary Prevention of Mental, Neurological and Psychological Disorders*. World Health Organization.

WHO (2002a). *Prevention and Promotion in Mental Health; Evidence and Research*. Geneva, Department of health and substance dependence.

WHO (2002b). *Prevention of Psychoactive Substance Use Selected Review of What Works in the Area of Prevention*. Geneva, World Health Organization.

WHO (2002c). *The World Health Report 2002; Reducing Risks, Promoting Healthy Life Style*, Geneva, World Health Organization.

WHO (2004b). *Promoting Mental Health. Concepts, Emerging Evidence, Practice, Summary Report*. Geneva, World Health Organization.

Williams. M. Jill *et al.* (2000), A Comprehensive model for Mental Health Tobacco Recovery, *Administrative Policy Mental Health*. New Jersy.

Winter, M.V., Donovan, R.J. and Fielder, J. (2008), Exposure of Children and Adolescents to Alcohol Advertising on Television in Australia. *Journal of Studies on Alcohol and Drugs, 69*, 676-683.

World Health Organization (WHO) (1981), *Global Strategy for Health for All by the Year 2000*, WHO.

World Health Organization (WHO) (1986), *Ottawa Charter for Health Promotion*, WHO and Canadian Public Health Association, Ottawa.

World Health Organization (WHO) (1992), *The ICD-10 Classification of Mental and Behavioural Disorders: Clinical Descriptions and Diagnostic Guidelines*, WHO, Geneva.

World Health Organization (WHO) (1997), *The Jakarta Declaration on Leading Health Promotion into the 21st Century*, WHO, Geneva.

World Health Organization (WHO) (1998), *Primary Prevention of Mental, Neurological and Psychosocial Disorders*, WHO, Geneva.

World Health Organization (WHO) (1999), *Strengthening Mental Health Promotion, WHO Fact Sheet No. 220*, WHO, Geneva.

10

Mental Health

Preventing Negative and Enhancing Positive

Garima Singh and *Anubhuti Dubey*

Introduction

Psychology has often than not stressed the shortcomings of individuals as compared with their potentials; the positive psychology approach focuses on the potentials. Positive mental health reflects mental health as a resource. It is crucial to our subjective well-being and to our ability to perceive, comprehend and interpret our surroundings, to adapt to them or to change them if necessary, and to communicate with each other and have successful social interactions. The present chapter is an attempt to analyze the phenomenon of mental health from a positive psychology perspective, focusing on the concept of positive mental health in the Indian perspective. It is of concern that most, not all, of the Indian research studies conducted in the field of mental health have focused primarily on the illness side of mental health and not the healthy side of it. In present, there is a greater need to shift our focus on the fact that the absence of mental disorder does not equal the presence of mental health, and individuals without a mental disorder may experience varying degrees of positive mental health.

Mental Health Conceptualization: Past and Present

The Past

1. *The Mental Hygiene Movement*: The origin of the mental hygiene movement can be attributed to the work of Clifford Beers in USA. In 1908, he published the book "*A mind that found itself*" based on his

personal experience of admissions to three mental hospitals. The book had a great upshot and in the same year a Mental Hygiene Society was established in Connecticut. Adolf Meyer suggested the term "mental hygiene" Beersby and enjoyed a quick popularity thanks to the creation in 1909 of the National Commission of Mental Hygiene. The internationalization of activities of this Commission in 1919 led to the establishment of some national associations concerned with mental hygiene as in France and South Africa (1920), and in Italy and Hungary (1924). From these national associations came up the International Committee on Mental Hygiene which was later succeeded by the World Federation of Mental Health. The mental hygiene movement in beginning was basically concerned with the improvement of the care of people with mental disorders. In the words of Beers "When the National Committee was organized, in 1909, its chief concern was to humanize the care of the insane: to eradicate the abuses, brutalities and neglect from which the mentally sick have traditionally suffered." Later, the Committee extended its programme with the exclusion of the "milder forms of mental disability" and a greater concern with preventive work. The rationale behind this modification was the belief that "mental disorders frequently have their beginnings in childhood and youth and that preventive measures are most effective in early life," and that environmental conditions and modes of living produce mental ill health.

By 1937, the US National Committee for Mental Hygiene stated that it pursued to achieve its purposes by: (a) promoting early diagnosis and treatment; (b) developing adequate hospitalization; (c) stimulating research; (d) securing public understanding and support of psychiatric and mental hygiene activities; (e) instructing individuals and groups in the personal application of mental hygiene principles; and (f) cooperating with governmental and private agencies whose work touches at any point the field of mental hygiene.

According to the group which launched it, the mental hygiene movement "visualized, not a single patient, but a whole community; and it considered each member of that community as an individual whose mental and emotional status was determined by definite causative factors and whose compelling need was for prevention rather than cure." The relation of Mental Hygiene Movement to psychiatry is similar to that of public-health movement to medicine in general. It is a systematized community response to a standard community need. On the other hand, it was also stated that: "At the present time both psychiatrists and mental hygienists are more than ever conscious that their objectives are in fact identical and that each group needs the other for the fulfilment of their common task."

2. *The World Health Organization (WHO)*: The WHO since its formation always had an administrative section especially committed to mental health. The first Report of the Director General of WHO refers to an administrative section called "Mental Health" in its English version and "Hygiene Mental" in the French version. Till the 1960s, we find "Hygiene" as the French translation of health in some WHO publications and in some instances we also find mental hygiene used interchangeably with mental health in the English versions. The ninth volume of the WHO's series Public Health Papers was published in 1961 with the title 'Teaching of Psychiatry and Mental Health'.

The Preamble of the WHO Constitution clearly states that "health is a state of complete physical, mental and social well-being and not merely the absence of disease or infirmity." This definition is clearly a holistic one, with three ideas central to the improvement of health: mental health is an integral part of health, mental health is more than the absence of mental illness, and mental health is intimately connected with physical health and behaviour. It should also be noted that the word mental in the definition of health (as well as physical and social) refers to dimensions of a state and not to a specific domain or discipline. Therefore, according to this concept, it is inappropriate to refer to physical health, mental health or social health. Should one wish to specify a particular dimension, the most appropriate noun to designate it should be well-being and not health (e.g. mental well-being or social well-being). This negligent use of the word health seems to have been also in operation when mental hygiene (a social movement, or a domain of activity) was replaced by mental health (originally intended to designate a state and later transformed in a particular domain or field of activity).

3. *The International Congress of Mental Health*: The First International Congress of Mental Health was organized in London by the British National Association for Mental Hygiene which was held from 16th to 21st August, 1948. Being an International Conference on Mental Hygiene, it ended with a series of recommendations on mental health. Throughout the proceedings of the conference, hygiene and health, succeeding mental, were used interchangeably. However, the pages of the recommendations of the conference used hygiene very sparingly. At the end of the Congress, the International Committee on Mental Hygiene was superseded by the World Federation for Mental Health.

In addition to the wording employed in the proceedings of that Congress, gradually replacing hygiene by health, some of its recommendations were also influential at other levels. An example is sixth recommendation to the WHO that "as soon as practicable, an advisory expert committee be established, composed of professional personnel in the field of mental health and human relations."

The Conference had been convened under the theme "Mental Health and World Citizenship". From a conceptual point of view, nevertheless, and perhaps reflecting an immediately post-war situation, discussions over world citizenship prevailed over those on mental health. Only one concept of mental health was put forward, by J.C. Flugel, Chairman of the Conference's Programme Committee: "Mental health is regarded as a condition which permits the optimal development, physical, intellectual and emotional, of the individual, so far as this is compatible with that of other individuals."

In a more detailed way, some delegates elaborated on what was summarized as the "four levels of mental health work: custodial, therapeutic, preventive and positive". It is not difficult to see a considerable overlapping between this proposal and the one already implemented by the mental hygiene movement.

At the closing session, O.L. Forel, Lecturer in Psychiatry at the University of Geneva, answering to criticisms that mental hygiene, as understood in that conference, went beyond the medical and scientific framework, made a clearly political (in Plato's sense) statement by saying that: "I dare hope to be your interpreter in expressing our pride that so many scientists came here not at all to develop their respective sciences, but to have them at men's service".

Reading through the proceedings of this Congress gives one a feeling of the tensions between a pragmatic approach, developed by the mental hygiene movement (basically defended by delegates from the USA), and a more politically-oriented approach, proposed by other participants, perhaps translating the experiences of some delegates from European countries, which had severely suffered from the war. In the end this latter approach prevailed, with the transformation of the mental hygiene movement into the mental health movement. Perhaps as a reflection of this basically political movement, in 1949 the National Institute of Mental Health started its activities in the USA.

Lastly, "mental health" could be believed to have its origins tracked back to developments in public health, in clinical psychiatry and in other branches of knowledge.

The Present

Mental health can be defined as a condition, subject to fluctuations due to biological and social factors, which enables the individual to achieve a satisfactory synthesis of his own potentially conflicting, instinctive drives; to form and maintain harmonious relations with others; and to participate in constructive changes in his social and physical environment. The Campbell's Dictionary of Psychiatry gives two meanings of mental health: first, as a synonym of 'mental hygiene' and second, as a state of psychological well-being. The Oxford English Dictionary defines 'mental hygiene as a set of measures to preserve mental health, and later refers to mental health as a state. However, a clear and widely accepted definition of mental health as a discipline was and is still missing.

Concept of Mental Health: There exist many misconceptions among the general public, politicians and even professionals regarding the concept of mental health. This is due to the fact that mental health is in many ways undervalued in our societies. The concept is often confused with severe mental disorders and associated with societal stigma and negative attitudes. It is also often the case that curative medicine focusing on health problems attracts more attention than public health questions of prevention and, even more so, of promotion. The positive value of mental health, contributing to our well-being, quality of life and creativity as well as to social capital, is not always seen.

Mental health as a concept reflects the equilibrium between the individual and the environment in a broad sense. In the so-called "structural" model of mental health, the determinants are grouped into four categories: individual factors and experiences, social support and other social interactions, societal structures and resources, and cultural values (Lahtinen *et al.*, 1999).

Mental Health Linked to Physical Health: Neither mental nor physical health can exist alone. Mental, physical and social functioning are interdependent. Furthermore, health and illness may co-exist. According to Sartorius (1990), they are mutually exclusive only if health is defined in a restrictive way as the absence of disease.

The fields of mental health and public health have a long history of weak interactions, despite the possibilities for a stronger working relationship (Cooper, 1990; Goldberg and Tantam, 1990; Goldstein, 1989). This relates mainly to the stigma of mental illness, and vagueness in the concepts of mental health and mental illness. The interest has grown recently for two main reasons. First, mental health is increasingly seen as fundamental to physical health and quality of life and thus needs to be addressed as an important component of improving overall health and well-being. The concept of health enunciated by WHO as encompassing physical, mental and social well-being is more and more seen as a practical issue for policy and practice. In particular, there is growing evidence to suggest interplay between mental and physical health and well-being and outcomes such as educational achievement, productivity at work, development of positive personal relationships, reduction in crime rates and decreasing harms associated with use of alcohol and drugs. It follows that promoting mental health through a focus on key determinants should not only result in lower rates of some mental disorders and improved physical health, but also better educational performance, greater productivity of workers, improved relationships within families and safer communities. Second, there is wide acknowledgement of an increase in mental ill-health at a global level. The authoritative work undertaken by WHO and the World Bank indicates that by the year 2020 depression will constitute the second largest cause of disease burden worldwide (Murray and Lopez, 1996).

Mental Health as Fitness and not Freedom from Illness: Until now, the prevailing stigma surrounding mental illness has encouraged the euphemistic use of the term "mental health" to describe treatment and support services for people with mental illness. This usage adds to confusion about the concept of mental health as well as that of mental illness. In recent times, the global focus on mental ill-health has sparked interest in the possibilities for promoting mental health as well as preventing and treating illness. There is a need to ensure that appropriate care and treatment is in place for those experiencing mental ill-health while at the same time developing a greater focus on promotion of mental health and prevention of illness.

In 2003, George Vaillant in the USA commented that mental health is too important to be ignored. Vaillant pointed out "Average mental health" is not the same as "healthy", for averageing always includes mixing in with the healthy the prevailing amount of psychopathology. What is healthy sometimes depends on geography, culture and the historical moment.

Contemporary Concept of Mental Health: After centuries of emergence of the concept of mental health, some developments can be purported. On a more general level, the WHO's very concept of health has been recently questioned; it is no longer felt by some as applicable to the current situation. On the whole, mental health continues to be used both to designate a state as a dimension of health and to refer to the movement derived from the mental hygiene movement, corresponding to the application of psychiatry to groups, communities and societies, rather than on an individual basis, as is the case with clinical psychiatry. However, mental health is, quite unfortunately, still viewed by many as a discipline, either as a synonym of psychiatry, or as one of its complementary fields.

A recent trend has been the addition of the contender public to either mental health or to psychiatry, as it can be seen in a WHO document entitled Public Mental Health. This is very much in line with the concept of mental health as a movement rather than a discipline. In 2001, the WHO dedicated its annual report (The World Health Report—Mental Health: New Knowledge, New Hope) to mental health. In the message from the WHO Director-General that opens that report, G.H. Brundtland summarizes the three main knowledge areas covered by the document: (a) effectiveness of prevention and treatment, (b) service planning and provision, and (c) policies to break down stigma and discrimination and adequate funds for prevention and treatment. If one allows for the semantic variations between the beginnings of the twentieth and the twentyfirst centuries, the same concerns of the origins of the mental hygiene movement can be found in the mental health content of the World Health Report. Perhaps the biggest difference between these two political platforms is the emphasis on the improvement of hospital care in the former (the only form of treatment available by then), and the contemporary emphasis on distancing mental health from psychiatric hospitals and placing it in the community.

However, one must state that, unfortunately what was prevalent in the past as an issue of improvement in the standards of mental health care and an eradication of the abuses to which people with mental disorders are usually subject, is still a major concern of the most progressive and advanced agendas of people interested in the promotion of mental health around the world.

The Emergence of Positive Psychology

The emergence of positive psychology brings a greater focus on the study of optimal human functioning (Seligman and Csikszentmihalyi, 2000; Seligman *et al.*, 2005), which includes studying positive psychological constructs such as optimism, love, emotional intelligence, creativity, hope, humour and a focus on positive subjective experiences, positive individual characteristics (strengths and virtues) and positive institutions and communities. Till today, much of the scientific endeavour has focused on individual-level interventions to increase happiness and enhance positive emotions and characteristics. While the focus on positive emotions, such as happiness, has indeed captured the public imagination, as Gable and Haidt (2005) point out that there has been a lack of progress in studying the positive institutions and social conditions necessary for flourishing and optimal functioning.

The Roots of Positive Psychology

Positive psychology has emerged only within the last 10 years or so. Peterson (2006) has remarked that positive psychology has a long history and a short past. He means that positive side of human nature has been of longstanding interest to both philosophers and psychologists, but it is only recently that the positive side of human behaviour has attracted serious and more widespread empirical study. In contemporary times positive psychology is an evolving mosaic of research and theory from various areas of psychology, centralizing the focus on positive aspects of human behaviour.

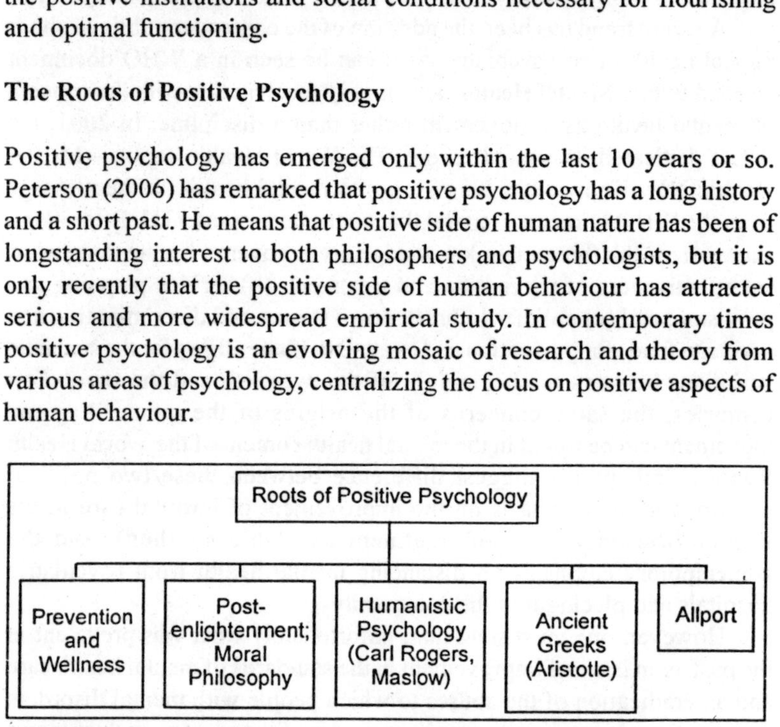

Fig. 10.1: Roots of Positive Psychology

Positive psychology is the study of the conditions and processes that contribute to the flourishing or optimal functioning of people, groups, and institutions. Defined in this way, positive psychology has a long history, dating back to William James's writings on what he termed "healthy mindedness" in 1902, to Allport's interest in positive human characteristics in 1958, to Maslow's advocacy for the study of healthy people in lieu of sick people in 1968, and to Cowan's research on resilience in children and adolescents (2000). However, the roots of positive psychology can be traced to the thoughts of ancient Greek Philosophers. Aristotle believed that there was a unique *daimon*, or spirit within each individual, that guides us to pursue things that are right for us. Acting in accordance with this '*daimon*' leads one to happiness. The question of happiness has since been picked up by hundreds of prominent thinkers, and gave rise to many theories, including Hedonism, with its emphasis on pleasure and utilitarianism, seeking the greatest happiness for the greatest number.

In the twentieth century, many prominent psychologists focused on what later became the subject matter of positive psychology. Amongst them were Carl Jung with his individuation, or 'becoming all that one can be' concept; Maria Jahoda, concerned with defining positive mental health and Gordon Allport, interested in individual maturity. Since then, the matters of flourishing and well-being were raised in the work on prevention and wellness enhancement.

The most notable of positive psychology's predecessors, however, was the humanistic psychology movement, which originated in the 1950s and reached its peak in the 60s and 70s. This movement placed central emphasis on the growth and authentic self of an individual.

Humanistic psychologists were critical of pathology oriented approaches to a human being. The most famous ones were Carl Rogers, who introduced the concept of the fully functioning person, and Abraham Maslow, who emphasized self-actualization. In fact it was Maslow who was the very first to use the term positive psychology.

Humanistic psychologists, however, did not only reject the dominant negative paradigm of psychology, they also believed that so-called 'scientific method' (good for studying molecules and atoms) helps little in understanding the human being in its complexity and called for more qualitative rather than quantitative (statistical, number crunching) research. This is where positive psychology disagrees with its major predecessor. Positive psychology thus distinguishes itself from humanistic psychology on the basis of methods, whereas the substance and the topics studied are remarkably similar. Rightly or wrongly, positive psychology tends to present itself as a new movement, often attempting to distance itself from its origins.

In January 2000, when Seligman and Csikszentmihalyi edited a special issue of American Psychologist devoted to positive psychology, they claimed that psychology was not producing enough "knowledge of what makes life worth living". In the second half of the twentieth century, psychology learned much about depression, racism, violence, self-esteem management, irrationality, and growing up under adversity, but had much less to say about character strengths, virtues, and the conditions that lead to high levels of happiness or civic engagement. In one metaphor, psychology was said to be learning how to bring people up from negative eight to zero but not as good at understanding how people rise from zero to positive eight.

Averting the Bad and Amplifying the Good

The most intimidating challenge to positive psychology stem from defining what actually is positive and the ambiguous line between *describing* something as "good" and *prescribing* it as "good" (Held, 2004). Positive psychology does not imply that the rest of psychology is negative, although it is understandable that the name may imply that to some people. In fact, the large majority of the gross academic product of psychology is neutral, focusing on neither well-being nor distress. Positive psychology grew largely from the recognition of an imbalance in clinical psychology, in which most research does indeed focus on mental illness. Despite the inequities, positive psychology's aim is not the denial of the distressing, unpleasant, or negative aspects of life, nor is it an effort to see them through rose-coloured glasses. Those who study topics in positive psychology fully acknowledge the existence of human suffering, selfishness, dysfunctional family systems, and ineffective institutions. But the aim of positive psychology is to study the other side of the coin—the ways that people feel joy, show altruism, and create healthy families and institutions—thereby addressing the full spectrum of human experience. Moreover, positive psychology makes the argument that these positive topics of inquiry are important to understand in their own right, not solely as buffers against the problems, stressors, and disorders of life.

According to positive psychologists, for most of its life mainstream psychology has been concerned with the negative aspects of human life. There have been pockets of interest in topics such as creativity, optimism and wisdom, but these have not been united by any grand theory or a broad, overarching framework. This rather negative state of affairs was not the original intention of the first psychologists, but came about through a historical accident. Prior to the Second World War, psychology had three tasks, which were to: cure mental illness, improve normal lives and identify and nurture high talent. However, after the war the last two tasks somehow got lost, leaving the field to concentrate predominantly on the first one. Given that psychology as a science depends heavily on the funding of governmental bodies, it is not hard to guess what happened to the resources after Second World War. Understandably, facing a human crisis on such an enormous scale, all available resources were poured into learning about and the treatment of psychological illness and psychopathology. This is how psychology as a field learnt to operate within a *disease model.* This model has proven very useful. Seligman highlights the victories of the disease model, which are, for example, that 14 previously incurable mental illnesses (such as depression personality disorder, or anxiety attacks) can now be successfully treated. However, the costs of adopting this disease model included the negative view of psychologists as 'victimologists' and 'pathologisers', the failure to address the improvement of normal lives and the identification and nurturance of high talent.

Positive Mental Health

Mental health has been variously conceptualized as a positive emotion (affect), such as feelings of happiness; as a personality trait inclusive of the psychological resources of self-esteem and mastery; and as resilience, which is the capacity to cope with adversity. Various aspects and models of mental health contribute to our understanding of what is meant by positive mental health.

The World Health Organization (WHO) defines health as being a complete state of physical, psychological and social well-being. Jahoda (1958) explained this by separating mental health into three domains. First, mental health involves "self-realization" in that individuals are allowed to fully exploit their potential. Second, mental health includes "a sense of mastery" by the individual over their environment and, lastly, positive mental health means "autonomy", as in individuals having the ability to identify, confront and solve problems.

Mental health can be described in two dimensions:

- Positive mental health considers mental health as a resource. It is essential to subjective well-being and to our ability to perceive, comprehend and interpret our surroundings, to adapt to them or to change them if necessary, and to communicate with each other and have successful social interactions.
- Mental ill-health is about mental disorders, symptoms and problems. Mental disorders are defined in the current diagnostic classifications mainly by the existence of symptoms. Mental symptoms and problems also exist without the criteria for clinical disorders being met (Lavikainen *et al.*, 2001).

Positive mental health is a set of key domains encompassing well-being and positive states of mind. It is an integral part of health, including positive physical health. It can co-occur with and influence the onset, nature and outcomes of physical and mental illnesses. The concept of positive mental health incorporates the abilities to develop psychologically, emotionally, intellectually, socially and spiritually. Empirical work (Keyes 2002, 2005; Huppert and Whittington, 2003) reported the points to the independence of positive and negative well-being and shows that mental health and mental disorders are not opposite ends of a single continuum, but rather constitute distinct, though correlated, axes. Thus, the absence of mental disorder does not equal the presence of mental health, and individuals without a mental disorder may experience varying degrees of positive mental health.

Indian Notion and Researches on Positive Mental Health

India is entering the new millennium with many challenges like promoting mental health of the population and developing mental services involving different social institutions. Professionals have been in the forefront to find solutions appropriate to the country and towards developing an Indian system of mental health care. There is need for a vision for the development of mental health that is broad-based, inclusive of all the needs of all the people. Positive psychology movement has an impact worldwide and has become an integrated fabric of psychology all over. Thus, the focus of Indian researches on positive mental health is the need of time.

The conceptualisation of the state of well-being is closer to the concept of mental health and happiness, life satisfaction and actualisation of one's full potential. Verma and Verma (1989) have defined *general well-being* as the subjective feeling of contentment, happiness, satisfaction with life's experiences and of one's role in the world of work, sense of achievement, utility, belongingness, and no distress, dissatisfaction or worry, etc.

The text of "*Taittiriya Upanishad*" has elaborated that happiness, joy and well-being are the moments when there is an unobstructed manifestation of *ananda* (bliss) which is our original or true nature. It is the opaqueness of our mental faculties that obstructs the manifestation and experience of *ananda*. The principle that is responsible for opaqueness, inertia, dullness, darkness, depression, etc. is called *tamas*. The principle that is responsible for brightness, illumination, transparency, etc. is called *sattva*. Greater is the transparency of the mental faculties, i.e. *sattva*, greater is the experience of *ananda* (Kiran Kumar, 2002). Thus, an ideal state of human functioning and constitutes health and well-being as a state of mind (somewhat equivalent to the concept of subjective well-being) which is peaceful, quiet, serene, and free from the conflicts and desires. Accordingly, a healthy person is of an auto-locus person (*svastha*) who flourishes on the recognition of life force derived from the material reality (*panch mahabhutas*) and, therefore, offers remedies for being healthy by opening a dialogue with its environment and recognition of order and cohesion (*dharma*) in the entire life world (*srishti*). The nutrition (*ahara*), world of leisure (*vihara*) and thoughts (*vichara*) need to be synchronized in proper order. Health and well-being are both personal as well as social. The desire for the well-being of everyone (*Kamaye duhkhtaptanam praninamartimshanam*) has been a core Indian concern that has panhuman relevance. Undoubtedly, such a conceptualization of health and well-being is significant in its own right (Sharma and Misra).

People with positive mental attitude have a significantly higher chance of survival and recovery. Subha *et al.* (2010) studied that a particular type of Positive Self Talk was developed from Frenchman Alexandre Simonnet to fight Panic Attacks. A study comparing people with chronic kidney disease with people kidney disease free showed that there was a significant difference between the groups. The kidney disease free group rated much higher in positive mental attitude. There was no difference found in spirituality and females with chronic kidney disease were found to be significantly more superstitious.

Positive orientation is another important cognition that has wide implications for recovery from any disease. In a study by Agrawal, Dalal, Agrawal and Agrawal (1995) positive life orientation emerged as an important predictor of medical, as well as, of psychological recovery of myocardial patients.

The study of health and well-being, however, is still an emerging area in psychology and in spite of all promises and possibilities the discipline has yet to mature as an independent enterprise in India. Although a few studies have their attention focused on the positive aspects of health. Mohan *et al.* (2007) studied dispositional forgiveness in relation to personality and spiritual well-being among Indian adolescents and reported positive correlations between dispositional forgiveness, spiritual well-being and personality dimensions of extraversion and social desirability and a negative correlation between dispositional forgiveness and personality dimensions of neuroticism as well as psychoticism. Similarly, Mohan *et al.* (2008) studied spiritual well-being among adolescents in relation to their emotions and the results indicated significant relationships emerged between spiritual well-being along with its components and positive emotions i.e., optimism, hope, happiness and negative emotions, state and trait anger, anger-in, anger-out and anger control.

Mohan *et al.* (2008) investigated relationship of psychological well-being with spiritual well-being and personality among adolescents and the results clearly revealed positive correlations between various dimensions of psychological well-being and spiritual well-being. Results also revealed negative correlations between various dimensions of psychological well-being and personality dimensions of neuroticism and psychoticism. Positive correlations were found between some dimensions of psychological well-being and personality dimensions of extraversion and social desirability.

Mohan *et al.* (2009) studied the structure of dispositional forgiveness in relation to happiness and well-being among Indian adolescents and the results revealed positive correlations between the dimensions of forgiveness, happiness and well-being. Two factors emerged significantly with Factor-I as a unipolar factor with significant loadings on forgiveness of self, happiness, life satisfaction, positive relations with others, self-acceptance, environmental mastery and positive affect. This implies that who are high on forgiving oneself are happier, experience more positive feelings, more accepting of one, share positive relations with others, seek environmental mastery, perceive their life to be purposeful and are satisfied with their life. Another factor emerged as a bipolar factor with significant loadings on all the three dimensions of forgiveness, i.e. forgiveness of self, others and situations, the dimension of autonomy and Negative affect which implies that people who are overall forgiving (oneself, others and situations) experience less negative feelings in day-to-day life. Mohan *et al.*, (2010) have compared males and females on the dimensions of interpersonal forgiveness and results clearly revealed that males are higher on the various dimensions of forgiveness.

Sehgal and associates (2010) have worked in the field of spiritual well-being and positive healthy ageing and psychological well-being, parental bonding and gratitude among adolescents. The keynote addresses by J. Mohan on Spiritual Psychology and well-being in Malaysia (2007), Eastern Viewpoints in well-being in U.K. (2009) and Challenges in Positive Psychology in India (2010, 2011 and 2012) highlighted the questions and the answers merging in this field.

Banth *et al.* (2011) compared the 24 character strengths in leaders in the Indian Army and Civilian Sector. Results revealed that both army officers and civilian managers scored high in all the character strengths, and there were significant differences among army officers and bank managers on 14 out of 24 character strengths that can be attributed to their disparate work environment and organizational expectations.

Banth *et al.* (2010) examined the relationship of *Anasakti* with well-being and the three distinct happiness orientations. *Anasakti*, a Sanskrit term for traits like non-attachment, equipoise, selfless duty orientation, and effort in the absence of concern for the outcome, can be regarded as a Hindu-ideal cluster of personality traits. It was explored through a study of 676 college students and a sample of 65 yogic practitioners in India. The findings revealed that the yogic practitioners were markedly higher in *Anasakti* than the secular population. For the yogic population, there was a large correlation between *Anasakti* and the Orientation to Meaningful Life, and it accounted for more than 20 per cent of the variance in the regression of *Anasakti* against all the measures of well-being. The yogic population's scores also correlated with several other measures of well-being. The scores of the secular population were less strongly related to the well-being scores; though, several correlation coefficients were statistically significant.

References

Agarwal, M., and Dalal, A.K. (1993). Beliefs about the world and recovery from myocardial infarction. *Journal of Social Psychology, 133*, 385-394.

Agarwal, M., Dalal, A.K. (1994). Patients in Indian hospitals: environmental stresses and affective reactions. *Indian Journal of Social Work, 55*, 41-46.

Agarwal, M., Dalal, A.K., Agarwal, D.K., and Agarwal, R.K. (1994). Positive life orientation and recovery from myocardial infraction. *Social Science and Medicine, 38*, 152-160.

Agarwal, M., and Naidu, R.K. (1988). Impact of desirable and undesirable life events on health. *Journal of Personality and Clinical Studies, 4*, 53-62.

Allport, G.W. (1955). *Becoming*. New Haven, CT: Yale University Press.

Banth, S., and Singh, P. (2011). Positive character strengths in middle-rung army officers and managers in civilian sectors. *Journal of Indian Academy of Applied Psychology, 37* (2), 320-324.

Banth, S., and Talwar, C. (2010). *Anasakti*, the Hindu Ideal, and its Relationship to Well-Being and Orientations to Happiness. *Journal of Religion and Health*. DOI: 10.1007/s10943-010-9402-3 (retrieved on 29-11-2011).

Boniwell, I. (2006). *Positive Psychology in a Nutshell*. Personal Well-being Centre, London.

Cowen, E.I. (1994). The Enhancement of Psychological Wellness: Challenges and Opportunities. *American Journal of Community Psychology, 22*, 149-179.

Dalal, A.K. and Mishra, G. (2006). Psychology of Health and Well-Being: Some Emerging Perspectives. *Psychological Studies, 2* (2-3).

Gable, S.L., and Haidt, J. (2005). What (and why) is positive psychology? *Review of General Psychology, 9*(2) 103-10.

Jahoda, M. (1958). *Current Concepts of Positive Mental Health*. New York, USA: Basic Books.

Johns Hopkins University. (2010). *Origins of Mental Health*. Retrieved from http://www.JHSPH.edu

Lewis, N.D. American psychiatry from the beginning to World War II. In: Arieti S., editor. *American Handbook of Psychiatry*, 2nd Ed. New York: Basic Books; 1974, pp. 28-43.

Mohan, J. (2007). Spiritual Psychology and Subjective Well-being. *Paper Presented in International Conference on Spiritual Psychology*, Malaysia.

Mohan, J., Sehgal, M., and Tripathi, A. (2008b). A study of dispositional forgiveness in relation to personality and spiritual well-being among adolescents. *Research Journal: Social Sciences*, Panjab University, *15*(1), 127-145.

Mohan, J., Sehgal, M., and Tripathi, A. (2009). The Forgiving personality: Identifying its structure in terms of Happiness and Well-being among Indian youth. *Journal of Well-being, 3*(2), 1-10.

Mohan, J., Sehgal, M., and Tripathi, A. (2010). Gender differences in offense specific and dispositional forgiveness among Indian adolescents. (*In the Edited book on Positive Psychology* by Prof. Jitendra Mohan).

Patel, V. and Prince, M. (1977). Global mental health—a new global health field comes of age. *JAMA, 303*, 1976-1977.

Seligman, M.E.P., and Csikszentmihalyi, M. (2000). Positive Psychology: An introduction. *American Psychologist, 55*(1).

Snyder, C. and Lopez, S. (1999). Handbook of Positive Psychology. New York: Oxford University Press.

Subha, T.G., and Mukherjee, Tilottama (September 2010). Optimism, superstitious beliefs and spirituality in chronic kidney disease. *Indian Journal of Community Psychology, 6* (2): 262-274.5-14.

World Health Organization. *Mental Health: Report on the Second Session of the Expert Committee*. Geneva: World Health Organization, 1951.

World Health Organization. (2001). *The World Health Report 2001: Mental Health: New Understanding, New Hope*. Geneva: WHO.

World Health Organization. (2002). *Prevention and Promotion in Mental Health*. Geneva: World Health Organization.

World Health Organization. (2005). *Promoting Mental Health: Concepts, Emerging Evidence, Practice*. Geneva: World Health Organization.

11

Values Beyond Boundaries

A Theoretical Analysis

Sunil K. Verma and *Pankaj Bharti*

The chapter aims to understand any concept, along with the dynamicity of culture, as culture free variable. This attempt is based on the basic debate of Cultural Psychology, viz. how to study culture/how is internalization different from importation? The questions or rather points raised in this write up can be understood by taking values as an example as values is one of the most diverse concepts which vary from society to society and individual to individual. In this process of understanding we will be taking up three theoretical models of values by Radha Kamal Mukerjee, Rokeach, and Schwartz, representing three cultures respectively. On the basis of these models, we will be trying to understand as to how cultures are similar and dissimilar. From these studies, it can be derived that preferences of means will differ in the different achieving goals. These differences are largely context and cultural specific. The above three models show the similarities across three cultures, mostly on basic needs and desire and in terms of biological, social, economical and spiritual values. So, across culture we can understand the commonness and uncommonness of any variable as individual level variable and explain it by socio-cultural explanation.

Psychology has its basic roots in Europe and modern psychology developed in America. Primarily America was the major source for the learning and circulation of knowledge, in terms of psychology. Scholars, who were trained in that tradition the methodology as well as tools and concepts in their own country to understand the social and cultural realities that were different to the American set-up. Adair (1992) calls the importation of knowledge. These theories or concepts studied were a major source of similarity or difference between different cultures, which together formed the base of Cross Cultural Psychology. However, with the changing times, either due to the problems faced in understanding the social as well as cultural realities or because of problems of the concepts or methodology voices emerged in favour of understanding concepts in the cultural specific context, which was later known as Indigenization. The main aim of Indigenization is to understand culture. According to Adair (1992) "an indigenous psychology gradually develops from blending of an imported discipline with increasing attention to unique elements within that culture." Indigenous psychology is regarded as an outcome that results from the interaction between two systems of psychological knowledge. Indigenization could be measured through a series of stages (Adair, 2006):

1. Importation (introduction of a discipline).
2. Implantation (conducting research emulating Western models).
3. Indigenization (identifying culturally unique variable/thoughts for study).
4. Autochthonization (process leading to emergence of a self-perpetuating discipline independent of imported source).

In this chapter an attempt is made to understand how we can understand any concept along with the dynamicity of culture or as a culture free variable. This attempt is based on the basic debate of Cultural Psychology. Overall in the journey of psychology two major points come to reckon:

1. How to study culture?
2. How is internalization different from importation?

The questions or rather points raised in this write up can be understood by taking values as an example. Why Values? Because values is one of the most diverse concepts that varies across societies and individuals. In this process of understanding we will be taking up three theoretical models of values which represent three cultures. On the basis of these models, we will be trying to understand as to how cultures are similar and dissimilar.

Values are defined as "cultural standard that influence the attitude, desire and needs. They are assessed in terms of the approved and non-approved behaviour out of the available means and ends." Values define the preferred behaviour. According to Paper (1950) values are the selective and preferred orientation of people in matters of desires, needs, means, aversions and attractions. Allport (1961) defined values as preferred behaviour in a cultural context. The preferred behaviour, in general, can be ordered on the basis of their relative importance in the social, cultural and time perspective (Schwartz, 1992; Schwartz & Bilsky, 1987, 1990; Triandis, 1994).

Parsons (1951) treats values as internalized cultural notions that influence the preferred behaviour of groups and individuals in a culture and facilitate the maintenance of the social equilibrium and integration in the society. The preferred behaviour of individuals and groups will contain affective component, liking. On that basis we can say that values have the component of shared cultural standards that define the preferences (means) of action and themes (ends).

For instance Singh (1977) had classified the values into two types, i.e. fundamental and instrumental values. The fundamental values are concerned with only ends themselves, but not means for the attainment of the ends. For example honesty, truth etc. are the fundamental values. The instrumental values are concerned with the means that are used in achieving certain ends. For instance, in the accumulation of money a person can be adventurist, capitalist or traditional capitalist. Thus, the instrumental values are closely related to social norms. Roy and Bhawan (1984) classified values as operative and moralistic. This classification comes closer to the classification of values provided by Yogendra Singh (1973). Rokeach's (1973) Instrumental and Terminal value comes closer to the classification of values provided by Singh (1973) and Roy and Bhawan (1984). Schwartz (1992) identified ten universal values, i.e. self-direction, stimulation, hedonism, achievement, power, security, conformity, tradition, benevolence and universalism. Thus, values are relatively stable and constitute sometimes the group ideology like class, ethnic group etc. Resher (1969) classified values on the basis of level of social unit into three types, i.e. personal, national, and social values. For instance justice and equality are treated as social values. What is important for a person only is known as personal values and that preferred by a nation are called as national values. Mukerjee (1965) proposed that values are mans' desires and interests, shaped and molded in its concrete content by the pattern of social and cultural condition. He described four types of values, in terms of basic desires and values, i.e. biological, economical, social and spiritual. Each basic desire and value has defined goals. That affects the ethics or norms at individual and societal level. The relationship propounded by Mukerjee (1965) is presented in Table 11.1.

Table 11.1: Affects the Ethics or norms at individual and societal level

Basic Desire, tendencies and values	*Goals*	*Ideals*	*Ethic of norms Individual*	*Social*
Biological: Hunger, Sex, Territory, Self-Preservation Rhythm of play and repose	Food, Marriage and family Territory, work, use and ownership of tools, Education, Protection, Leisure recreation	Human Individuality	Improvement and survival of the psychogenetic personality	Bio-ecologic Co-operation for continuity of race and habitat.
Economic: Appropriation, Possession, curiosity constructiveness, Maturation Movement	Wealth, domicile, and dress, property, competition, cooperation contracts, technology, efficiency of labour, employment, training and apprenticeship security	Security and Standard of living	Development of occupational personality	Maximum satisfaction and minimum sacrifice.
Social: Aggression and sympathy, Response, recognition (status) security, dominance and submission, imitation suggestion.	Mobility, freedom of association and movement, privilege, power, honour, prestige	Status	Development of status personality	Justice
Spiritual: The creative impulses, curiosity, anxiety, phantasy compensation, reparation	Knowledge, Art, religion	Character	Development of Spiritual personality	Universal personalism, personal equality, freedom and solidarity.

Rokeach (1975) described values as terminal and instrumental.

Table 11.2: Values as terminal and instrumental

Instrumental values	*Terminal values*
A comfortable life	Ambitious
An existing life	Broadminded
A sense of accomplishment	Capable
A world at peace	Cheerful
A world of beauty	Clean
Equality	Courageous
Family security	Forgiving
Freedom	Helpful
Happiness	Honest
Inner harmony	Imaginative
Mature love	Independent
National security	Intellectual
Pleasure	Logical
Salvation	Loving
Self-respect	Obedient
Social recognition	Polite
True friendship	Responsible
Wisdom	Self-controlled

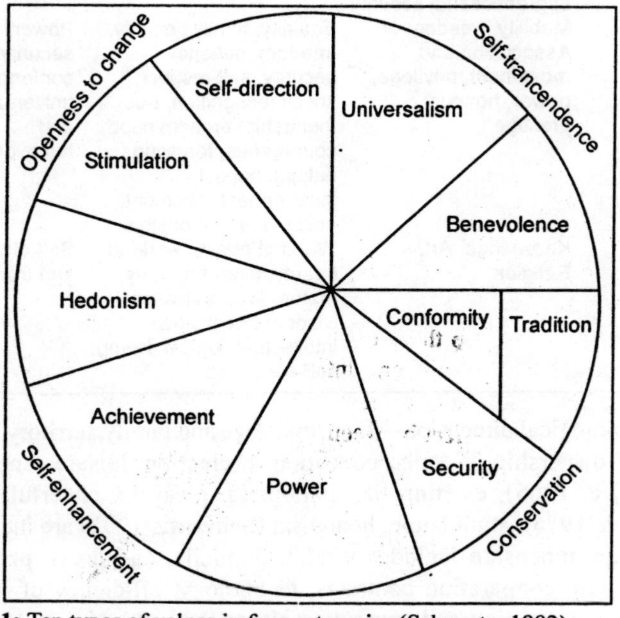

Fig. 11.1: Ten types of values in four categories (Schwartz, 1992)

However, Schwartz (1992) categorized ten types of values in four categories, i.e.: Self-transcendence, Openness to change, Self-enhancement and Conservation (Fig. 11.1).

The above three models have emphasized on the basic goals, desires and tendencies that can be categorized into biological, economic, social, and spiritual dimension.

Table 11.3: Biological, economic, social and Spiritual Dimension

Dimension	*Mukerjee*	*Rokeach*	*Schwartz*
Biological	Food, Marriage and family territory, work, use and ownership of tools, Education, Protection, Leisure recreation	Existing life, happiness, pleasure, cheerful, clean	Stimulation, hedonism
Economical	Wealth, domicile, and dress, property, competition, cooperation contracts, technology, efficiency of labour, employment, training and apprenticeship security	A comfortable life, a sense of accomplishment, ambitious, capable	Achievement
Social	Mobility, freedom of Association and movement, privilege, power, honour, prestige	Equality, family security, freedom, national security, self-respect, social recognition, true friendship, broadminded, courageous, forgiving, helpful, honest, independent, obedient, polite, and responsible	Power, security, conformity, universalism and benevolence
Spiritual	Knowledge, Art, Religion	World at peace, world at beauty, inner harmony, mature love, salvation, wisdom imaginative, intellectual, logical, loving, self-controlled.	Self-direction and traditions

In biological dimension—food, marriage and family, territory, work, use and ownership of tools, education, protection, leisure recreation (Mukerjee, 1965), existing life, happiness, pleasure, cheerful, clean (Rokeach, 1975), stimulation, hedonism (Schwartz, 1992) are included. Economic dimension includes wealth, domicile, and dress, property, competition, cooperation contracts, technology, efficiency of labour, employment, training and apprenticeship security (Mukerjee, 1965), a comfortable life, a sense of accomplishment, ambitious, capable (Rokeach, 1975). Social dimension incorporates mobility, freedom of association and movement, privilege, power, honour, prestige (Mukerjee, 1965), equality, family security, freedom, national security, self-respect, social recognition, true friendship, broadminded, courageous, forgiving, helpful, honest, independent, obedient, polite, and responsible (Rokeach, 1975), power, security, conformity, universalism and benevolence (Schwartz, 1992). In Spiritual dimension some of the similar values as in these three models are included like knowledge, art, religion (Mukerjee, 1965), world at peace, world at beauty, inner harmony, mature love, salvation, wisdom imaginative, intellectual, logical, loving, self-controlled (Rokeach, 1975), self-direction and traditions (Schwartz, 1992).

The behavioural manifestation of fulfilment of goals can be comprehended in the following ways: The fulfilment of biological needs and desires enhances the biological human individuality; economic security enhances the quality of living and social status and spiritual character (Mukerjee 1965). Rokeach (1973) classified values as instrumental means for the achievement of certain goals that are terminal in nature and are intrinsic in nature. In character, i.e. the morale or fundamental values. Schwartz had arranged the ten identified universal values in terms of high to low conservation, high to low self-transcendence.

The above three models differ not only on preferences of goals and desires, but also differ on the preferred type of goals (like food: food is a means to fulfil one's own appetite, but what type of food, how to get it, where to eat? comfortable life, knowledge etc.). If individual gives priority to self in matter of biological, social, economic and spiritual goals then he/she develops, psychogenetic personality, occupational personality, status personality, and spiritual personality. If he gives more preference to society, then he develops Bio-ecologic Co-operation for continuity of race and habitats, i.e. maximum satisfaction and minimum sacrifice, for example Justice, Universal personalism, personal equality, Freedom and Solidarity (Mukerjee, 1965).

Thus, both Mukerjee and Schwartz identified preferences in terms of self-centredness and other centredness. Second trend relates to the debate of individualism and collectivism. The dimension of individualism and collectivism resembles the concept of Association versus Community given by Tonnies (1887/1957). The concept of Individualism and Collectivism acquired significance after the publication of *Culture Consequences.* Individualism emphasizes on "I" consciousness, i.e. autonomy and emotional independence, individual initiative, right to privacy, pleasure seeking, financial security, need for specific friendship and universalism. Collectivism on the other hand stresses on "We" consciousness, i.e. collective identity, emotional dependence, group solidarity, sharing duties and obligations, need for stable and pre-determined friendship, group decisions and particularism (Hofstede, 1980). Sinha and Tripathi (1988, 1994), found that both the values exists in through are dichotomies but coexists as figure and ground in Indian context. One of the values emerges as figure while the other recedes into the background. Indians emphasize more on collectivistic values in terms of building relationships in long-term perspective. The evaluation process is not based on instant gain and loss (Roland, 1988). According to Sinha (1990 b) "the heightened expectancy to care or be cared for at times creates tension and frustration but keeps the person embedded with other members in the group. Positive emotions like mutual caring, involvement, social networking and emotional affinity; also found in the Indian context (Kakar, 1982). Verma (1992 b) observed that 'contractual' relationships were given lesser importance in collectivistic orientated society. Trust and positive emotions were the most preferred values in collectivistic societies and many resulted in favouritism and nepotism (J.B.P. Sinha, 1990 b).

Conclusion

Thus, a comparison of the above three models shows that similarity across the three cultures is mostly on basic needs and desires, i.e. in terms of biological, social-economical and spiritual values. However, the preferences of means will differ in the different achieving goals. These differences are largely context and cultural specific. So across cultures, we can understand the commonness and uncommonness of any variable as individual level variable and explain by socio-cultural explanation. As points of reference one could move beyond the general larger values as Social and Economic values that could be considered as 'psychological universals'. Such universal values exist in a continuum, where cultures could be arranged as less collectivist and more individualists or *vice versa* rather than as purely collectivist and individualist. However, the more specific goals formulated may be flavoured by culture specific ingredients. For instance Achievement as a value could be expressed differently in a highly individualist society leading to more competition that is quite contrary to preference for achievement as may be evident in the Japanese management principles for collective achievement.

References

Adair, J.G. (1992a). Empirical studies of indigenization and development in developing countries. In S. Iwawaki, Y. Kashima and K. Leung (Eds.), *Innovations in Cross-cultural Psychology* (pp. 62-74). Amsterdam: Swets & Zeitlinger.

Adair, J.G. (2006). Creating Indigenous Psychology: Insights from Empirical studies of the science of Psychology. In Kim, U., Yang, S.K. and Hwang, K.K. (2006). *Indigenous Psychology and Cultural Psychology: Understanding People in Context*. New York: Springer.

Allport, G.W. (1961). *Pattern in Growth in Personality*. New York: Holt, Rinehart & Winston.

Hofstede, G. (1980). *Culture's Consequences: International Differences in Work Related Values*. Beverly Hills, CA: Sage.

Kakar, S. (1982). *Shamans, Mystics and Doctors: A Psychological Enquiry in to India and its Healing Traditions*. Bombay: Oxford University Press.

Mukerjee, R. (1965). *The Social Structure of Values*. S. Chand & Company: New Delhi.

Parsons, T. (1951). *The Social System*, New York: Free Press.

Pepper, S. (1958). *The Source of Value*. Berkely, University of California Press.

Raland, A. (1988). *In Search of Self in India and Japan: Towards a Cross Cultural Psychology*. Princeton. N5: Princeton University Press.

Resher, N. (1969). *Introduction to Value Theory*, Eaglewood. Cliffs, N.J. Prentice Hall.

Rokeach, M. (1973). *The Nature of Human Values*. New York: Free Press.

Roy, S. and Bhawan, S.K. (1984) Indian managers and their values. *Indian Journal of Industrial Relations*, *19*(3), 367.

Schwartz, S.H. (1992). Universal in the content and structure of values: A theoretical advances and empirical test in twenty countries. In M. Zanna (Ed.) *Advances in Experimental Social Psychology* (Vol. 25). Orlando, F.L.: Academic.

Schwartz, S.H. and Bilsky, W. (1987). Towards a Psychological Structure of Human Values. *Journal of Personality and Social Psychology*, *53*, 878-891.

Singh, Y. (1977). *Modernization of Indian Tradition*. Thompson Press, Faridabad.

Sinha, D. and Tripathi, R.C. (1994). Individualism in a Collectivistic Culture: A Case of Coexistence of Opposites. In U. Kim, H.C. Trandis, C. Kagitibasi, S.C. Choi and G. Yoon (Eds.). *Individualism and Collectivism: Theory, Method and Applications* (pp. 123-126), Newbury Park, C.A.: Sage.

Sinha, J.B.P. (1990b). The Salient Indian Values and their Socio-ecological Roots. *Indian Journal of Social Science, 3*(4), 477-488.

Tonnies, F. (1957). *Community and Society* (C.P. Loomis, Ed. and Trans). New York: Harper & Row. (Original work published in 1887).

Triandis, H.C. (1994). *Culture and Social Behaviour*. New York. McGraw-Hill.

Verma, J. (1992b). Allocentrism and Relationship Orientation. In S. Iwawaki, Y. Kashima and K. Leung (Eds.) *Innovations in Cross Cultural Psychology* (pp. 152-163). Lisse: Swets and Zeitlinger.

12

Promoting Mental Health, Quality of Work Life and Productivity of Employees in India

The Application of Positive Psychology

Suhas Shetgovekar

Employees can be termed as most important resource in any organization. Promoting their mental health, quality of work life and productivity in order to enhance the organizational production and productivity thus becomes significant for any organization. Organizations, therefore, need to take necessary measures in this direction. One way in which the mental health, quality of work life and productivity of employees can be promoted is by applying the principles of positive psychology. Positive psychology as a branch of psychology has been making rapid developments over the years and has found its application in varied fields like counselling and psychotherapy, education, health and industries. In the present chapter, how the principles and tenets of positive psychology can be applied in order to promote mental health, quality of work life and productivity amongst the employees in Indian context will be discussed along with empirical evidences. The challenges and problems that can arise while applying positive psychology will also be dealt. The chapter will also highlight the criticisms of positive psychology and future prospects.

Positive psychology has flourished over the years as a branch of psychology. It was first introduced as an area of study by Seligman at the time of his inaugural address to the American Psychological Association in 1998 (Seligman, 1999). Psychology made rapid strides after Second World War. However, before the World War, psychology mainly dealt with mental illnesses and selecting and training employees for specific jobs. Positive psychology to a greater extent based on the principles of humanistic approach. Though the term positive psychology is relatively new, but its essence was always present in the theories proposed by the philosophers like Aristotle and Plato and thinkers in psychology like Freud, Rogers, Adler, Jung and Maslow who spoke about terms like pleasure, actualization, wholeness, good life and so on (Duckworth *et al.*, 2005; Ryff, 2003).

Positive psychology can be defined as "the study of strengths, virtues, excellence, thriving, flourishing, resilience, optimal functioning in general, and the like" (Donaldson, 2011). As described by Lopez & Snyder (2003), the essence of positive psychology is "to develop the strengths and manage the weaknesses". Positive Psychology can also be defined as "the study of the conditions and processes that contribute to the flourishing or optimal functioning of people, groups, and institutions" (Gable and Haidt, 2005).

According to Seligman (2002), the main goal of positive psychology is promoting happiness and subjective well-being, which can be described as positive feelings. Happiness according to Seligman has three main parts, that is, pleasure, engagement and meaning (Kulshreshtha, 2014). Pleasure is described as the good feeling that is part of the happiness. Engagement has to do with leading a better life with regard to work, family and so on. Meaning has to deal with how an individual's strengths can be used adequately. According to Seligman, though all three, are relevant, engagement and meaning, are the most important in promoting well-being of the individuals. On the other hand, subjective well-being can be described as an cognitive and affective evaluation of one's life by an individual (Diener, Lucas, and Oshi, 2002: 63).

As stated by Andrew Fleming (2006), the three main principles or tenets of positive psychology are "Positive emotions that have to do with happiness, contentment, well-being, optimism, and others; positive personal characteristics: resilience, goal setting, engagement, and virtues; and positive institutions and communities. Elements of the environment include families, schools, and communities and these are considered to support the development and maintenance of mental health."

Positive Psychology also focuses on the optimal human functioning. This optimal human functioning entails a study of various psychological aspects like hopefulness or optimism, emotional intelligence, hope, love, humour, creativity, subjective experiences that are positive, positive individual characteristics as well as positive institutions and communities (Seligman and Csikszentmihalyi, 2000; Seligman *et al.*, 2005). A major assumption of Positive Psychology is that individuals can achieve their full potential even when they are undergoing a problem.

The principles of Positive Psychology can be applied to varied fields and can help individuals in leading better life and achieve their potential. It has found its application to various fields like education, counselling/ psychotherapy, clinical psychology and even industrial and organizational psychology. Some of the key terms that are included under positive psychology are happiness, optimism, mindfulness, strengths, hope, resilience and positive thinking and these can be relevant and have a positive impact on the way individuals lead their lives, carry out activities and interact with people. Ignored to understand how positive psychology can have an influence on mental health, quality of life and productivity of employees, understanding these terms are significant. These terms are discussed in details in the next section of this chapter.

Mental Health, Quality of Work Life and Productivity

Mental health, quality of work life and productivity are three important terms when we talk about employees in an organizational context. These terms and relevant empirical evidences with regard to these terms need to be discussed in order to understand them in a better way and discuss how principles of positive psychology can be effectively applied to enhance them. There has been a growing concern about mental health of individual in society in general and of employees in specific. There is growing stress that is experienced by the employees as a result of work load and complexities of the work activities. There is also growing stress at family level. Further, due to various pressures, societal, environmental, familial and personal, employees are also prone to various mental health problems and illnesses. Technological developments and advancements have also contributed to development of stress and subsequent development of major psychological problems amongst employees. This can have a negative impact on the overall productivity and performance of the employees and thus can have a detrimental effect on the production and profitability of the organization. Therefore, mental health of the employees needs to be focused on and necessary measures need to be undertaken to promote positive mental health amongst the employees.

The WHO (2004) describes mental health as "a state of well-being in which the individual realizes his or her own abilities, can cope with the normal stresses of life, can work productively and fruitfully, and is able to make a contribution to his or her community." Mental health is a broad concept that encompasses psychological, emotional as well as social well-being of individuals. Mental health is relevant at every developmental stage from childhood to the old age. Though there can be some differences in what kind of mental health issues are of concern at different developmental stages. Mental health issues can range from stress, anxiety, depression to various major psychological disorders like personality disorders, schizophrenia and so on. Physiological factors, personal life experiences and even family history can contribute to the development of mental health problems.

Employees suffering from mental health problems will not be in position to function optimally and perform to their fullest potential. There are also chances of increased accidents, absenteeism and increased conflicts. Mentally healthy employees are in better position to cope with stress, work effectively and contribute qualitatively to their organization.

When discussing about mental health, mental health problems and mental disorders also need to be focused on. Mental health problems can be described as symptoms that are related to mental disorders, but their severity is not sufficient enough to be diagnosed as a mental disorder (World Health Organization Report, 2005). They can be described as minor psychological problems. Though mental health problems may or may not lead to development of mental disorders amongst individuals, they can interfere with one's work performance and quality of work life.

"Mental disorders on the other hand can be described as conditions that are clinically significant. They can be characterized with altered thoughts, emotions and behaviour with associated distress or impaired functioning" (World Health Organization, 2001). When mental health is discussed in an organizational context, the factors as well as the effects of mental health problems and mental disorders need to be considered. Further, benefits of promoting mental health amongst employees also need to be focused on.

Various studies have been carried out on mental health of employees in India, though the studies mainly focus on employees in call centres and IT professionals. There is also a need for studies to be carried in various organizational set-ups in India so as to understand the nature of problems and issues that the employees face that can lead to development of mental health problems and mental disorders. Suitable intervention can thus be developed in order to help employees deal better with the situation. To mention some of the studies, a study was carried out by Machado, Sathyanarayanan, Bhola and Kamath (2003) on the psychological vulnerability, burnout, and coping among employees of a business process outsourcing organization. The results indicated that 38 per cent of the sample displayed psychological distress. The study also stressed on the need for mental health professionals in corporate sector. Stress and work overload can have detrimental effects on overall health of the employees as well. Another study carried out by Pandey (2003) on professionals in advertising indicated that some of the major health problems that these professionals suffered from were headache, backache and stomach related disorders and so on and these were attributed to extended working hours, relationship with clients as well as work environment. The study also reflected a need for healthy workplaces as well as need for suitable human resource policies in order to promote mental health amongst the employees. A survey was carried out by Data Quest on BPO/Call Centre industry in India in the year 2003, revealed that the employees reported job stress as well as other ailments that were related to work activities. This resulted in high rate of attrition and lack of motivation amongst employees. Another survey carried out by Data Quest in the year 2005 indicated lack of sufficient holidays, low motivation due to repetitive nature of work, work load and work shift (night shift) as factors contributing to stressful working conditions (as cited in Pandey, 2008: 175). A study carried out by Jain, Bhatia and Mathur (2012) on workplace stress and suicide in public sector organizations highlighted that stress was premier reason contributing to suicides amongst employees. Another research was carried out by Jayashree (2010) on stress management with special reference to public sector bank employees in Chennai. The study indicated presence of stress amongst the employees in public sector banks. A large number of participants of the study reported suffering from ailments that were related to stress. They also reported suffering from psychological problems. The stress was seen to be as a result of work pressure as well as work-life balance. The study stressed the need for initiatives on the part of the management in order to help employees deal with stress and its effects. Besides stress, there can also be other concerns in organizational set-up like substance abuse and other major psychological problems that need attention.

The term quality of work life has caught major attention in recent times. Quality of work life was introduced for the first time by Louis Davis. Quality of work life has been defined as "a process by which an Organization responds to employee needs by developing mechanisms to allow them to share fully in making the decisions that design their lives at work." (Robbins, 1989 as cited in Jayakumar and Kalaiselvi, 2012: 141). It can also be defined as "the quality of relationship between the employees and the total working environment" (Pugalendhi, Umaselvi and Santhil Kumar, 2010). According to Davis, quality of work life refers to "favourable or unfavourable of the job environment for public".

Quality of work life can simply be described as relationship between employees and overall work environment. It also concerns how employee needs are been taken care by the organization. The main objectives of promoting quality of work life amongst employees are not only to generate a positive attitude towards work activity but also to increase productivity and bring about improvement in overall standard of living of the employees. Some of the factors that contribute to quality of work life are income, job security, job stress, relationships at workplace, opportunities for growth and promotion and so on. Enhanced quality of work life can not only enhance productivity and increase job satisfaction amongst the employees but also help organizations in retaining talent and maintaining a positive organizational culture in the organization. There are various factors that are related to quality of work life like workload and perception of the employee, motivation and relationship amongst employees in an organization, productivity and performance, job performance, health and safety facilities, working conditions, communication in the organization, organizational climate and support, flexible arrangements in work environment and activities, rewards, benefits and compensation and so.

Pugalendhi, Umaselvi and Santhil Kumar (2010) carried out a study on the perception of quality of work life amongst college teachers. The study stressed that the responsibility of quality of work life is not only of the management and employees but society as well. It also indicated that in order to improve quality of work life, it is necessary to first identify and satisfy the needs of the employees in work environment. The study also revealed significant relationship between quality of work life and quality of life and indicated that the college teachers had lower quality of work life. The study concluded that in order to improve quality of work life, necessary modifications need to make in the work environment. Another study was carried out by Sandhu and Prabhakar (2012) on factors influencing the quality of work life in the Indian banking industry. The data was collected from professional from banking industry. The results indicated that five factors that have an influence on quality of work life, namely, remuneration, opportunities for personal growth, supportive leadership and structures, work environment and work-life balance. The study implied that these factors need to be taken into consideration when policies are drafted for retention programmes in banking industry. A study, carried out by Sinha (2012), studied the factors that influence quality of work life in Indian organizations revealed their main factors of relationship—sustenance orientation, futuristic and professional orientation, and self-deterministic and systemic orientation. These factors were found to be playing important role in fulfilling the needs of the employees. A study was also carried out on linkage between quality of work life and two important aspects of job satisfaction and performance revealed that the outcome of quality of life like positive attitude, commitment and satisfaction. The results indicated that relationship does exist between quality of life and job satisfaction, which in turn can have a positive impact on performance of the employees (Gayathiri and Ramakrishnan, 2013).

Discussing the term productivity, any organization makes use of various resources including raw material, finance, technology and human resource in order to achieve its goal. However, one of the most important resources is the human resource or the employees that make use of all the other resources. Thus, this particular resource requires the utmost attention ignored to maintain its productivity. Productivity as defined by Kopleman is "the relationship between physical output of one or more of the associated physical inputs used in production" (as cited in Singh and Kamlesh, 2013:66). But when we talk about Employee productivity, also referred to as workforce productivity, it denotes the efficiency of the employee. It is thus related to the performance of the employee on the job. It is to be kept in mind that the employees will perform better when they are motivated, are satisfied with their jobs, are able to manage stress, are mentally healthy and are comfortable in the work environment. Both the personal characteristics as well as characteristics of the work environment will play a role while determining the productivity of the employees. Selecting right employees is thus important in this regard as if the employee is not fit or right match for the job, he/she may not be able to perform it well or is going to be dissatisfied and de-motivated in carrying out the work activity. Besides a work environment that is not safe or comfortable enough or which is very rigid can also have detrimental effects on the productivity of the employees.

Productivity of the employees will also depend on the training with regard to both technical and behavioural skills provided to them and thus due care needs to be taken to regularly train the human resource in any organization not only in technical skills required for the job but also in behavioural or soft skills. Employees need to be trained in manageing stress, time, and emotions along with effective communication, team work, and leadership skills and so on.

Though employee productivity seems to a concern of any organization, its benefits are twofold. It will not only benefit the organization by helping it in direction of achieving the organizational goals, it can also be advantageous to the employee. A productive employee will have better self-esteem and self-respect, will display job satisfaction, will be intrinsically motivated and committed to the work activity. He/she will also enjoy doing the work activity and will develop belongingness towards the organization that will go a long way as far as the relationship between the organization and employee is concerned.

All the three variables discussed above are also interrelated, as a positive mental health and better quality of work life can promote productivity of the employees. Next what is relevant is how the principles of positive psychology can be adequately used in order to promote all the three, that is mental health, quality of life and productivity. The same can be determined by focusing on the significance of positive psychology in workplace and then discussing how its principles can be applied effectively.

Positive Psychology in Organizations: Significance and Application

Over the years, the role and work activities of the employees in an industrial set-up have changed. This is also as a result of changes in society, globalization, changes in job market, and developments in technology and so on that have influenced the organizations in a big way. This has further resulted in various complexities and problems for the employees that can have a negative impact on the well-being and performance of the employees and thus can affect output and profitability of the organization. Further, the work itself has become complex and demands more from the employees. The situation can serve as a challenge to the employee and he/she may find it difficult to cope with the situation.

As discussed above there are various factors like globalization, developments in technology, increased urbanization and higher migration rates that have an impact not only on the work activities and demands of the job but also on the overall health (including mental health) of the employees. This is especially true of developing countries like India. The challenges thrown by these factors can have further detrimental effect due to lack of basic infrastructure and facilities available to deal with the problems like mental health issues and deteriorating quality of work life of the employees. This in turn can affect the organizational outcomes and profitability.

The first and the foremost challenge is that of globalization. World Health Report (2005: 10) refer to globalization as "*the progressive integration of economies and societies*". Globalization on one hand can bring strides of rapid developments by bringing about improvements in national economy. However, it also gives rise to competition and can impact the working conditions in negative manner. The advents of multi-national companies in India have on one hand have brought increased job opportunities, but this has not resolved the issues related to mental health and quality of work life of the employees. Increased competition and strenuous working conditions can have a negative impact on overall well-being of the employees.

Development in technology is yet another challenge in the workplace. Advancement in technology has resulted in complex work activities for which there is a high demand for skilled employees. Developments in technology on one hand has reduced requirement of manpower, cost of production, and reduced the errors and wastage of raw material. But on the other hand, it has also lead to decrease in job positions and increased demand for skilled employees that can create problems in developing countries. There is also increase in stress and development of other psychological disorders due to reduced social interactions as a result of improved technology. Further, continuous use of technology can also have negative effect on health of the employees.

Increased urbanization and migration are other challenges. There has been increasing shift in the population from rural to urban areas. A number of employees leave their skilled jobs in their villages due to lack of adequate income and migrate to urban areas for better prospects. However, they may not be able to either get suitable jobs, or may land in jobs in unorganized sectors. In organized sector, they may not be termed as skilled employees. Thus, they need to be educated and suitably trained to take up the new jobs. Migration also can lead to increased stress and psychological problems as the employees are away from their families and may not be able to cope with the demands of the job and the urban setting. They can also experience stress, depression and other major psychological problems due to financial and societal pressures.

Thus, keeping in mind these challenges and many more that develop over a period of time, the organizations need to ensure that conducive environment is created at the workplace in order to help employees deal and cope better with the everyday challenges and stressors and work with their full potential.

To discuss about workplace and human resources, the approach of management towards human resource, over the years, is largely based on negativity. The whole approach focuses on finding quick solutions to problems rather than investing on long-term basis that can deliver maximum benefits and over a long period of time. When there are more serious concern regarding production and profitability, promoting happiness and optimism amongst employees may indeed seem to be trivial. The organizations often refrain from investing in unwell employees or employees who are not in a position to perform and thus such employees may be replaced. The focus is not on the well-being of the employees, but on their performance that contributes to the organizational output. This is also as a result go high demands, pressures, financial issues and competitions that the organization has to face. But as a raw material that is substandard in quality will produce a product that is substandard, if the human resource is not adequately treated, the whole process of production and the output will suffer. Further, the managers and supervisors are not adequately trained to motivate the employees or provide them with suitable feedback with regard to their performances. The organizations need to change their strategies from taking shortcuts to investing in human resource for long-term gains. As unhappy, dissatisfied, stressed employees can in fact have negative effects on the profits as well as decrease in market shares of the organization (Spreitzer & Cameron, 2012). Further, the characteristics of employees today have also changed. They no more look for jobs that would last till retirement but seek continuous growth and development. They give relevance to personal growth as well as their personal life and family.

The employees can experience high level of stress due to workload and high demands of the job. Various studies have been carried out in this context. A study carried out by American Psychological Association in 2007 indicated that almost 74 per cent of the employees reported experiencing stress due to work which even led them to miss their work. A study carried out by Kleppa, Sanne, and Tell (2008) indicated increased anxiety and depression amongst workers who worked overtime, when compared to workers who worked for normal hours.

The employee-employer relationship has also become shorter compared to what it was a few years back. The turnover in various organizations has increased. In this scenario, retaining employees is also one of the significant challenges that an organization has been facing. Organization needs to develop suitable strategies in order to retain talented employees. Also since the employee-employer relationship is becoming shorter.

Further, the main focus of the organizations is not on whether the employee is carrying his/her work or not. Rather, the focus is on how he/she can carry out the work in a better manner by functioning fully. For this, the necessary support, opportunity as well as suitable organizational climate needs to be provided to the employees. The organizations also want the employees to be more creative and involve in lateral thinking so as to adequately deal with the complexities of work activities.

There is also the issue of work-life balance that need stop be dealt with. Employees today value their family life as much as their work activities. An employee who is satisfied with personal, family life will in a way be able to contribute better to the work activities. Thus, the employees need to be provided suitable help in maintaining work-life balance.

Manageing human resource in India is strongly influenced by social, cultural and economic factors. These factors can contribute to uncertainties and can create issues and problems while manageing human resource. According to Sparrow and Budhwar (1997) in India social and cultural norms greatly influence the work climate as well as the behaviour and performance of employees. Various researchers have also indicated resistance to any change, lack of discipline, lack of willingness to accept any authority and lack of initiative in taking independent decision and so on are some of the characteristics of human resource in India that can interfere with effective management of human resource or employees (Sharma, 1984; Sparrow and Budhwar, 1997). At the same time, Indians can also be described as being hardworking, ambitious, materialistic and resourceful (Tayeb, 1996). It is significant that these aspects need to be taken into consideration while manageing human resources in Indian context. Determinants like culture, age and nature of the organization including its size also need to be taken into consideration (Budhwar and Varma, 2011). Paul, Garg and Pooja (2014) carried out a study on healing human resources through positive psychology. The study discussed the role of principles of positive psychology in dealing with issues related to human resource management. The study also focused on how emerging trends can also be dealt with the help of concepts like resilience, subjective well-being, hope and optimism, termed as positive psychological traits. Besides social, cultural and economic factors, one needs to take political situation in India as well into consideration. The policies and laws related to human resource and industries are also relevant. The human resource in India is also unique due to its demographic characteristics as youth constitute considerable section of the Indian population and are available to be employed. India being a country with diverse cultures, the employees in any organization also belong to diverse cultures. Indian organizations constitute employees from diverse cultures, speaking different languages, having distinct beliefs and values and food habits working together. Diversity can be advantageous in an organizational set-up as it brings different perspectives and help deal with complexities of work. However, the employees need to accept and respect this diversity and should be willing to work as a team. If diversity is not adequately managed then there can be detrimental effects on the organizational culture and climate.

Till date organizations in India not only lack counselling facilities but many of the organizations even do not have a proper human resource department or personnel departments. Human resource is not yet valued as any other resource. Given these circumstances and the strenuous working conditions combined with low income and lack of facilities can have an impact on the overall well-being of the employees? Further, there are various challenges that can have a negative effect on the organization as a whole and determine the focus of the organization on the well-being and welfare of the employees.

Given the above challenges and issue in the workplace, positive psychology can play an important role in dealing with them mainly by creating a conducive environment for the employees and helping them achieve their full potential. Positive psychology can play a significant role in these contexts whether to promote employee satisfaction, help them deal with stress and anxiety or promoting effective team work. Further, principles of positive psychology can also help in promoting high performance amongst the employees. Positive psychology can be applied to workplace in order to make employees more productive, become aware about their strengths, and nurture their talents so that they can achieve their full potential, motivate them and improve their mental health. It can also be helpful in reducing conflicts in the organization.

According to Lewis (2013), the two main concepts of positive psychology that are relevant when we speak about employees are, positivity and strength. Positivity denotes the ratio of positive and negative emotions experienced by individuals. Whereas, strengths have to do with an individual's inherent abilities that are result of physiological or hereditary as well as environmental influences. The application of positive psychology at workplace focuses on the optimum functioning or functioning of the employee to the fullest and promoting well-being of the employees. The employees should be encouraged to develop resilience, optimism and become aware about their strengths which in turn will help them cope with situations and they will be less prone to suffering from anxiety and depression. It will also help them maintain relationships at work and at home in a better manner, maintain health and be productive. A research was carried out on employee commitment and its impact on sustained productivity of employees in Auto component industry in India (Dixit and Bhati, 2012) indicated that the sustained productivity was influenced by employee commitment, namely affective, continuance and normative. Thus, it can be said that if the employee commitment is increased, the employee productivity can also be improved and sustained.

As discussed earlier, the focus of psychology has been on mental illnesses and disorders rather than positive mental health. However, with developments in positive psychology there has been a shift towards positive functioning of individuals. Thus, the concept of psychological well-being is not just absence of illness but presence of constructs in an individual like positive emotions, life satisfaction, and acceptance of self and personal development. Well-being can be enhanced and symptoms of depression can be reduced with the help of positive psychology interventions (Sin and Lyubomirsky, 2009).

The techniques of positive psychology can also help individuals deal with depression. Techniques like writing and sending gratitude letters, the exercise of 'writing three good things in life', exercising optimism, identifying strengths indeed helped the participants in ameliorating the symptoms of mild depression (Seligman *et al.,* 2005).

Principle of positive psychology can also be applied to improving the quality of work life of the employees. Work environment is relevant in order to promote job satisfaction, motivation, productive work related behaviours and even productivity. When employees are optimistic, happy, and resilient and are aware about their own strengths, the quality of work life will definitely improve. Further, when the employees are convinced that the organization is making efforts towards their well-being, a sense of gratitude and responsibility will also develop amongst the employees. Better quality of work life will in turn help retain employees and attract talented employees. A study by Donaldson and Bligh (2006) on rewarding careers applying positive psychological science to improve quality of work life and organizational effectiveness indicated that application of positive psychology can contribute to enhancing quality of work life and organizational effectiveness as well. Positive psychology can also enhance organizational citizenship (Luthans, 2002).

It was mentioned earlier that positive psychology is based on humanistic approach. Some of the main assumptions of humanistic approach are that each individual is unique and his/her unique way of looking at the world. It also assumes that individuals have the potentiality and can take their own decisions. These assumptions need to be applied to the employees in an organizational set-up. Employees need to be seen as beings that have capacities and potential, are unique and can take their own decisions, grow to their fullest potential and even solve their own problems. However, as Carl Rogers states in the context of psychotherapy, a 'conducive environment' needs to be created for these employees. Thus, the focus again shifts on the work environment that constitutes not only the space and the machinery and technology but more importantly people, who are managers, supervisors, colleagues, subordinates. Positive psychology needs to be applied at all levels of hierarchy for positive results.

Some of the techniques of positive psychology that can be used with the employees are as follows:

One of the techniques of positive psychology is helping employees nurture their relationships at home and at work. Conducive environment needs to be created in order to help employees build and nurture relationships. At work, events and programmes, formal and informal, can be organized so that there are opportunities for the employees to interact with each other and build relationships. This will also help build high performing teams and achieve the organizational goals. Further, employees should be provided suitable opportunities to spend time with their families. This will in long-term promote life satisfaction amongst the employees. Communication is an important part of any relationship. Positive communications should also be promoted amongst the employees, besides having open communication in an organization.

Yet another technique is that of helping employees become aware about their strengths and to use them adequately. With the help of awareness programmes the employees can be helped to become aware and recognize their strengths. The employees also need to be motivated to perform their best by regular encouragement and performance feedback, especially, from their immediate superiors. This will also help maintain positive mental health amongst the employees.

Flow is one of the techniques that can help employees lead an engaged life. Flow can be described as an individual's subjective experience of getting involved in challenges that are manageable and that can be dealt with, with the help of series of goals, regular feedback and modifying one's actions based on the feedback. The technique can be incorporated in the day-to-day activities of the employees. The employees should also be encouraged to practice optimism. Being positive is one of the tenets of positive psychology and can be imbibed in the employees. Employees can be encouraged to carry-out exercises that focus on positive things and people in one's life. They can be asked to write positive conclusions to difficult situations that they have been facing. Optimism can help develop positive mood in employees and thus enhance mental health and can also have a positive impact on physical health of an individual.

Employees can also be encouraged to get involved in pro-social behaviours. This can also be linked with social responsibility activities of the organization. These acts of kindness can provide satisfaction to the employees and a sense of contribution to the community and society. The self-esteem of the employees can also be enhanced. Any organization is also a part and parcel of the society and has certain commitments towards the society in which it exists. Encourageing pro-social behaviours amongst the employees will serve both the purposes. It will on one hand promote well-being of the employee and on the other contribute positively to the society and community. Further, promoting employee well-being can also be seen as a part of overall social responsibility of the organization that can benefit society as a whole (Cameron, Dutton, & Quinn, 2003).

The employees should be encouraged to regularly encourage employees in expressing gratitude to their colleagues, superiors, subordinates and even family members. They can also be encouraged to maintain a gratitude journal, where they could write at least three positive things or experiences of the day. Further, gratitude visits to people who have supported or helped employees in their lives can also be encouraged.

Mindfulness is one of the significant techniques in positive psychology. It mainly denotes awareness, about one's self as well as one's surrounding. Mindfulness can play a significant role in promoting positive mental health as well as improve the quality of work life of an employee. Mindfulness can alleviate depressive symptoms and is significantly correlated with well-being, life satisfaction and positive emotions (Sephton *et al.*, 2007; Ortner, Kilner and Zelazo, 2007). The employees can be trained in exercising mindfulness that in turn will help them cultivate positive emotions, enhance their relationships and perform better in their work activities. It can also help employees become better team members, deal with conflict and enhance their creativity.

It is important to note here that activities related to positive psychology are incorporated in human resource management and development activities or employee welfare activities. Further, it is also important that human resource managers and supervisors are trained in order to carry out these activities. Workshops and training programmes with reference to the techniques of positive psychology can be regularly organized. Also though the techniques of positive psychology may seem simple, they can be difficult to implement. Positive psychology can also be incorporated with the various processes of human resource management and development, like training, performance appraisal, career development programmes, mentoring and coaching. Activities in this regard can be organized at individual levels as well as with groups. For example, certain employees who display signs of stress, anxiety, depression or any other mental health problems can be provided interventions including techniques of positive psychology. On the other hand, managers, workers can be involved in group activities and exercises related to techniques of positive psychology. Programmes can also be organized for the family members, including spouses, children and parents of the employees. This will further ensure job involvement, reduce absenteeism, increase productivity and improve the overall quality of life of the employees.

However, for these techniques to be successful, the employees need to have a positive attitude towards them and need to practice them sincerely and seriously. The human resource managers/personnel managers/managers/supervisors should ensure this for the successful application of principles of positive psychology at the workplace.

Application of Positive Psychology: Issues, Problems and Challenges

Some of the issues, problems and challenges in applying positive psychology to HRM are as follows:

The Role of Human Resource Managers/Personnel Managers is one of the challenges. Human resource managers/personnel managers play an important role in application of principles of positive psychology. They should be first convinced about the benefits of positive psychology so as to implement them successfully. The relevance of promoting mental health and quality of work life should be foremost. However, the pressures of achieving organizational goals and enhancing profitability can divert the focus of these managers. In fact, the importance of promoting mental health, for example, amongst employees has been upheld by the international organizations like European Union and World Health Organization and considerable attention has been paid in this regard in many developed countries. However, in India, the overall awareness about the relevance and the concept of mental health is low (Pandey, 2001). Once the human resource managers/personnel managers develop right attitude towards positive psychology, they also need to develop the necessary skills. They themselves should be able to practice the techniques like optimism, expressing gratitude, mindfulness and so on before preaching the same to other managers and employees.

Yet another challenge is the role and attitude of management. Management as well need to develop a positive attitude towards positive psychology, this will in turn promote a positive attitude amongst the managers as well as employees. Positive psychology can also be incorporated in the policies related to human resource management and activities and programmes should be planned and organized in this direction. The management should also be willing to allow such an innovative practice to be applied in the organizational set-up and should work closely in this regard with the human resource department/personnel department. Further, there also has to be a sense of patience as there might not be immediate results, but there will be long-term benefits.

It is also important to focus on the role and attitudes of the managers/supervisors. The managers need to be trained in developing the skill of empathy so that they are able to understand their employees in a better manner. Open communication needs to be promoted in the organization. The managers in this context need to develop the skill of listening. They should also be helped to develop suitable attitude and skills regarding positive psychology. Practicing positive psychology can also help managers/supervisors develop effective leadership skills.

Any change or modification or a new practice is often perceived as a threat by the employees. Such a perception can interfere with the application of positive psychology. Any apprehensions on the part of the employees need to be clarified and they should be prepared to engage in the new practices. Further, in developing countries like India where individuals and organizations face an imminent challenge of financial crunch, focus on happiness, optimism, resilience and so on may seem impractical and also excessively difficult. Further, employees may have very basic needs of food and shelter, without which most of the terms in positive psychology will not make sense. The main goal of the employee is earning to fulfil basic needs of himself/herself and his/her families. In such a situation, the employee may not be open to the ideas of positive psychology.

Nature and type of the organization can also be an issue while implementing positive psychology. There are different types of organizations in India like Multi-National Companies, Public Sector Units, smaller industries and organizations and so on. A large number of organizations in India may barely have a human resource department or personnel management department that could take care of human resource and employee welfare, leave alone application of principles of positive psychology. Though there are organizations like Central Board for Worker's Education and various private consultancies from where experts in the field of positive psychology can be outsourced to at least carry out workshops and programmes. There is also unorganized sector where application of positive psychology has no existence and may not see the light of the day for years to come.

Lack of resources is yet another challenge. Resources imply not only finance, but also experts in the field and time. Accommodating the workshops, programmes, activities and events related to positive psychology in the busy production, manufacturing and work schedule can be a challenge. Many organizations may not be able afford such activities due to financial constraints. Further, organizations would be more interested in allocating finances to buying raw material and better technology than investing on the human resources. This is again a challenge while promoting application of positive psychology to workplace.

There is also a lack of awareness about positive psychology. Many managers, including human resource managers may not be aware about positive psychology and its benefits or its application in industrial set-up. Besides, even if the managers are aware about positive psychology, they also need to possess suitable skills to implement principles of positive psychology. This is yet another challenge, as if the managers including human resource managers/personnel managers do not have suitable skills to implement principles of positive psychology, the whole idea of applying positive psychology will fail.

Issues can also crop is due to the gap between theory and practice. The principles and techniques of positive psychology are theoretically easier to understand. However, problems may crop up while actually implementing them. Also the person who implements them needs to have a strong background knowledge and skills in positive psychology for its successful implementation.

Despite the challenges discussed above and the criticisms that will be discussed later in the chapter, considering the benefits of the application of positive psychology, its principles and techniques can be gradually introduced and implemented in Indian organizations.

Application of Positive Psychology: Critical Analysis and Future Prospects

With all the research and empirical evidence highlighting the advantages and benefits of positive psychology, there are also criticisms that need to be considered. The critics seek stronger empirical evidences with regard to application of positive psychology. Further positive psychologists have also been criticized for terming the field of positive psychology as being new, whereas there are evidences that the concepts covered under the term have been used since long time (Duckworth *et al*., 2005; Ryff, 2003). Even in Indian context the tenets like resilience, optimism etc. that have been discussed and passed over generations.

Further, the critics also feel that illnesses and disorders cannot be dealt with by just being optimistic, for instance. Principles of positive psychology can be promoted based on the needs of the individual, but not by compromising the main line of treatment that the individual is undergoing. Growing awareness about the field has also lead to sprouting of happiness *gurus* and positive psychology experts who give lessons in optimism, happiness, resilience and so on. They may not be necessarily trained in positive psychology; however, they flourish due to high demand from the societies and communities. Thus, there has been increased commercialization of the field but without strong empirical backing. The general public is also not completely aware about the field as a whole and thus can be deprived of benefits of suitably practicing the techniques. Further, the techniques of positive psychology need to be used as per the needs of the individuals. The techniques cannot be generally applied to a group as the needs of each individual will vary. In such a scenario, teaching the techniques of positive psychology can even backfire. One of the critics of positive psychology is Lazarus. Positive psychology has been criticized by him for being too simple in its approach to emotions and realities of life (Lazarus, 2003).

There is definitely a trend in the stride of positive psychology and openness to certain extent on part of the general public. However, this is where the experts and the proponents of positive psychology should come in and ensure that the lacunas and criticisms in the field are dealt with and taken care of. Research on application of positive psychology should be promoted amongst not only the students of psychology, but amongst human resource managers/personnel managers. Research can not only provide empirical evidences but also make way for further developments in the subject area. Further, it is necessary to critically evaluate the research carried out in the field. It is also necessary to uphold the ethical issues while applying the principles of positive psychology in any field, whether counselling and psychotherapy, education or in workplace.

In India, there is no review board or an organization that can take care of licensing to practice psychology. Rehabilitation Council of India just takes care of clinical psychologist and that too is not compulsory, nor guarded by legal implications. Suitable measures need to be taken in to consideration in this direction. This will ensure that the principles and techniques of psychology in general and positive psychology in specific are practiced by individuals with necessary expertise.

Conclusion

To conclude, positive psychology can be applied to workplace to promote the well-being of the employees and effectively achieve the organizational goals. Despite the number of challenges and criticisms, strong empirical evidences and further research will help in both developing better understanding about the field as well as evaluating its efficacy in different settings. Though the basic ideas about positive psychology are not new, the subject has been in limelight only since a few decades. The subject has a long way to go and a lot to contribute to individuals and society.

References

Budhwar, P.S., and Verma, A. (2011). Emerging HR management trends in India and the way forward. *Organizational Dynamics, 40*, 317-325.

Cameron, K., Dutton, J., and Quinn, R. (2003). Foundations of positive organizational scholarship. In Cameron, K., Dutton, J., and Quinn, R. (Eds.), *Positive Organizational Scholarship: Foundations of a New Discipline* (pp. 3-13). San Francisco, CA: Berrett-Koehler Publishers, Inc.

Chatterjee, S.R. (2007). Human Resource Management in India: 'Where From' and 'Where To?', *Research and Practice in Human Resource Management, 15*(2), 92-103.

Dixit, V. and Bhati, M. (2012). A Study about Employee Commitment and its Impacton Sustained Productivity in Indian Auto-Component Industry. *European Journal of Business and Social Sciences, 1*(6), pp. 34-51.

Davis, K. (1981). *Human Behavioural Work.* Tata McGraw-Hill Publishing Company, New Delhi.

Diener, E., Oishi, S., and Lucas, R.E. (2002). Subjective well-being: The science of happiness and life satisfaction. In C.R. Snyder and S.J. Lopez (Ed.) *Handbook of Positive Psychology.* New York: Oxford University Press.

Donaldson, S.I. and Bligh, M.C. (2006). Rewarding careers applying positive psychological science to improve quality of work life and organizatior effectiveness. In S.I. Donaldson, D.E. Berger and K. Pezdak (Eds.) *Apr Psychology: New Frontiers and Rewarding Careers* (pp. 277-295). Ya NJ: Lawrence Erlbaum Associates.

Donaldson, S.I. (2011). Determining What Works, If Anything. In S.I. Donaldson, M. Csikszentmihalyi and J. Nakamura (Eds.) *Applied Positive Psychology: Improving Everyday Life, Health, Schools, Work and Society*. Routledge.

Duckworth, A.L., Steen, T.A., and Seligman, M. (2005). Positive psychology in clinical practice. *Annual Review of Clinical Psychology, 1*, 629-651.

Fleming, A.W. (2006). Positive Psychology "Three Good Things in Life" and Measuring Happiness, Positive and Negative Affectivity, Optimism/Hope, and Well-Being, *Counsellor Education Master's Theses*. Paper 32. State University of New York College at Brockport.

Gable, S.L., and Haidt, J. (2005). What (and Why) Is Positive Psychology? *Review of General Psychology, Vol. 9*, 103-110.

Jain, M., Bhatia, R., and Mathur, T.N. (2012). Work Place Stress and Suicide: A Study with reference to Public Sector Organization. *International Journal of Multidisciplinary Research, Vol. 2* (7), 186-196.

Jayakumar, A. and Kalaiselvi, K. (2012). Quality of Work Life—An Overview. *International Journal of Marketing—Financial Services & Management Research, 1*, 34-39.

Jayashree, R. (2010). Stress Management with Special Reference to Public Sector Bank Employees in Chennai. *International Journal of Enterprise and Innovation Management Studies (IJEIMS), Vol. 1*, (3), 34-35.

Jayawickreme, J., Pawelski, J., and Seligman, M. (2008). Positive Psychology and Nussbaum's Capabilities Approach. Conference Presentation: Subjective Measures of Well-Being and the Science of Happiness: Historical Origins and Philosophical Foundations, Birmingham AL.

Kleppa, E., Sanne, B. and Tell, G.S. (2008). Working overtime is associated with anxiety and depression: the Hordaland Health Study. *Journal of Occupation and Environmental Medicine, 50*(6), 658-666.

Kulshreshtha, S. (2014). Talent Management and Positive Psychology: Some Thoughts assessed on 24.11.2014 on http://www.positivepsychologyindia.org.

Lazarus, R.S. (2003). The Lazarus manifesto for positive psychology and psychology in general. *Psychological Inquiry, 14*(2), 173-189.

Lewis, S. (2013). Positive Psychology – A Useful Tool for HR directors assessed on 21/11/2014 on http://www.hrzone.com/topic/business-lifestyle/positive-psychology-useful-tool-hr-directors/135996

Lopez, S.J. and Snyder, C.R. (2003). *Positive Psychological Assessment: A Handbook of Models and Measures*. Washington, DC: American Psychological Association.

Luthans, F. (2002a). The need for and meaning of positive organizational behaviour. *Journal of Organizational Behaviour, Vol. 23*, 695-706.

Luthans, F. (2002b). Positive Organizational Behaviour: Developing and Manageing Psychological Strengths. *Academy of Management Executive, Vol. 16*, 57-72.

Machado, T., Sathyanarayanan, V., Bhola, P. and Kamath, K. (2003). Psychological vulnerability, burnout, and coping among employees of a business process outsourcing organization. *Indian Psychiatry Journal, 22*, 26-31.

Ortner, C.N., Kilner, S.J., and Zelazo, P.D. (2007). Mindfulness Meditation and Reduced Emotional Interference on a Cognitive Task. *Motivation and Emotion, 31*(4), 271-283.

Pandey, S. (2008). Work Stress and Mental Health: Issues and Concerns for HR Managers. In I.S. Singh (Ed.) *Recent Trends in Human Resource Management* (pp. 174-187), Mahatma Gandhi Labour Institute, Ahmedabad.

Paul, H. and Garg, P. (2014). Healing HRM through Positive Psychology: An Outlook. Procedia—Social and Behavioural Sciences Volume 133, 15 May, 2014, pp.141-150 International Conference on Trade, Markets and Sustainability (ICTMS-2013).

Pandey, S.C. (2003). Work Stress in Advertising Professionals of India: A HRD Perspective. In Chiraprapha T. Akaraborworn, Aahad Osman Gani and Gary N. McLean (Eds.) *Human Resource Development in Asia: National Policy Perspectives*. National Institute of Development Administration, Bangkok, Thailand.

Programme on Mental Health. (1997). World Health Organization 1997 assessed on 25/11/2014 on http://www.who.int/mental_health/media/68.pdf

Pugalendhi, S.B., Umaselvi, M. and Senthil Kumar, N.(2010). Quality of Work Life: Perception of College Teachers. *Indian Journal of Commerce and Management Studies, Vol. 2* (1), 47-65.

Ryff, C.D. (2003). Corners of Myopia in the Positive Psychology Parade. *Psychological Inquiry, 14*(2), 153-159.

Sandu, N. and Prabhakar, R. (2012). Factors Influencing the Quality of Work Life in the Indian Banking Industry: An Empirical Study, DOI: 10.7763/ IPEDR. V55. 23, 115-119.

Sarikwal, L. and Gupta, J. (2014). The Relationship between High Performance Work Practices and Organizational Citizenship Behaviour: The Role of Positive Psychological Capital assessed on 26/11/2014 on http://ssrn.com/ abstract=2391596.

Seligman, M.E.P. (1999). The President's Address. *American Psychologist, 54*, 559-562.

Seligman M.E.P. and Csikszentmihalyi, M. (2000) Positive Psychology: An Introduction. *American Psychologist, 55* (1) 5-14.

Seligman M.E.P. (2002). *Authentic Happiness: Using the New Positive Psychology to Realize Your Potential for Lasting Fulfilment*. New York: Free Press.

Seligman M.E.P., Steen, T.A., Park, N. and Peterson, C. (2005). Positive Psychology Progress: Empirical Validation of Interventions. *American Psychologist, 60* (5) 410-21.

Sharma, I.J. (1984). The Culture Context of Indian Managers. *Management and Labour Studies, 9*(2), 72-80.

Sinha, C. (2012). Factors affecting Quality of Work Life: Empirical evidence.

Australian Journal of Business and Management Research, Vol. 1 (11), 31-40.

Sin, N.L., and Lyubomirsky, S. (2009). Enhancing Well-being and Alleviating Depressive Symptoms with Positive Psychology Interventions: A practice-friendly meta-analysis. *Journal of Clinical Psychology*: In Session, *65*, 467-487.

Sparrow, P.R. and Budhwar, P. (1997). Competition and Change: Mapping the Indian HRM Recipe against the World Wide Patterns. *Journal of World Business, 32*, 224-242.

Spreitzer, G. and Cameron, K. (2012). Applying a POS lens to bring out the best in organizations. *Organizational Dynamics, 41*, 81-85.

Sephton, S.E., Salmon, P., Weissbecker, I., Ulmer, C., Floyd, A., Hoover, K., and Studts, J.L. (2007). Mindfulness Meditation Alleviates Depressive Symptoms in Women with Fibromyalgia: Results of a Randomized Clinical Trial. *Arthrites Care and Research, 57*(1), 77-85.

Tayeb, M. (1996). India: A Non Tiger of Asia. *International Business Review, 5*(5), 425-445.

World Health Organization. (2001). *The World Health Report 2001: Mental Health: New Understanding, New Hope*. World Health Organization.

World Health Organization. (2004). Promoting Mental Health: Concepts, Emerging Evidence, Practice: Summary Report.

World Health Organization. (2005). *Mental Health Policies and Programmes in the Workplace*.

Yoder, S. (2013). "Is America Overworked?" *The Fiscal Times*. 16 February, 2012. Web. 4 March, 2013.

13

Positivity

Strength of Human Resources for Mental Health

Subhash Meena

Mental health is defined as a state of well-being in which every individual realizes his or her own potential, can cope with the normal stresses of life, can work productively and fruitfully, and is able to make a contribution to her or his community. The positive dimension of mental health is stressed in WHO's definition of health as contained in its constitution "Health is a state of complete physical, mental and social well-being and not merely the absence of disease or infirmity" (WHO, 1947).

Mental Health: Strengthening Our Response

Mental health and well-being are fundamental to our collective and individual ability as humans to think, emote, interact with each other, earn a living and enjoy life. Hence, the promotion, protection and restoration of mental health can be regarded as a vital concern of individuals, communities and societies throughout the world.

- Mental health is a central element of health; undeniably, there is no health without mental health.
- Mental health is more than the absence of mental disorders.
- Mental health is determined by socio-economic, biological and environmental factors.
- Cost-effective public health and intersector strategies and interventions exist to promote, protect and restore mental health.

Determinants of Mental Health

Multiple social, psychological, and biological factors determine the level of mental health of a person at any point of time. For example, persistent socio-economic pressures are recognized risks to mental health for individuals and communities (Adler *et al.*, 1994; Kawachi and Berkman, 2001). The clearest evidence is associated with indicators of poverty, including low levels of education (Patel and Kleinman, 2003). Poor mental health is also allied with rapid social change, stressful work conditions, and gender discrimination, social exclusion, and unhealthy lifestyle, risks of violence, physical ill-health and human rights violations.

There are also specific psychological and personality factors that make people vulnerable to mental disorders. Lastly, there are some biological causes of mental disorders including genetic factors which contribute to imbalances in chemicals in the brain.

Positive Emotions Enhances Mental Health and Life Satisfaction

When experiencing an episode of depression, there are often some triggering events that lead to a perpetual downward spiral of emotional and physical health. People become more and more engulfed and stressed, and begin to shrink emotionally, physically, and socially, eventually becoming whacked, depressed, and hopeless. Likewise, many negative emotional states lead to a restricted and constricted view of coping strategies and behaviour. Such as, when experiencing fear, stress, or anxiety, the fight or flight response may be the foremost focus of dealing with the emotions. This may be imperative if the person is in immediate danger, but by no means improves mental health when stress and anxiety are chronic. Thus, the big question is.....If negative emotions lead to a narrow view of problem-solving and coping, and when chronic, tend to prompt a downward spiral in mood, could there also be an upward spiral that expands thinking and problem-solving capabilities from experiencing positive emotions? Some of the most enthralling research in positive psychology has come from Barbara Fredrickson (2001) in examining this concept.

Broaden-and-build Theory of Positive Emotions

Fredrickson, best known for her Broaden-and-Build Theory of Positive Emotions, proposes, "that the positive emotions broaden an individual's momentary mindset, and by doing so help to build enduring personal resources" (Fredrickson, 1998, 2003). The experience of positive emotion leads to novel thoughts, activities, and relationships, which in turn provides more personal resources, such as social support, improved skills, and resilience to overcome obstacles (Fredrickson, and Joiner, 2002).

The Broadening Effect: Positive emotions, such as joy, curiosity, hope, and contentment, can broaden the cognitive capacity to be more flexible and receptive to new ideas and novel possibilities. People may be more creative and open-minded, be willing to seek out social support, and develop greater emotional and intellectual resources for problem solving.

The Building Effect: As positive emotions increase and broaden possibilities, relationships, and behaviour, it leads to building greater personal resources. Specifically, have improved health, greater hope, optimism, and better quality relationships. Individual's that discover novel approaches are able to incorporate and establish these resources through expanding social support, learning new skills, increasing knowledge, and applying these when coping with struggles.

The Upward Spiral: The benefits of positive emotions don't stop with broadening options and building resources. They also lead to greater life satisfaction. Because of the growing and enduring resources people start to develop, it leads to greater health, fulfilment, and overall better functioning, which in turn leads to a perpetual upward spiral of positive emotions. In general, people will be in a better situation and more contented, hence leading to more opportunities and the capability to experience more positive emotions. In the culmination of the broadening and building effects of positive emotions on social, physical, and mental resources one is able to build a framework for later use to adequately manage life's threats and obstacles, as well as having more outlets for increasing emotional well-being and finding fulfilment.

How to Increase Positive Emotions Little by Little: Although positive emotions are natural, but it can be quite difficult at times to experience them. However, the researchers suggest that there are a number of things which one can incorporate in one's life to improve the state of mind. Some of them may watch a funny movie and laugh; Write down 5 good things that happened to you today; Engage in an activity or hobby that provides you pleasure; Have fun and talk with friends; Read an inspiring book; Play board games instead of watching television; Start practicing meditation; Doing random acts of kindness; Count your blessings; Exercise.

By starting any of these things one can start experiencing more positive emotions and even such an ordinary boost up can be helpful in the long-run. However, the other side of the coin is the question 'Can people be too happy'.

Can People Be Too Happy? (Oishi, Diener, and Lucas, 2007)

Everyone goes through life in search of happiness. We work to relieve pain, experience pleasure, and reach our goals to be satisfied with our life. But what if we are already pretty happy? Does it serve a purpose to work to find ultra-happiness?

Many believe that success leads to happiness. This sends us on a mission to achieve more, be more, and do more in the name of happiness and living life to the fullest. Research has shown that satisfaction with life is a major indicator of success (Pavot, and Diener, 1993), or in other words, happier people tend to be more successful in certain life domains. Though on closer observation, very high levels of satisfaction can actually limit the achievement of our full potential in certain domains. One research article reveals that the happiest people tend to be most successful when it comes to relationships and volunteer work (Boehm, and Lyubomirsky, 2008; Diener, and Ryan, 2009), but those who were a little less happy were more successful in terms of income, education, and political participation.

So, the question becomes what is success and where do we derive happiness? For some, success is related to income, education and prestige and for others; success is about performing and nurturing meaningful and positive relationships. Our level of satisfaction in these different domains can impact our happiness. For instance, aspiring more and not being fully satisfied is a good motivating force to raise income, education, and political participation. However, when it comes to intimate relationships, desiring more tends to cause problems. Thus, happiness is not always better, or at least complete satisfaction with life, is not always better. It depends on our goals and aspirations. If I desire a meaningful and deep relationship, being satisfied is important to stay committed and passionate; otherwise we will always be looking for something "better". If my desires are for wealth, professional influence, and money, being somewhat dissatisfied will serve me well to stay motivated and striving for progress. In due course, we can merge these findings and find common ground between what we expect from relationships and what we expect in a professional and financial aspect of life.

Do You Have "Complete" Mental Health? (Compton, 2005)

Mental health has long been defined as the absence of psychopathologies, such as depression and anxiety. However, the absence of mental illness is only a minimal outcome from the perspective of positive psychology. The absence of mental illness does not necessarily constitute complete mental health. Someone may not have a mental illness but they may not be satisfied with their life or striving to reach his/her potential. Such people may be surviving, but not thriving.

According to the World Health Organization (2004), mental health is defined as "a state of well-being in which the individual realizes his or her own abilities, can cope with the normal stresses of life, can work productively and fruitfully, and is able to make a contribution to his or her community."

This definition gives an emphasis on the idea of living optimally and gainfully, which relates to a term applied to complete mental health called flourishing. Someone who is flourishing is living with optimal mental health and may be experiencing subjective well-being in most or all of three general domains. These domains of well-being include emotional, psychological, and social.

***Emotional Well-being*:** This is when people are satisfied with their life as a whole. They feel a positive affect and experience high levels of positive emotions. They are cheerful, in good spirits and seem full of life.

***Psychological Well-being*:** Someone with positive psychological functioning would have a sense of purpose and meaning in life; would have self-confidence and feel positively about one's abilities and who they are as a person. There would be argue to persist on personal growth and development, and engage in the world through personal values and convictions.

***Social Well-being*:** Positive social functioning involves having a sense of belonging and acceptance of the world around us. Having a positive attitude toward others and society, and taking an approach that society can be improved and engageing in the world with this motivation.

Mental Illness and Subjective Well-being

Even with these areas of well-being in mind, we cannot overlook the mental and emotional distress that emerges in our life. A model developed by Keyes and Lopez (2002) explains how mental illness and subjective well-being can be examined concurrently by categorizing their prevalence into four basic dimensions:

I. ***Flourishing*** – Someone who is high on subjective well-being and low on mental illness.

II. ***Languishing*** – Someone who is low on subjective well-being and low on mental illness.
III. ***Struggling*** – Someone who is high on subjective well-being, but also high on mental illness.
IV. ***Floundering*** – Someone who is low on subjective well-being and high on mental illness.

Research data to date indicates that flourishing, a fundamental element of complete mental health and is a looked-for stipulation that any community, corporation, or government would want to protect or promote in its citizens. Results from studies by Keyes (2004, 2005a) reported that adults with a mental illness who also had either moderate mental health or flourishing reported more workdays missed or more work cutbacks than languishing adults (Keyes, 2004). Overall there is a low prevalence of flourishing in the American adult population. Adults who were completely mentally healthy had the lowest number of chronic physical conditions at all ages and the youngest adults who were languishing had the same number of chronic physical conditions as older flourishing adults.

Why Happiness is a Journey, Not a Destination (Mauss *et al.*, 2011)

When asked to people what their biggest motivation is, what would be the answer? Would it be to be successful, to have loving relationships, to make a difference in the world, or to be wealthy? Maybe it's all of the above—though there is one common denominator for all of these, i.e. to be happy. We all want to be happy?

Some would say the search for happiness is the greatest motivator of humankind. For many people this is the prime goal of their life. We do what we do in the hopes that we will ultimately find greater happiness. It is instinctive to think that if we cherish happiness so much, we would eventually be happier. Unfortunately, when happiness is our end goal and we approach it this way, it may lead to less happiness. There is a paradoxical effect between the goal and our evaluation of the outcome. The more we value happiness the more likely we are to expect happiness and to set higher happiness standards that are difficult to obtain. Place a high value on happiness leads to be disappointed because our level of happiness won't meet our expectations. This is particularly true in situations where there is little stress and where happiness would seem to be most in reach. There is nothing to attribute our lack of happiness to, and we may assume "I should be happier!" This only takes away from our potential of experiencing greater joy, contentment, and pleasure.

So, what does this mean if we want to flourish and experience greater happiness? Should you just neglect this natural tendency and not worry about what happens in life? Certainly not, but it will entail learning and developing a happiness plan. A plan where anyone can stick on to deliberate actions and make mindful attempts to alter the way of one's life. There are five interventions that may help in developing a greater quality of life.

Learning to be Grateful– Research indicates that 'grateful' appears to be highly valued trait to people and gratitude is important to people (Gallup, 1998). In a study of over 800 descriptive trait words 'grateful' was rated in the top four per cent terms of likeability (Dumas, Johnson, and Lynch, 2002). Focusing on what you're grateful or thankful for is a major way to begin experiencing more happiness. People who keep a gratitude and appreciation diary generally see a rise in their happiness within a few weeks. The idea is simple. Just write down 3-5 things that you appreciate, and hope to see continue. Write a brief note about how those good things came about. Try to make an entry every few days, or at least once or twice a week.

Building on Strengths – Peterson, and Seligman (2004) developed a list of virtues or personal strengths. These core virtues are widely valued (Dahlsgaard, Peterson, and Seligman, 2005) with nearly universal acceptance. These virtues are: wisdom, courage, humanity, justice, temperance, and transcendence. Research now suggests if you develop your strong areas, you will be more productive and happy. Write each night about what you did to work on your strengths. Pick the top two or three strengths in yourself and do something each day that "plays to" that strength.

Lifestyle Skills – There is a strong relationship between diet, physical activity, sleep and mood (Fox, 1999). If you want to be happier get adequate sleep, eat a well balanced diet and avoid drugs, alcohol, and caffeine, spare time to exercise at least three times per week, even if it is just going for a walk for 20-30 minutes.

Random Kindness – In our high-speed, high pressure society we are encouraged to take care of ourselves and not worry about others. This has become such a habit that we have forgotten how to be kind to strangers for the sheer pleasure of helping a fellow human being (Baskerville *et al.*, 2000). Otake and associates (2006) reported that kind people experience more happiness and have happier memories. Simply by counting the acts of kindness for one week, people appear to have become happier and more grateful.

Meditation – Meditation can help in relaxation, stay in the moment, and be more mindful of thinking and emotions. Many people use meditation to treat stress and stress-related conditions, as well as to promote general health. Meditative techniques are categorized as emphasizing "mindfulness", "concentration" and "automatic self-transcendence." After reviewing 17,801 citations, Goyal and associates (2014) included 47 trials with 3,320 participants and reported that mindfulness meditation programmes had moderate evidence to improve anxiety at 8 weeks; depression and pain at 8 weeks; and low evidence to improve stress/distress and mental health-related quality of life (Goyal *et al.*, 2014). However, developing a meditation practice can be a great way to cope with a fast-paced life and cultivate more positive emotions.

Mental Health Care and Treatment

In the context of national efforts to develop and implement mental health policy, it is vital to not only protect and promote the mental well-being of its citizens, but also address the needs of persons with defined mental disorders. Knowledge of what to do about the escalating burden of mental disorders has improved substantially over the past decade. There is a growing body of evidence demonstrating both the efficacy and cost-effectiveness of key interventions for priority mental disorders in countries at different levels of economic development. Examples of interventions that are cost-effective, feasible, and affordable include:

- treatment of epilepsy with anti-epileptic drugs;
- treatment of depression with (generically produced) anti-depressant drugs and brief psychotherapy;
- treatment of psychosis with older anti-psychotic drugs plus psychosocial support; and
- Taxation of alcoholic beverages and restriction of their availability and marketing.

A range of effective measures also exists for the prevention of suicide, prevention and treatment of mental disorders in children, prevention and treatment of dementia, and treatment of substance-use disorders. The WHO Mental Health Global Action Programme (MHGAP, 2001) has produced evidence based guidelines for non-specialists to enable them in identification and management of mental health priority conditions.

Mental Health and Psychosocial Support (MHPSS)

Composite term used to describe any type of local or outside support that aims to protect or promote psychosocial well-being and/or prevent or treat mental disorder (IASC, 2007). This may include support interventions in the health sector, education, community services, and protection and in other sectors.

The ways in which people experience and respond to loss, pain, disruption and violence vary significantly and in various ways affect their mental health and psychosocial well-being or increase their vulnerability to develop mental health problems. Often, reactions to disruptive situations are normal and can be overcome with time. Many individuals will be able to cope with these difficult experiences, and even build resilience, if a supportive family and community environment is available.

Some people may develop negative coping mechanisms that may be reinforced while they struggle to meet basic needs. Some will newly develop mental disorders while others with pre-existing mental disorders may experience exacerbation of their symptoms. The usual systems for providing mental health care may be negatively affected, leaving people with mental disorders without adequate treatment. Mitigating immediate and long-term risks and consequences for mental health and psychosocial well-being of individuals, families and communities are an integral part of protection mandate.

MHPSS problems in humanitarian contexts can be addressed through activities such as supporting communities' resilience, promoting mechanisms for social support, and offering services to individuals with more complex mental health needs. Adopting an MHPSS approach means providing a humanitarian response in ways that are beneficial to the mental health and psychosocial well-being of whole nation. This is relevant for all actors involved in the protection of and assistance to individuals who are facing mental health problems. MHPSS interventions consist of activities with a primary goal to improve the mental health and psychosocial well-being of peoples. MHPSS interventions are usually implemented in the sectors for health, community-based protection and education.

Mental Health Services

Services offered with the goal of improving individuals and families' mental health and functioning with a particular focus on mental disorders.

Services may include psychotherapy, medication, counselling, behavioural treatment etc. In many national health systems the term 'mental health services' include services for people with neurological disorders such as epilepsy and dementia.

Psychosocial: The term psychosocial suggests the shared relation involving psychological factors (the way an individual feels, thinks and acts) and social factors (related to the environment or context in which the person lives: the family, the community, the state, religion, culture) (PSW, 2003). Psychosocial is an adjective that needs to be followed by a noun, e.g. a psychosocial problem, a psychosocial intervention, a psychosocial approach.

Psychosocial Support (PSS): Psychosocial support incorporates entire processes and actions that uphold the holistic well-being of people in their social world. It comprises the support bestowed by family, friends and the wider community. It can be employed to illustrate what people (individuals, families and communities) do themselves to care for their psychosocial well-being, and to describe the interventions by outsiders to serve the psychological, social, emotional and practical needs of individuals, families, and communities, with the goal of protecting, promoting and improving psychosocial well-being.

Guiding Principles to Utilize Mental Health Resources

1. ***Use Rights-based, Community-based and Participatory Approaches***: Government, NGOs and other partners need to make certain that people with mental health problems and as well as other groups including children, youth, women, older persons, sexual and other minorities, groups with specific needs, are engaged in various steps of design and execution of the MHPSS activities. A participatory approach that try to link-up people's participation to programme design, and feedback; a community-based approach that acknowledges the resilience, capacities, skills and resources of the peoples, and concentrates on spotting and developing community capacities for self-protection; a rights-based approach that needs to vigorously functioning towards the awareness of human rights of peoples, looking for rectifying discriminatory practices and unfair distributions of power that hamper the development progress and make sure that plans, policies and processes of development are fasten in a system of rights and corresponding commitments

set up by international law. The relevant agencies should consult the community and people with mental and psychosocial problems when designing services. Community consultation should be the norm rather than the exception when designing and implementing interventions for mental and psychosocial problems. Moreover, advocacy for the economic and social rights of people with mental health and psychosocial problems should also be done.

2. ***Ensure Equity of Care and Access***: All concerned persons should have right to use to quality mental health and psychosocial support. This must be make available to recipient in ways that are similar to the services available to the rest of the population and with no less than quality and at similar or lower costs and devoid of discrimination within the community. There may be reasons like stigmatization, shame, social marginalization and lack of information; why people with mental and psychosocial problems would not receive the assistance they need. In addition, the monitoring of which group access to services and which do not is also required. The concerned agencies should also ensure that people have information about available services and supports for mental health and psychosocial problems. This can be done by taking appropriate steps to inform the target population about the availability and location of these services and support. People with mental disorders and psychosocial problems and their families may fear that seeking help for such problems makes them vulnerable to discrimination and rejection in the communities. In the design of services, it is important to minimize any interventions that may cause stigma and discrimination. For example, ensure confidentiality using designated consultation rooms and provide MHPSS promotion messages in non-stigmatizing language. Ensure that people with specific MHPSS needs are able to access basic services. In some cases, it may be necessary to conduct outreach to excluded groups, who may be unaware of MHPSS services, or may not have access due to physical or social barriers. Examples of potential measures are: Arrange for peer-support if children have difficulties to access education, for example because a child or parent is too afraid of the walk to an educational facility; include messages of equal access to services in any sensitization messages in the community; advocate for medication for chronic

mental, neurological or substance use (MNS) conditions that are affordable to all, by making them either free of charge or available at subsidized rates.

3. ***Assess Needs and Resources***: MHPSS programmes should be based on systematic and inclusive assessment of needs. This includes the perspectives of various stakeholders including girls and boys, youth, women, men, older people and different cultural, religious and socio-economic groups. Assessments with a narrow perspective, such as focusing only on one mental disorder such as Posttraumatic Stress Disorder (PTSD), do not provide the data needed to design a salient and comprehensive MHPSS programme. Hence, to use a broad definition of mental health and psychosocial problems is appropriate as well as the collection and analysis of existing information leads to avoid duplicating assessments. Uses of the tools that are appropriate to the specific community setting also provide useful information. Usually, qualitative methods are best suited to quickly get an understanding of the most urgent problems and the way various stakeholders perceive these problems. To increase the likelihood that any humanitarian response builds on the supports, resources and capacities that are already there, assessment of available resources for MHPSS, both formal and informal resources is important.
4. ***Use a Systems Approach***: MHPSS programmes should be conceptualized through a systems-based approach with multiple layers of complementary supports with functional referral systems between the different layers. Different people will have different types of needs (ranging from preventive and promotion services to specialized treatments), and it is crucial that the diversity of needs are taken into consideration. It is equally important to promote a balanced and justified use of resources. Therefore, MHPSS activities should be developed within a system of multiple layers of complementary supports with referral systems.

Conclusion

Positive emotions, such as joy, curiosity, hope, and contentment, can broaden the cognitive capacity to be more flexible and receptive to new ideas and novel possibilities. Adopting an MHPSS approach means providing a humanitarian response in ways that are beneficial to the mental health and psychosocial well-being of whole nation. This is relevant for all actors involved in the protection of and assistance to individuals who are facing mental health problems. As positive emotion increase and broaden possibilities, relationships, and behaviour, it leads to building greater personal resources. Specifically, have improved health, greater hope, optimism, and better quality relationships. Individual's that discover novel approaches are able to incorporate and establish these resources through expanding social support, learning new skills, increasing knowledge, and applying these when coping with struggles.

References

Adler, N.E., Boyce, T., Chesney, M.A., Cohen, S., Folkman, S., Kahn, R.L., and Syme, S.L. (1994). Socio-economic status and health: the challenge of the gradient. *American Psychologist, 49*(1), 15.

Baskerville, K., Johnson, K., Monk-Turner, E., Slone, Q., Standley, H., Stansbury, S., and Young, J. (2000). Reactions to random acts of kindness. *The Social Science Journal, 37*(2), 293-298.

Boehm, J.K., and Lyubomirsky, S. (2008). Does happiness promote career success? *Journal of Career Assessment, 16*(1), 101-116.

Compton, W.C. (2005). *An Introduction to Positive Psychology*. Belmont, CA. Wadsworth, Cengage Learning.

Dahlsgaard, K., Peterson, C., and Seligman, M.E.P. (2005). Shared Virtue: The convergence of valued human strengths across culture and history. *Review of General Psychology, 9*, 209-213.

Diener, E., and Ryan, K. (2009). Subjective well-being: A General Overview. *South African Journal of Psychology, 39*(4), 391-406.

Dumas, J.E., Johnson, M. and Lynch, A.M. (2002). Likableness, familiarity, and frequency of 844 person-descriptive words. *Personality and Individual Differences, 32*, 523-531.

Fox, K.R. (1999). The influence of physical activity on mental well-being. *Public Health Nutrition, 2*(3a), 411-418.

Fredrickson, B.L. (2001). The role of positive emotions in positive psychology: The broaden-and-build theory of positive emotions. *American Psychologist, 56*(3), 218.

Fredrickson, B.L. (1998). What good are positive emotions? *Review of General Psychology, 2*(3), 300.

Fredrickson, B.L., and Joiner, T. (2002). Positive emotions trigger upward spirals toward emotional well-being. *Psychological Science, 13*(2), 172-175.

Fredrickson, B.L. (2003). The Value of Positive Emotions. *American Scientist, 91*(4), 330-339.

Gallup, G. (1998). Gallup survey results on "gratitude", adults and teenagers.

Emerging Trends, 20 (4-5), 9.

Goyal, M., Singh, S., Sibinga, E.M., Gould, N.F., Rowland-Seymour, A., Sharma, R., and Haythornthwaite, J.A. (2014). Meditation programmes for psychological stress and well-being: A systematic review and meta-analysis. *JAMA Internal Medicine, 174*(3), 357-368.

IASC (2007). *IASC Guidelines on Mental Health and Psychosocial Support in Emergency Settings*. Geneva: Inter-Agency Standing Committee.

Kawachi, I., and Berkman, L.F. (2001). Social ties and mental health. *Journal of Urban Health, 78*(3), 458-467.

Keyes, C.L.M. and Lopez, S. (2002). Toward a science of mental health: Positive directions in diagnosis and treatment. In C.R. Snyder and S.J. Lopez (eds.), *The Handbook of Positive Psychology* (pp. 45-59). New York: Oxford University Press.

Keyes, C.L.M. (2004). The nexus of cardiovascular disease and depression revisited: The complete mental health perspective and the moderating role of age and gender. *Ageing and Mental Health, 8*, 266-274.

Keyes, C.L.M. (2005a). Chronic physical conditions and ageing: Is mental health a potential protective factor? *Ageing International*, 30, 88-104.

Mauss, I.B., Tamir, M., Anderson, C.L., and Savino, N.S. (2011). Can Seeking Happiness Make People Unhappy? Paradoxical Effects of Valuing Happiness. *Emotions, 11* (4), 807-815.

Oishi, S., Diener, E., and Lucas, R.E. (2007). The Optimum Level of Well-Being: Can People Be Too Happy? *Association for Psychological Sciences, 2*(4), 346-359.

Otake, K., Shimai, S., Tanaka-Matsumi, J., Otsui, K., and Fredrickson, B.L. (2006). Happy people become happier through kindness: A counting kindnesses intervention. *Journal of Happiness Studies, 7*(3), 361-375.

Patel, V., and Kleinman, A. (2003). Poverty and common mental disorders in developing countries. *Bulletin of the World Health Organization, 81*(8), 609-615.

Peterson, C., and Seligman, M.E. (2004). *Character Strengths and Virtues: A Handbook and Classification*. Oxford University Press.

Pavot, W., and Diener, E. (1993). Review of the satisfaction with life scale. *Psychological assessment, 5*(2), 164.

PSW (2003). *Psychosocial Intervention in Complex Emergencies: A Framework for Practice*. Edinburgh: Psychosocial Working Group: The Psychosocial Working Group Centre for International Health Studies Queen Margaret University College, Edinburgh. EH12 8TS United Kingdom. http://www.forcedmigration.org/

WHO and UNHCR. (2013). *Assessment and Management of Conditions Specifically Related to Stress*.mhGAP Intervention Guide Module. Geneva: World Health Organization and United Nations High Commissioner for Refugees.

World Health Organization. (2004). *Promoting Mental Health: Concepts, emerging evidence, practice* (Summary Report). Geneva: WHO.

14

Wellness Among Elderly

A Study in Institutionalized Homes

Archana Shukla and *Shilpa Singh*

Old age is considered to be the evening phase of life. But few can understand the beauty of this quiet evening. There are numerous joys which only an elderly can enjoy. The utmost satisfaction from life, a relaxed routine, joy of being a grandparent, knowledge and experience only years can give and last, but not the least, a wiser mind and peaceful solitude—these are the advantages only elderly can enjoy. However, today not only youth, even elderly pay more attention to deteriorating health, and cope with feelings of being unproductive, unwanted (especially by children) and dejection from society.

Life is a beautiful journey spanning across various stages. Out of all the stages, childhood and old age are considered to be the most crucial ones. And the reason is quite obvious; in both these periods, a human being is vulnerable and needs care and support from others to sustain himself; both physically and emotionally. An individual who in his youthful days, acts as a financial and emotional supporter of his family, becomes a responsibility for the family himself in his old age. During later years of life, it becomes the duty of the whole family to look after elderly physical as well as psychological requirements, which remain overtly unproductive in the eyes of the family and society at large.

Across the world, declining fertility and increased longevity have jointly resulted in higher numbers and proportions of older persons 60 years and above. This trend will continue as the estimated 737 million older persons in 2009 (United Nations, 2009) is likely to increase to two billion by 2050 at which time the population aged 60 and above will outnumber children (0-14 years of age). The oldest-old age segment (80 years and above) is the fastest-growing segment and by 2050, about 20 per cent of older persons will be 80 years and above. The coming decades, therefore, are characterized by ageing of the aged (Subaiya and Bansod, 2011).

Not only around the globe, ageing population has led to the birth of grave concerns in India also, where it is one of the fastest growing sections of the population. In India, the proportion of the population aged 60 years and above was 7 per cent in 2009 and was projected to increase to 20 per cent by the year 2050. In absolute numbers, the elderly population in 2009 was approximately 88 million and is expected to sharply increase to more than 315 million by 2050 (Subaiya and Bansod, 2011).

An overview of the above aspects of ageing suggests that an elderly goes through a lot of problems which are unique to old age. Majority of them face challenges like physical helplessness, economic insecurity, unsatisfactory living conditions, problems in making new friends and in developing new leisure activities, lesser involvement in community activities and easily targeted for being victimized (Hurlock, 1989). All these problems, if eradicated, can enhance an elderly spheres of health, well-being, social and attitudinal behaviour, spirituality etc. which lead to a lifelong development and fruitfully results in overall wellness.

Wellness: The Western Perspective

The term wellness is used by various people and organizations since the sharp rise in health care costs, diabetes and obesity during the past decade. Traditionally, wellness has been viewed as freedom from disease, however, in modern times, this perspective is changing. Wellness doesn't remain mere absence of disease, rather it is a proactive, preventive approach designed to achieve optimum levels of health, social and emotional functioning. It indeed is a positive approach to living—an approach that emphasizes the whole person.

Wellness has a very important work to do. It integrates mind, body and spirit of an individual to produce a balanced lifestyle (Pufal, 2001). A wellness oriented lifestyle encourages adopting habits and behaviours that promote better health and an improved quality of life. In every stage of life, wellness plays an important and influential role. However, it becomes much more crucial during old age. During this stage of life, the age related changes put a major impact on an individual's overall behaviour and the strategies of coping with life.

Wellness is easily misunderstood with the term well-being. In fact well-being is only a part of wellness. Wellness is a 7 dimensional process and a state of well-being while well-being is "*a subjective perception of vitality and feeling well... can be described objectively, experienced and measures... and can be plotted on a continuum*" (Hood and Leddy, 2002). However, wellness becomes much more important issue than others because it focuses on an overall growth of individual towards a positive living.

The term wellness is used in everyday language; however, it is not an easy concept to define. Larson (1999) states that the WHO (1948) was the first to give a holistic definition of health and many subsequent conceptualizations of wellness include this central concept. Oliphant (2001) explains that suggestions by WHO (1967) that health has a positive component led to the now widely used term 'wellness'.

However, the terminology of wellness was introduced by Dunn (1961) in the book "High Level Wellness" (Ardell, 1984). He defined wellness as an "integrated method of functioning which is oriented towards maximizing the potential of which, the individual is capable. It requires that the individual maintains a continuum of balance and purposeful direction within the environment where he is functioning" (Dunn, 1961). He emphasized wellness as a positive state, one that is beyond simply non-sickness, the detailed, the interconnected nature of wellness of the mind, body and environment, which exists as a dynamic equilibrium as one tries to balance between each. After Dunn (1961), many others came up with their own definition of the term.

To summarize, despite the term wellness becoming increasingly popular and applied for, there is interestingly, no universally acceptable definition of wellness. That said, a definition by Corbin (2002) can be overviewed—"wellness is a multi-dimensional state of being, describing the existence of positive health in an individual as exemplified by quality of life and a sense of well-being."

The wellness of an individual is affected by various influential factors. As the term wellness has multidimensional aspects like physical, mental, social, emotional etc., the factors affecting wellness are also of different categories.

Factors Affecting Wellness

1. *Physical Wellness Factors*—heredity, regular exercise, stress, living style, progressive overloading, balanced diet, smoking and drugs, rest, recreation and relaxation and environment.
2. *Social Wellness Factors*—peer acceptance, attachments/bonds

with others, and social skills (communication, assertiveness, conflict resolution), quality and extent of one's social network (Durlak, 2000), nature of relational styles and patterns, focusing on one's attitude toward relationships and seeking help from others (Crose *et al.*, 1992).

3. *Emotional Wellness Factors*—coping and manageing skills, emotional stability, self-esteem, maintaining optimistic dispositions, friendship network and personal stress management/reduction behaviour.
4. *Intellectual Wellness Factors*—critical thinking, ability to adapt to change, ability to access resources, problem solving, creativity, mental status and abilities or challenges, education and learning goals (*UBC Health and Wellness Guide*, 2010).
5. *Environmental Wellness Factors*—(i) Positive Factors (source of nutrition, water, ozone layer, sanitation/waste recycling, air quality, space for exercise and recreation) and (ii) Negative Factors (environmental disruptions, human changes, disruption caused by war and violence).
6. *Spiritual Wellness Factors*—purpose and meaning in life, unifying interconnectedness and private religious practices (Gill, Minton and Myers, 2010).

Wellness: An Indian Perspective

Wellness, considered to be a recently introduced term in West, has been rooted since ancient times in the Hindu culture. The Indian perspective of wellness has been discussed next to gain a clearer understanding of the origin of the terminology.

In India, wellness is a concept which has been in vogue since ancient times. This term, despite being in prominent usage in the Western culture, has its roots in India. Traditional, medicinal and health practices like Ayurveda and yoga, which are believed to be born in the foothills of the Himalayas and practiced by sages and monks, have propounded the concept of mental and bodily wellness.

Most of the ancient wellness concepts have largely focused on the basic needs of an individual within the need hierarchy, namely a focus on health, nutrition and relaxation. However, with the progress of time, wellness as a concept has taken up a multi-dimensional definition, encompassing the individual's desire for social acceptance, exclusivity and collective welfare. In recent years, the notion of "wellness" has increasingly become more ingrained as part of a healthy lifestyle, complementing scientific and medical approaches to health.

It has been observed that the term 'wellness' was introduced in the West rather recently in the early 60s (Dunn, 1961). However, the Indian ancient culture and manuscripts depict a wide usage of terms which all lead to wellness, without using the term directly. For example, health is a concept widely and deeply studied in the Indian culture. It is considered to be the first prerequisite for all attainments of life (Ratan, 1997).

Our ancient scriptures also mention health as fruits of one's '*Karmic deeds*' while disease is the consequence of evil deeds (*Chanakyaneeti*, 300 B.C.; *Yajurveda*; ch.1; 20). The Vedic period construed health more as '*kalyan*' (well-being). In one of the Vedic *mantras*, health is defined as:

> सर्वे भवन्तु सुखिनः सर्वे सन्तु निरामयाः।
> सर्वे भद्राणि पश्यन्तु मा कश्चिद्दुःख भाग भवेत।।
> *Sarve Bhavantu sukhinah, sarve santu niramayah,*
> *sarve bhadrani pashyantu, ma kashchid dukha bhag bhavet.*
> (One should claim for well-being for all, in everyone's well-being lies our well-being. Hence, we should aspire for well-being of humanity and mankind; this will itself bring well-being, peace and health to all of us.)

In every stage of life, wellness plays an important and influential role. However, it becomes much more crucial during old age. During this stage of life, the age related changes put a major impact on an individual's overall behaviour and the strategies they apply for coping with life. The challenges aggravate when elderly are forced to spend later years of life in an old age home.

Elderly Life in Institutionalized Homes

Indian society has traditional informal support systems such as joint family, kin and community. Here, family is idealized as an institution that could take care of the older persons. However, due to modernization and globalization, the capacity of the traditional informal support system is gradually weakening and is not in a position to fulfil even the basic needs of the elderly (Dube, 1999). A lot of reasons emerge which lead elderly to reside in institutions like migration of the younger generation, lack of proper care within a family, insufficient housing especially in urban area, economic hardships and breakup in joint family system.

While the Western countries have a fairly well organized network of institutions for the care of elderly, the growth and development of these facilities in India, which began as early as 1901, still remain inadequate. In 1998, India had 728 old age homes, but as per recent statistics, there are 1018 old age homes in India. Out of these 427 homes are free of cost while 153 old age homes are on a pay and stay basis, 146 homes have both free as well as pay and stay facilities and detailed information is not available for 292 homes. A total of 371 old age homes all-over the country are available for the sick and 118 homes are exclusive for women. A majority of old age homes are concentrated in the developed states. As far as Delhi is concerned, it has more than 40 old age homes, besides 2 in Noida, 3 in Faridabad and 1 in Ghaziabad. Most of them are pay-and-stay homes run by either government or by NGOs (*Directory of Old Age Homes in India*, 2002).

As is evident, the needs and issues of elderly population have been immense. A lot of physical and psychosocial problems emerge in the later years of life. However, the situations get worsened when due to circumstances, elderly are forced to leave the secure boundaries of their abode and loved ones to live their sunset years in an old age home.

Wellness Across Institutionalized Homes: A Research Report

To study the level of wellness of elderly in institutionalized homes, a study was conducted in some reputed institutionalized homes of Delhi. The basic framework was to explore wellness among institutionalized elderly with the help of a wellness measure on 200 elderly (100 males, 100 females).

A glance at the results depicted a profound level of wellness for both the genders. Further, moving on towards dimensions that make-up wellness, similar trend for both males and females emerged on most of the dimensions. However, in case of physical and social wellness, gender differences were observed.

Physical wellness includes physical activity, nutrition, and self-care, and involves preventative and proactive actions that take care of one's physical body. As revealed by the results, male elderly were mentioned to be more advantaged with physical wellness as compared to female elderly (Chou & Chi, 1999; Smith & Baltes, 1998). Males were observed to accomplish higher intensity physical activity than women. While women pass their time in smaller groups, engageing in household activities, male form larger groups and engage in more active things like walking and social work etc. In a cultural context, Indian females are conditioned from an early age to pay more attention towards the male members of the family, either it be father, brother, husband or son. This leads to a self-implicated neglect towards maintaining their health. Costa and McCrae (1980) also state that the people who grow older are inclined to maintain the same habits, personality and style of life they developed in earlier years.

As far as social wellness is concerned, it encompasses the degree and quality of interactions with others, the community, and nature and includes the extent to which a person works towards supporting the community and environment in everyday actions, such as volunteer work etc. Males were reported to be higher also on social wellness as compared to females. The findings are in strong contradiction of the previous findings and the popular beliefs (Benenson *et al.*, 2013). In an attempt to arrive at a probable outcome of the finding, it may be stated that in an institutionalized setting, males gradually understand the importance of social ties to avoid a state of isolation and loneliness. Also, as females suffer from poorer physical health, they are unable to connect socially at a great extent, despite of being intrinsically more socially active than males. Therefore, males get an advantage of better health as compared to females. In the Indian scenario, males are increasingly becoming aware of being isolated if they don't extend an effort towards maintaining fulfilling social relationships. The results find a theoretical base in the *Subculture of Ageing Theory* (1962) which states that elderly, when excluded from younger age groups, form strong communities with people who share a common background.

Moving further, no significant gender differences were observed for emotional wellness, environmental wellness, spiritual wellness, intellectual wellness and overall wellness. In other words, gender was found to play an insignificant role in the level of wellness among institutionalized elderly on a major basis.

Emotional wellness is conceptualized as awareness and control of feelings, whereas intellectual wellness is the degree to which one engages in creative and stimulating activities. Renger *et al.* (2000) have put special emphasis on the importance of environmental wellness which considers the nature of an individual's reciprocal interaction with the environment on a global level including home, work, community, and nature. Lastly, spiritual wellness is the process of seeking meaning and purpose in existence and includes the appreciation of the depth and expanse of life.

Conclusion

Overall, the emerged picture further strengthens the fact that wellness plays an influential role in the life of institutionalized elderly. Males portrayed higher wellness and their lives were enriched with physical and social wellness. They were found to be cautious and self-regulatory towards their physical health and fitness. Also, despite being isolated and rejected, they have managed to maintain their social relationships to a satisfactory extent. Taking up miniature steps, they have tried to maintain various aspects of wellness in their day-to-day life.

Implications

In the present social scenario, wellness has emerged as the prime requisite for elderly on a universal basis and not specifically for the institutionalized elderly. The geriatric population is facing a lot of challenges—socially as well as emotionally. Therefore, issues related to upholding wellness among the institutionalized elderly are of prime importance. Findings of the present research can be fruitfully applied to facilitate the overall enhancement of wellness during later years of life. Plans and policies may be formed in terms of increasing the wellness and executing researches and programmes focusing towards the geriatric population. The need of the hour is not just to add more theoretical research but to provide some intervention and action research on elderly. Researches of applied orientation would provide a platform for social scientists, paramedical, counsellors and social workers to provide handholding to the elderly. Sixty-seven years of Indian Independence has brought about medical advancements, increased longevity and health, but increasing level of social negligence and breaking joint family system has led them to go for options like institutionalized homes, a concept not much appraised in the Indian society. An institutionalized home can provide a physical environment and surrounding but cannot fill up for the voids created by the distance from the most loved people of life—those who constitute family. An initiation from the significant others in life is required to help elderly deal with negative circumstances of life. There is no hiding from the fact that these economically independent, educated and elite elderly who have lived all their life in worldly comforts and sometimes in luxury are left alone devastated and isolated by the younger generation. And therefore, as a matter of fact, it is the young generation who must understand that elderly are the backbone of the family and without these experienced and seasoned roots, we would not survive in the long run.

During the sunset phase of life, elderly, often considered 'unproductive mouths to feed', lack flexibility and have firm beliefs and thought process. However, providing unconditional positive regard can help minimize the feeling of isolation and lack of worthiness.

References

Adams, T., Bezner, J., and Steinhardt, M. (1997). The Conceptualization and Measurement of Perceived Wellness: Integrating balance across and within dimensions. *American Journal of Health Promotion, 11*, 208-218.

Ardell, D.B. (1984). Perspectives on the History and Future of Wellness. Wellness Perspectives: *Journal of Individual Family and Community Wellness*, *1*(1), 3-23.

Ardell, D.B. (2010). The History of Wellness Models retrieved from, http://www.seekwellness.com/wellness_models.htm

Benenson, J.F., Markovits, H., Hultgren, B., Nguyen, T., and Bullock, G., *et al.* (2013). *Social Exclusion: More Important to Human Females than Males*. PLoS ONE 8(2): e55851. doi:10.1371/journal.pone.0055851

Chou, K.L. and Chi, I., (1999). "Determinants of life satisfaction in Hong Kong Chinese elderly: A longitudinal study." *Ageing and Mental Health*, Vol. 3, pp. 328-335.

Corbin, C.B. *et al.*, (2004). Definitions: Health, Fitness and Physical Activity. In C.B. Corbin *et al.* (Eds.) *Toward a Better Understanding of Physical Fitness and Activity, Selected Topics,* Volume II. Scottsdale, AZ: Holcomb Hathaway.

Costa, P.T., and McCrae, R.R. (1980). Influence of Extraversion and Neuroticism on Subjective Well-being: Happy and Unhappy People. *Journal of Personality and Social Psychology, 38*, 668-678.

Crose, R., Nicholas, D.R., Gobble, D.C., and Frank, B. (1992). Gender and Wellness: A multidimensional systems model for counselling. *Journal of Counselling and Development, 71*, 149-156.

Directory of Old Age Homes in India (2002). Help Age India, Research and Strategic Development Department, Help Age India, New Delhi.

Dube, A.K. (1999). The Angst of Ageing. Nutrition. A Quarterly Publication of NIN, *ICMR. 33* (4), 22-25.

Dunn, Halbert L. (1961). *High Level Wellness*. Arlington, VA: R.W. Beatty, Ltd.

Durlak, J.A. (2000). Health promotion as a strategy in primary prevention. In D. Cicchetti, J. Rappaport, I. Sandler, and R.P. Weissberg (Eds.), *The Promotion of Wellness in Children and Adolescents* (pp. 221-241). Washington, DC: CWLA Press.

Gill, C.S., Minton, C.A.B., and Myers, J.E. (2010). Spirituality and Religiosity: Factors affecting wellness among low-income, rural women. *Journal of Counselling and Development*, *88*, 293-302.

Hettler, W. (1979). *Six Dimensions of Wellness*. Stevens Point, WI: National Wellness Institute, University of Wisconsin.

Hood, L.O. and Leddy, S.K. (2002). Leddy and Peppers Conceptual Basis of Professional Nursing, 5th edition Philadelphia, Lippincott Williams and Wilkins.

Hurlock, E.B., (1989). *Developmental Psychology: A Life Span Approach*, 5th edition, Tata McGraw Hill, 1981.

Larson, J.S. (1999). The Conceptualization of Health. *Medical Care Research and Review*, Vol. *56* (2), 123-136.

Oliphant, L.E. (2001). Toward a Uniform Definition of Wellness: A Commentary. *Research Digest Series 3*, 15.

Pufal, S.L. (2001). *Enhancing the Wellness of Reserve Forces: A Strategic Challenge*. Strategy Research Project, USAWC Qadri.

Renger, R.F., Midyett, S.J., Mas, F.G., Erin, T.E., McDermott, H.M., Papenfuss, R.L., Eichling, P.S., Baker, D.H., Johnson, K.A., and Hewitt, M.J. (2000). Optimal Living Profile: An inventory to assess health and wellness. *American Journal of Health Promotion, 24*(6) 403-412.

Smith, J. and Baltes, M.M. (1998). The Role of Gender in Very Old Age: Profiles of Functioning and Everyday Life Patterns. *Psychological Ageing. 13*(4), 676-695.

Subaiya, L. and Bansod, D.W. (2011). *Demographics of Population Ageing in India: Trends and Differentials,* BKPAI Working Paper No. 1, United Nations Population Fund (UNFPA), New Delhi.

UBC Health and Wellness Guide (2010). UBC division of health care communications, Vancouver BC.

United Nations (2009). *World Population Prospects: The 2008 Revision*. New York: United Nations.

Witmer, J.M. and Sweeney, T.J. (1992). A Holistic Model for Wellness and Prevention Over the Lifespan. *Journal of Counselling and Development, 71*, 140-148.

WHO (1948). Preamble to the Constitution of the World Health Organization as adopted by the International Health Conference, New York, 19-22 June, 1946; signed on 22 July 1946 by the representatives of 61 States (Official Records of the World Health Organization, No. 2. p.100) and entered into force on 7 April, 1948.

WHO (1967) Shodhganga. infibnet.ac.in/[spui/bitstream/10603/124/11_chapter 2.pdf

15

Mental Health and Death Anxiety in Old Age

Bharat H. Mimrot

Mental Health is important at every stage of life. Over the course of life, if anyone experiences mental health problems, his/her thinking, mood, and behaviour could be affected. The times in which we live in are the "age of anxiety", but probably every era of human history could be designated on the same way. Anxiety, fear and worry seem to be permanent parts of the human condition. Research evidences had established the relationship between mental health and death anxiety. Death anxiety essentially lead to either or both implicit and explicit fear components to a varying degree that differentially play a part to the actual experience. The present chapter is based on an empirical study in which the relationship between mental health and death anxiety among old age elderly is ascertained.

In the mid-nineteenth century, William Sweetzer was the first to clearly define the term "mental hygiene" which can be seen as the precursor to contemporary approaches to work on promoting positive mental health. Dorothea Dix (1802-1887) was an important figure in the development of "mental hygiene" movement. Dix was a school teacher who endeavoured throughout her life to help those suffering from mental illness, and to bring to light the deplorable conditions into which they were put. This was known as the *"mental hygiene movement"*. Before this movement, it was not uncommon that people affected by mental illness would be considerably neglected, often left alone in awful conditions, barely even having sufficient clothing. Dix's efforts were so great that there was a rise in the number of patients in mental health facilities, which sadly resulted in these patients receiving less attention and care, as these institutions were largely understaffed. At the beginning of the twentieth century, Clifford Beers founded the National Committee for Mental Hygiene and opened the first outpatient mental health clinic in the USA. The mental hygiene movement, related to the Social Hygiene Movement, had at times been associated with advocating eugenics and sterilization of those considered too mentally deficient to be assisted into productive work and contented family life. After year 1945, references to mental hygiene were gradually replaced by the term 'mental health'.

Concept of Mental Health

Mental Health is the level of psychological well-being, or an absence of a mental disorder, it is the "psychological state of someone who is functioning at a satisfactory level of emotional and behavioural adjustment". Mental Health includes our emotional, psychological, and social well-being. It affects how we think, feel, and act. It also helps determine how we handle stress, relate to others, and make choices. From the perspective of positive psychology or holism, mental health may include an individual's ability to enjoy life, and create a balance between life activities and efforts to achieve psychological resilience.

According to WHO (2003) Mental Health includes "subjective well-being, perceived self-efficacy, autonomy, competence, intergenerational dependence, and self-actualization of one's intellectual and emotional potential, among others." WHO further states that the well-being of individual also encompasses the realization of their abilities, coping with normal stresses of life, productive work and contribution to their community? However, cultural differences, subjective assessments, and competing professional theories all affect how "mental health" is defined:

> WHO (WHOm 2001a) has proposed that mental health is:... a state of well-being in which the individual realizes his or her own abilities, can cope with the normal stresses of life, can work productively and fruitfully, and is able to make a contribution to his or her community. Many factors contribute to mental health problems including biological factors, such as genes or brain chemistry; life experiences, such as trauma or abuse; family history of mental health problems.

Positive mental health allows people to realize their full potential; cope with the stresses of life; work productively; make meaningful contributions to their communities. Ways to maintain positive mental health include getting professional help if you need it; connecting with others; staying positive; getting physically active; helping others; getting enough sleep and developing coping skills.

Mental Changes in Old Age

Older people are more cautious about learning, need more time to integrate their responses, are less capable of dealing with new material that cannot readily be integrated with earlier experience, and are less accurate than younger people. Ageing-induced biological factors are a prominent source of individual differences in cognitive plasticity in very old age (Singer, Lindenberger, and Baltes, 2003). Deterioration in vocabulary is very slight in old age because elderly people constantly use words most of which were learned in childhood or adolescence. Learning new words in old age is more infrequent than frequent.

There is a general reduction in the speed with which the individual reaches a conclusion in both inductive and deductive reasoning, this is partly the result of the tendency to become increasingly cautious with age (Nettelbeck and Burns, 2010).

Many older people tend to lack the capacity for, or interest in, creative thinking. However, Fisher and Specht (2000) found that creative activity contributes to successful ageing by fostering a sense of competence, purpose, and growth. Artistic creativity also facilitates successful ageing by encourageing the development of problem-solving skills, motivation, and perceptions that translate into a practical creativity in the way these individuals manage their everyday lives.

Older people tend to have poor recent memory but better remote memory. This may be partly to the fact that they are not always strongly motivated to remember things, partly to lack of attentiveness and partly to not hearing clearly and distinctly what other say. In the domain of episodic memory, available evidence shows that cognitively healthy older adults are able to acquire skilled episodic memory performance through instruction and training of mnemonic strategies (Verhaeghen *et al.*, 1992) and show less improvement and lower performance asymptotes than do younger adults (Singer, Lindenberger, and Baltes, 2003; Verhaeghen *et al.*, 1992). In normal ageing, declines are evident in episodic memory, source memory, working memory and prospective memory, but not in semantic, implicit or procedural memory.

Recall is affected more by age than recognition many older people use cues, especially visual, auditory, and kinesthetic one, to aid their ability to recall (Craik, and McDowd, 1987). The tendency to reminisce about the past become increasingly more marked with advancing age find how much the individual reminisces depends mainly on how pleasant or unpleasant the elderly find their living condition now.

Mental rigidity sets in during middle age; it tends to become more pronounced with advancing age partly because the elderly learn more slowly and with more difficulty than they did earlier and partly because they believe that old values and ways of doing things are better than new ones.

Death Anxiety

Death anxiety refers to the fear and apprehension of one's own death. It is the neurotic fears of loss of self which in intense state parallels feelings of helplessness and depression. Man's awareness of his own death produces anxiety that can only be dealt with by recognizing one's individuality. According to former an existential analysts, man's awareness of death gives him the responsibility of finding meaning in life.

Death is a biological, personal, socio-cultural and existential phenomenon. The biological death distinguishes between the process of ageing and the ending called death. Yet, when the actual time comes, and the individual faces death alone, the psychological reactions appear to be remarkably similar. Kubler (1969) had found that in the majority of people, almost regardless of age, the personal reactions to imminent death pass through five phases—denial, anger, bargaining, depression and acceptance (although not every individual achieves the final phase).

Dying and death, like other major aspects of human life, are also very important cultural and social phenomena. Even less than a century ago, death was a common and familiar event in everyday life. There was no widespread technology to control infection and medicine could not do much for most diseases. Among the poor classes the death at young and tender age was at an appalling rate. And the old die in their time, and generally they all die at home. The average person had been in the immediate presence of dead bodies at least half a dozen times before reaching adulthood. Against this background, death was in former years much more a part of life than it is today.

The death can be fully understood only if it is viewed as one of the central meanings of human existence. An idea of the centrality of one's own death can be gathered if individuals could be made to contemplate seriously the possibility of their own death (McCarthy, 1980). As death is the final stage of life cycle, it can be approached naturally by dying individuals and their families. Death and dying can be seen as part of the life process, or they can be viewed as a dramatic, painful, tortured experience both for the patients and the families. Increasingly, more research reports are being presented on the nature of death and dying. Research on exactly when death occurs, how the dying should be treated, and how their families might better cope will continue for many years.

In old age, people confront the possibility of their own death as well as the death of loved ones. Death may also be considered in statistical terms, which supply us with significant figures and facts. Even though death most commonly occurs in later years, it may happen at any stage in life. Accidents and suicides are the major causes of death among younger persons, and continue to be so in later years, although their relative significance declines, often death is associated with some special psychological stress, it may be acute mourning, or an anniversary or some particular loss of status or self-esteem.

Death is sometimes defined as the absence of certain clinically detectable vital signs. A person is dead "if his heart stops beating and he quits breathing for an extended period of time, his blood pressure drops as low as to be unreadable his pupils dilate, his body temperature begins to go down, and so forth. This clinical definition has been used over the centuries, both by physicians and laymen. More recently, death has sometimes been defined as the lack of brain wave activity still others say that death can only be defined as a bodily state which represents an irreversible loss of vital functions and from which the individual cannot passively be revived. According to the concept of terminal drop, death can be predicted from certain dramatic changes in cognitive function in the period preceding demise. This is significant changes both in personal adjustment and performance may serve as indicators of impending death (Riegal and Riegal, 1972).

Robert Longs has described three forms of death anxiety. It has been the practice to treat death anxiety as a uniform or single entity without recognizing the existence of an underlying typology. The importance of refining the concept comes from clinical findings that different types of traumatic events lead to different forms of death anxiety, each of which is experienced and responded by humans in a distinctive manner. These responses are both conscious and unconscious, i.e. within or outside of direct awareness. The former are generally well known and include traumatic and post-traumatic stress syndromes and responses to cancer and other types of grave illness. But it is not generally appreciated that death anxiety is prompted by every type of traumatic event and that it can register and operate entirely outside of awareness. The effects nonetheless, are powerful and devastating, and always include a lightening of communicative defences in an effort to obliterate the conscious recognition of the various ways that a given trauma is impacting on the individual and the extent to which death related anxieties have been activated.

The three forms of death anxiety are:

1. ***Predatory Death Anxiety:*** The unicellular organisms have receptors that have evolved to react to external dangers and they also possess self-protective, responsive mechanisms designed to insure survival in the face of chemical and physical forms of attack or danger. In humans this form of death anxiety is evoked by a variety of dangerous situations that put the recipient at risk or threatens his or her survival. These traumas may be psychological and or physical. Predatory death anxieties mobilize an individual's adaptive resources and lead to fight or fight active efforts to combat the danger or attempts to escape the threatening situation. These responses also may take mental and/or physical forms and include both conscious and unconscious processing and modes of adapting.
2. ***Predation Death Anxiety*:** This form of death anxiety arises when an individual harms others physically and/or mentally. The arousal of this type of anxiety often involves unconscious rather than conscious realizations and processing. The primary reaction to this type of anxiety is that of conscious and unconscious guilt, which, in turn, motivates a variety of self-punitive decisions and actions by the perpetrator of harm to others whose deeper sources go unappreciated.
3. ***Existential Death Anxiety*:** This is the most powerful form of death anxiety and its activation is based in humans on the definitive, conscious awareness and anticipation of the inevitability of personal demise. This expectation and the anxieties it evokes are the result of human language acquisition, which led to a definitive awareness of the distinction between self and others, a full sense of personal identity, and the ability to anticipate the future. Humans defend against this type of death anxiety through denial, which is effected through a wide range of mental mechanism and physical actions? Many of which also go unrecognized. While limited use of denial tends to be adaptive its use is usually excessive and proves to be costly emotionally.

Previous Studies

Madnawat and Kachhawa (2007) had examined the effect of age, gender, and living circumstances on elderly individuals' death anxiety. For this purpose, 299 persons attending public parks (average age = 70 years) were interviewed. The findings revealed that relatively older women, and those living with family were significantly more anxious about the word "death". The gender and age results in this Indian sample are similar to that in some Western samples. Those living with family have significantly higher death anxiety are not in agreement with past Western studies and may reflect cultural differences in anxiety about death. Aday (2006) had looked into the key variables associated with death anxiety among a group of ageing prisoners. The regression analysis showed that age, inmate social supports, and a number of health related variables were important predictors of death fear. The findings revealed that fear of death is slightly higher among older prisoners than for similar age groups in the community. The personal narratives illustrated that some inmates perceive death as an escape, whereas others expressed fears of dying in prison or the stigma associated with imprisonment. Reactions of Chinese elderly people towards specific death-related issues were discussed with regard to Chinese cultural beliefs by Wu, Tang, and Kwok (2002). The cognitive and emotional reactions of Chinese elderly people toward death was examined and results revealed that a high level of death anxiety was associated with younger age, a high level of psychological distress, and the presence of recent stressors but was unrelated to number of physical disorders, gender, personal income, marital and employment status, and religious affiliations.

Suhail and Akram (2002) had investigated the effect of gender, age, and religiosity on death anxiety on a Pakistani sample. The findings indicated that women, older participants, and less religious participants were found to be more scared of their impending death. Women and less religious people reported to experience greater anxiety than their respective counterparts on different dimensions of death, for example, the shortness of life, total isolation of death, fear of not being, and disintegration of body after dying. The findings of the current work indicate that the general predictors of death anxiety, gender, age, and religiosity reported in Western, predominantly Christian samples also hold in an Eastern, Muslim sample.

Fortner, Robert and Neimeyer (1999) reviewed the literature on death anxiety and summarized 49 published and unpublished research studies concerning the relationship between death anxiety and age, ego integrity, gender, institutionalization, physical and psychological problems, and religiosity in older adults. Results indicated that lower ego integrity, more physical problems, and more psychological problems are predictive of higher levels of death anxiety in elderly people. Naidu and Sinha (1992) investigated impact of four metaphysical beliefs (existence of god, afterlife attributes of God, and attributes consequences of suffering) on death anxiety. Pictures depicting death and non-death scenes were constructed to measure death anxiety. A sample of 120 householders (60 heads of unsettled and 60 heads of settled families) had participated in the study. Half of them lived in high exposure to death sight areas and the other half lived in low exposure areas. Subjects from only low exposure areas revealed significant relationships between beliefs and death anxiety. Beliefs play functional roles that are different for people with different needs.

White and Handal (1991) had examined relationship between death anxiety and mental health distress and found that high death-anxious females were statistically and clinically more distressed and were significantly less satisfied with life than low death-anxious females. Hickson, Housley, and Boyle (1988) had examined Rotter's Internal-External locus of control concept in relation to life satisfaction and death anxiety in aged population. Analysis revealed significant correlations between the variables of life satisfaction and death anxiety, regardless of the Ss' control orientation.

Shukla and Rishi (2014) investigated the relationships among psychosocial, spiritual well-being and death anxiety among advance stage cancer patients. Data was collected from sample of 80 advance stage cancer patients, from six exclusive cancer hospitals of western and central zones of India. Results revealed negative correlation between psychosocial well-being and death anxiety and spiritual well-being and death anxiety. It indicates that enhancing the psychosocial and spiritual well-being of cancer patients can reduce their death anxiety and promote better quality of life. Ardelt and Koenig (2006) studied the hospice patients and relatively healthy older adults and path analyses showed that a sense of purpose in life rather than religiosity had a direct positive effect on subjective well-being and a direct negative effect on death fear after controlling for physical health and demographic characteristics. Intrinsic religiosity had an indirect positive effect on subjective well-being and a strong direct positive effect on approach acceptance of death. Extrinsic religiosity, however, was positively related to death anxiety and, for hospice patients, negatively related to approach acceptance of death. McClain-Jacobson *et al.* (2005) assessed afterlife beliefs, spiritual well-being and psychological functioning at the end of life among terminally ill cancer patients. Belief in afterlife appeared to be associated with lower levels of end-of-life-despair (desire for death, hopelessness and suicidal ideation), but not with levels of depression or anxiety. When controlled for spirituality the effect of afterlife beliefs disappeared. The authors conclude that instead of beliefs held about afterlife it is rather spirituality that has a powerful effect on psychological functioning.

Objectives of the Study

The major objective of the study is to find out the relationship between mental health and death anxiety of old age elderly as well as to find out the gender differences in mental health and death anxiety of old age elderly.

Sample: The present study is conducted on old people who were living in the family and institutions in Aurangabad city. The sample of the present study consists of 200 old persons. These old persons belong to both the sexes of various families and institutions and only ex-service holder in civil and corporate sector employees were chosen for study in Aurangabad city. The age group of old person is above sixty. Random sampling technique was used for the selection of the respondents. The total sample of old age men are 100 and old age women are 100 selected for the study.

Tools: As per scope of problem, the researcher of the study has selected two psychological tests related to death anxiety and mental health:

1. *Death Anxiety Scale*—This scale was constructed and developed by Upinder Dhar, Savita Mehta and Santosh Dhar. This scale consists of 10 items. The split-half reliability coefficient was = 0.87. In order to determine validity from the coefficient of reliability (Garrett, 1981), the reliability index was calculated. The later has indicated high validity on account of being 0.93.
2. *Mental Health Questionnaire*—This questionnaire in Hindi is developed and standardized by O.N. Srivastava and V.K. Bhat. Reliability was calculated by the split-half method from the scores of the medical students Group. The split-half reliability of the whole test (i.e. between the first 24 items *vs* the next 24 items) was 0.70. Validity was found that the M.H.Q. scores differentiate the neurotics from the normal at a statistically highly significant level.

Procedure of Data Collection—For administering the scales, the

Ss were called in small groups. Their seating arrangement was made in the recreation hall of the institutions. All the scales used in the study were group scales; hence, they were administered on small groups of subject. Selected number of the Ss was asked to assemble in the recreation hall. At a time only 15 to 20 Ss were invited. They were asked to sit in chairs kept at sufficient distance from each other, for the reason than one cannot see what the other had written in the answer sheet. Researcher explained the purpose of the study in brief. Through informal talk rapport was established and the Ss were requested to answer the items of two scales sincerely and honestly. They were assured that their responses would be used strictly for research purpose only, and would not be disclosed to others. Their written documents would be treated as confidential.

Statistical Analysis: In present study the researcher had analyzed data with the help of descriptive statistics, "*t*" test and product movement correlational method has been carried out for statistical analysis.

Table 14.1: Co-efficient of correlation between mental health and death anxiety of old age people (N = 200)

Variables	*Mean*	*SD*	*r*	*Sig.*
Mental Health	47.50	12.124	0.071	NS
Death Anxiety	5.72	1.204		

An attempt has also been made to observe the relationship between mental health and death anxiety. In terms of the present mental health inventory high score indicate neurotic traits. The correlation between mental health and death anxiety was not found significant.

Table 14.2: The difference between old age men and women on death anxiety

Variable	*Group*	*Mean*	*SD*	*t*
Death Anxiety	Old age Men (N = 100)	5.68	1.127	0.469
	Old age Women (N =100)	5.76	1.280	

Table 14.2 indicates that there was no significant difference emerged in old age men (M = 5.68, SD = 1.127) and old age women (M = 5.76, SD = 1.280) on their level of death anxiety. Old age men and women are facing similar problems of death anxiety.

Table 14.3: The difference between old age men and women on mental health

Variable	*Group*	*Mean*	*SD*	*t*
Mental Health	**Old age men (N = 100)**	43.37	12.20	5.106**
	Old age women (N = 100)	51.62	10.59	

Note = P >.01** P > .5**

Table 14.3 shows that there were significant differences found in old age men (M = 43.37, SD = 12.20), and old age women (M = 51.62, SD = 0.595) in their mental health. The mean values suggested that the old age women were showing neurotic tendency than old age men.

Discussion

Death is a very significant issue for mental health and it is an undeniable event for every human.

Mental Health and Death Anxiety

The findings showed in Table 14.1 indicate that there is no relationship between mental health and death anxiety. However, since the low score on mental health scale indicates good mental health, it reveals that Ss having poor mental health experience more death anxiety because when people have good mental health they are generally free from anxiety of death. From the above findings researcher suppose that sound mental health of old age people keep away from death anxiety.

The concept of death develops from our childhood. Religions have influence on this concept where they are practiced. But such an important concept in human life is rarely approached scientifically. Death is the end of life. But Muslims believe death is an event between two lives, not an absolute cessation of life. This is same as Hindus believe. Religiosity as a criterion of Muslims influenced the quality of adjustment with death positively (Hossain and Siddique, 2008). Science has very little approaches about death in comparison to its impact on human life. In contrast different religions have tried to elaborate death and death anxiety is managed at both the individual and cultural levels. Research evidences suggest that people from various Eastern cultures tend to have less measured death anxiety than their Western counterparts (McMordie and Kumar, 1984; Schumaker *et al.*, 1988; Westman & Canter, 1985). Kubler-Ross (1975) provides a theoretical basis for the findings of the present study based on the view that Eastern systems of religious belief more effectively assuage fear of death.

Gender Differences in Death Anxiety

Women may be subjected to distinct socio-cultural experiences and cultural conditioning than men. Studies have uncovered that female gender has been associated with higher death anxiety in adolescent populations and in cross-cultural research (Adbel-Khalek, 2004, 2005; Cotter, 2003; Pierce, 2007; Singh Madnawat, and Singh Kachhawa, 2007). In a large sample of older individuals aged 61 to 80 years, elderly females have significantly higher death anxiety than males (Hickson, Housley, and Boyle, 1988).

Erikson's psychosocial theory asserts that people progress through a series of predicament as they age. The theory puts forward that in the later stages of life "ego integrity" is attained. That is, a person finds meaning to, and acceptance of, their lives. Erikson proposed that when a person arrives at late adulthood he/she start a review of his/her life. If a person finds meaning or purpose in his life, he has integrity and if a person witnesses his/her life as a series of missed opportunities, the person does not attain the ego integrity (Belsky, 1999). Given Erikson's theory, older adults who find ego integrity should have lower death anxiety.

Some studies have found no age differences in death anxiety scores. Goebel and Boeck's (1987) study found no relationship between death anxiety and age, but the participants used in this study were over the age of 70. A theory that could be considered from the Goebel and Boeck (1987) research is that older adults experience less death anxiety, but age is not a significant factor in determining the degree of death anxiety when examining only late adulthood. In another study examining the relationship between death anxiety and age, Rasmussen and Johnson (1994) suggested that the differences in death anxiety might be due to a third variable, psychosocial maturity. If one can equate psychosocial maturity with ego integrity, her findings could be considered to support Erikson's studies. After the examination of the various studies and findings, it is the contention of the present researcher that ego integrity, or a personal sense of accomplishment and fulfilment, whether founded in religion or some other measure of fulfilment and accomplishment, is probably the biggest factor in death anxiety.

The findings of the present research showed that old age women are showing neurotic tendency and old age men showing good mental health.

MacDonald (1997) stated that psychiatric care of elderly people can be more interesting than that of younger patients. Important biological symptoms of depression in old age are change in sleep patterns (especially reduced sleep and early morning awakening); decline in appetite and weight loss; regular variation of mood over day (especially worse in early morning); constipation; physical and mental slowing not accountable by other disorders; and suicidal thoughts. He concludes that old age women are prone to general problems, e.g. anxiety, irritability, suicidal ideas, hypochondriacally ideas, withdrawal, decline in self-care, desire to change life radically. Hence, it can be concluded that the mental health of old age men is better than old age women. WHO's Report (2005) stated that gender is a critical determinant of mental health and mental illness. The morbidity associated with mental illness has received substantially more attention than the gender specific determinants and mechanisms that promote and protect mental health and foster resilience to stress and adversity. Gender determines the differential power and control men and women have over the socio-economic determinants of their mental health and lives, their social position, status and treatment in society and their susceptibility and exposure to specific mental health risks. Gender differences occur particularly in the rates of common mental disorders—depression, anxiety and somatic complaints. These disorders, in which women predominate, affect approximately 1 in 3 people in the community and constitute a serious public health problem.

Conclusion

No significant relationship observed between mental health and death anxiety. Old age women experience more death anxiety than old age men and old age men have good mental health than old women.

References

Abdel-Khalek, A.M. (2004). Does war affect death anxiety level? Seven readings of measurements (1988-2002) before and after the Iraqi invasion of Kuwait. *Omega, 49*, 287-297.

Abdel-Khalek, A.M. (2005). Death anxiety in clinical and non-clinical groups. *Death Studies, 29*, 251-259.

Aday, R.H. (2006). Ageing prisoners' concerns toward dying in prison. *OMEGA-Journal of Death and Dying*, *52*(3), 199-216.

Ardelt, M. and Koenig, C.S. (2006). The role of religion for hospice patients and relatively healthy older adults. *Research on Ageing, 28*(2), 184-215.

Barlow, D.H., Durand, V.M., Steward, S.H. (2009). *Abnormal Psychology*: An integrative approach (Second Canadian Edition). Toronto: Nelson, p.16.

Cotter, R.P. (2003). High risk behaviours in adolescence and their relationship to death anxiety and death personifications. *Omega, 47*, 119-137.

Craik, F.I., and McDowd, J.M. (1987). Age differences in recall and recognition. *Journal of Experimental Psychology: Learning, Memory, and Cognition, 13*(3), 474.

Fisher, B.J., and Specht, D.K. (2000). Successful ageing and creativity in later life. *Journal of Ageing Studies, 13*(4), 457-472.

Fortner, V., Robert, A. and Neimeyer, B. (1999). Death anxiety in older adults: A quantitative review. *Death studies, 23*(5), 387-411.

Goebel, B.L., and Boeck, B.E. (1987). Ego-integrity and fear of death: A comparison of institutionalized and independently living older adults. *Death Studies, 11*(3), 193-204.

Hickson, J., Housley, W.F., and Boyle, C. (1988). The relationship of locus of control, age, and sex to life satisfaction and death anxiety in older persons. *The International Journal of Ageing and Human Development. Vol. 26* (3), 191-199.

Hossain, M.S., and Siddique, M.Z. (2008). Does religiosity help Muslims adjust to death?: A research note. *OMEGA-Journal of Death and Dying, 57*(1), 113-119.

Jahoda, M. (1958): *Current Concepts of Positive Mental Health*, New York; Basic Books.

Keyes, C. (2002). The mental health continuum: From languishing to flourishing in life. *Journal of Health and Social Behaviour, 43* (2), 207-222.

Kubler-Ross, E. (1969). *On Death and Dying*. New York: MacMillan.

Kubler-Ross, E. (1975). *Death: The Final Stage of Growth*. Englewood Cliffs, NJ: Prentice-Hall.

Madnawat, A.S., and Kachhawa, P.S. (2007). Age, gender, and living circumstances: Discriminating older adults on death anxiety. *Death Studies, 31*(8), 763-769.

McClain-Jacobson C., Rosenfeld B., Kosinski A., Pessin H., Cimino J.E., and Breitbart W. (2004). Belief in afterlife, spiritual well-being and end-of-life despair in patients with advanced cancer. *General Hospital Psychiatry, 26*, 484-486.

MacDonald, A.J. (1997). ABC of mental health. Mental health in old age. *British Medical Journal, 315*, 413-417.

McMordie, W.R. and Kumar, A. (1984). Cross-cultural research on the Templer/McMordie Death Anxiety Scale. *Psychological Reports, 54*, 959-963.

Naidu, R.K., and Sinha, A. (1992). Metaphysical beliefs as predictors of death anxiety. *OMEGA-Journal of Death and Dying, 25*(2), 95-107.

Nettelbeck, T., and Burns, N.R. (2010). Processing speed, working memory and reasoning ability from childhood to old age. *Personality and Individucl Differences*, *48*(4), 379-384.

Pierce, J.D. (2007). Gender differences in death anxiety and religious orientation among U.S. high school and college students. *Mental Health, Religion, and Culture, 10*, 143-150.

Shukla, P. and Rishi, P. (2014). A Correlational Study of Psychosocial and Spiritual Well-being and Death Anxiety among Advanced Stage Cancer Patients. *American Journal of Applied Psychology*, *2*(3), 59-65.

Rasmussen, C. and Johnson, M. (1994). Spirituality and religiosity: Relative relationships to death anxiety. *Omega*, *29*, 313-318.

Riegal, K.F. and Riegal, R.M. (1972): Development drop and death. *Development Psychology, Vol. 6*, 306-319.

Schumaker, J.F., Barraclough, R.A., and Vagg, L.M. (1988). Death anxiety in Malaysian and Australian University Students. *Journal of Social Psychology, 128*, 41-47.

Singer, T., Lindenberger, U., and Baltes, P.B. (2003). Plasticity of memory for new learning in very old age: A story of major loss? *Psychology and Ageing*, *18*(2), 306.

Suhail, K. and Akram, S. (2002). Correlates of death anxiety in Pakistan. *Death Studies*, *26*(1), 39-50.

The World Health Report 2001—*Mental Health: New Understanding*, New Hope. WHO. Retrieved 4 May, 2014.

Verhaeghen, P., Marcoen, A., and Goossens, L. (1992). Improving memory performance in the aged through mnemonic training: A meta-analytic study. *Psychology and Ageing, 7*, 242-251.

Westman, A.S. and Canter, F.M. (1985). Fear of death and the concept of extended self. *Psychological Reports, 56*, 419-425.

White, W., and Handal, P.J. (1991). The relationship between death anxiety and mental health/distress. *OMEGA-Journal of Death and Dying*, *22*(1), 13-24.

Wu, A.M., Tang, C.S. and Kwok, T.C. (2002). Death anxiety among Chinese elderly people in Hong Kong. *Journal of Ageing and Health*, *14*(1), 42-56.

16

Mental Health, Well-being and Quality of Life as Correlates of Successful Ageing

Harshita Shukla and *Anubhuti Dubey*

Population ageing is one of the most significant emerging demographic phenomenon in the contemporary world. Remarkable improvements in healthcare, medicine, and living conditions have led to a dramatic increase in the number of persons reaching old age. By 1990, a clear majority (58%) of the world's population aged 60 years and above were already to be found living in developing countries. By 2020, this proportion would probably reach to (67%). The Indian aged population is currently the second largest in the world after China (100 million). The demographic profile of India has changed significantly towards an ageing population since 1950. The population aged 60 plus in India as per the 1991 census was 56.7 million, which shows an increase from 26 million in 1961, that clearly indicates a doubling-up of the elderly population in the last thirty years. The proportion of the elderly has been going up steadily in each census, though at varying rates. The 1991 Census indicated that 6.58 per cent of the total population belonged to the 60 plus age group. This proportion was expected to go up to 7.08 per cent by 2001 and 9.87 by 2021. Consistent with this large increase in number of persons reaching old population, ageing is the most significant emerging demographic phenomenon in the world. Simultaneously, with the growth in the field of gerontology and geriatric medicine, an astonishing amount of research relating to ageing came forward. Ageing is a natural process and what family thinks or expects of older people—what they say and how they relate, alongside personal narrative—all that affects them. Some elderly may be in touch with the fullness of life, while others are a part of emptiness, and may be little depressed. Introduction to the study of human ageing has typically emphasized changes in demography, focusing on the 'ageing of population—a trend', which has characterized industrial societies throughout the twentieth century, but in recent decades has become a world-wide phenomenon.

Ageing can generally be described as the process of growing old and is an intricate part of the life cycle. The ageing process is of course a biological reality which has its own dynamic, largely beyond control. Like every other period in the life span, old age is characterized by certain physical and psychological changes. The elderly population is extremely diverse, ranging from fit, active and healthy octogenarians to extremely frail, totally dependent people with chronic diseases and severe disabilities. The age of 60 or 65, roughly equivalent to retirement ages in most developed countries, is said to be the beginning of old age. Chronological age is commonly used to define an age band of older adults. Old can be subdivided into young-old (60s), middle-old (70s), and old-old (80s+ years) or young old (65-75 or 80), old-old (75-80 or 90), and very old (90+). An additional way of defining age is to use *Functional age*—to assign a person's functional age depending on their performance in relation to age graded norms. Thus, a person might have a chronological age of 70 (be 70 years old), but have a functional age of 50 for reaction time and of 60 for speed of information processing. The term related to *Biological age*—may be used to relate individual function to age based norms of physiological functions and similarly. *Social age* – may be used to refer to societal norms of how people should behave at particular age. Although there is no general agreement on the age at which person become old. Lacking an acceptable definition, in many instance the age at which a person became eligible for statutory and occupational retirement pension has become the default definition. Being elderly is an unpreventable process that has biological, chronological and social aspects and problems.

Ageing is a multidimensional change involving the physical, psychological as well as social aspects for an individual. It can be described as a progressive deterioration of the physical and mental functions resulting in a simultaneous decline in both the capacity of the body to maintain homeostatic balance as well as the adaptability of the individual to various stressors thereby consequently increasing the chances of illness and mortality. Many changes occur as people enter old age and these changes decrease quality of life. The needs and problems of the elderly vary significantly according to their age, socio-economic status, health, living status and other such background characteristics (Siva Raju, 2002).

Ageing in India: According to Hindu Mythology, *"Vridhatyam—Jarasa Vina"*, which means, let the old age be without senility or disability (poet Kalidasa, Second century B.C.), there is some evidence that older people may be becoming decreasingly satisfied, lonelier and more depressed and, due to demographic changes, there are increasing numbers of older people, many of whom are living with low levels of life satisfaction and well-being. Older adults typically face many life stressors, retirement, death of close family member and friends, increasing health problems and disability. Old age brings fear to many because of the seemingly inescapable decline of health. Keeping the body and mind healthy, and maintaining good relationships, are paramount to attaining positive ageing, those who engage in various activities, like meeting friends, attending social gathering, waking and exercising, are happier and more satisfied of their age than those who only sit at home. Monitoring, maintaining and promoting health and well-being with age is critical for older people, their families, communities and for wider economic and social planning. The ageing of a person presents various problems to the individual as well as those around them. With age mental faculties become weak and ailing, hence making it difficult for them to stay in a happy state of mind.

Old age is a time with significant challenges, especially for those with health problems. In traditional Indian society, the informal support systems of family, kinship and community are considered strong enough to provide social security to its members, including older people. Urbanisation, industrialisation and the ongoing phenomenon of globalisation have cast their shadow on traditional values and norms within society. The status of older people is closely correlated with social class, power, wealth and previous achievement; the more the person acquires these attributes during adulthood and the more they are successful in maintaining them in old age, the more likely they maintain their status in old age. When older people are no longer able to fend for themselves they become a 'burden' and are of no further value. Older people often sense a lack of interest in them as significant person, both from professional groups and even from their own family. However, many older adults experience good health and much joy and satisfaction in their achievements and the achievements of those they love. Now-a-days, the role of families in case of older person has declined due to structural changes which have taken place in the Indian society and the concomitant disintegration of the joint family system, which results in the rejection or neglect of the aged. Thus, the elderly citizens are in need of urgent attention.

Factors affecting the elderly: Granieri (1990) suggested that factors affecting the elderly can be categorized into primary, secondary, and tertiary.

Primary factors are the result of the normal ageing process. In communication, this might include changes in vocal quality and respiratory reserves, slight increases in active word-finding problems, increased response time, and possible problems in understanding long, complex written or spoken passages.

Pathological factors are secondary ageing factors. Elderly people are more prone to conditions such as stroke, heart disease, arthritis, impaired vision, and hearing loss. Additionally, the elderly person is likely to suffer from more than one of these conditions.

Tertiary factors are those that result from social, psychological, and environmental changes. The social and support network of the elderly client is often reduced from retirement, death of peers, children moving away, and loss of mobility. The elderly couple may be on a fixed income, with illness further reducing their financial resources. When these factors combine, it is not unusual for the older person to experience depression. If both the client and the spouse are elderly, the ageing factors affecting each must be considered.

Psychosocial Theories of Ageing

Everyone encounters problem in everyday life and for some people the problem can become too much to deal with on their own. Several psychosocial theorists have identified stage and task for each age group. Erik Erikson's (1963) work is well known. The stage pertaining to older adult is Ego integrity *versus* Despair. The work of this stage is to accept one's life as meaningful. The older person who reaches ego integrity looks back with satisfaction, and has an acceptance of life and death. Death is seen as a part of life, if this stage is not adequately abridged, the person is in a state of despair—which is failure to accept the meaningfulness of one's life. When one is in despair, there are feelings of anger, bitterness, depression, inadequacy, failure and fear of death. However, even older adults who achieve a high degree of integrity may feel some despair at this stage as they contemplate their past. No one makes it through life without wondering if another path may have been happier and more productive.

Two major theories which explain the psychosocial aspects of ageing in older adults are Disengagement Theory and Activity Theory.

1. ***Disengagement theory***—views ageing as a process of mutual withdrawal in which older adults voluntarily slow down by

retiring, as expected by society. Proponents of disengagement theory hold that mutual social withdrawal benefits both individuals and society. However, Tornstam (1989) had argued that what social gerontologists describe in negative terms and label "disengagement" is in reality often a positive development towards gero-transcendence. This latter can be described as a shift in meta-perspective from a materialistic and rational view to a more cosmic and transcendent one, normally followed by an increase in life satisfaction. To understand the nature of gero-transcendence gerontologists have to make a meta-theoretical shift from a traditional positivist view to a view where disengagement is phenomenologically comprehended.

2. ***Activity theory***—sees a positive correlation between keeping active and ageing well. Menec (2002) reported the findings of the regression analysis indicated that overall activity level is related to successful ageing. Social and productive activities are positively related to happiness, function and mortality whereas solitary activities like handwork and hobbies are related to happiness only. To date, research has not shown either of these models to be superior to the other. Growing old means different things to different people and individuals who led active lives as young and middle adults will probably remain active as older adults, while those who were less active may become more disengaged as they age.

Reminiscence in Older Adults

As older adults approach the end of their life span, they are more apt to conduct a life review. In their quest to find life's meaning, older adults often have a vital need to share their reminiscence with others who care, especially family. Reminiscence is the recalling of the memories of past experiences is a multi-dimensional process which occurs in people of all ages. Reminiscence has been identified as an important contributor to adaptation in later life by gerontologists, developmental theorists and clinical practitioners. Older adults use reminiscence for many different purposes than younger ones. Older adults tend to use past memories as entertainment whereas younger ones' use as problem solving tool (Revere and Tobin, 1980). Wang and Watt (1991) had developed taxonomy of six types of reminiscence—integrative, instrumental, transmissive, narrative, escapist, and obsessive. Research findings suggest that successful agers show significantly more integrative and instrumental forms of reminiscence which primarily functions as reconciliation of the past, sense of self worth and problem solving (Watt, and Cappeliez, 2000; Wong and Watt, 1991). A number of authors also argued that reminiscence plays a crucial role in search of meaning of life and build or rebuild a sense of identity and coherence (Ruth & Mader, 1999; Parker, 1995).

Reminiscence (or life review) therapy is one intervention which has been developed to offer a substitute to the traditional approaches to psychotherapy with older adults. The proposal that reminiscence performs an important function in successful ageing (Butler, 1974) has obtained popularity among researchers and practitioners. The rapid changes in traditional values, mobility of the younger generation, changes in family structure and role of caregivers are a factor to a 'crisis in caring' for the elderly.

There is a need to focus on ageing issues and to take effective measures for improvement in the quality of life of elderly. Older people's reaction to events and situations are no different to that of the rest of the population and their capacity to cope will vary from person to person. Older person is likely to have multiple and/or chronic health problems, a reduced social network, financial restrictions and sensory deficits. The impact of ageing can be emotive for old ones. They may fear growing old, isolation or abandonment, or have our own personal fears, anxieties. Physically, as our bodies change, our quality of sleep may decline. Self-acceptance may be in short supply. Many older people feel awkward discussing their problems and concerns with friends or members of their family and so an older person may benefit from talking to a trained and experienced counsellor. Taking to people about their problems and difficulties, which is what counselling is about, has intended to be undervalued, and even neglected. There are a number of issues, which many older people encounter:

Bereavement: Many older people have been with their spouse or partner for a considerable amount of time and it is likely that each partner will have a strong attachment to the other. When a spouse dies it is often difficult for the widow/widower to adjust. Also as we get older the number of deaths of close friends and family members increases and so older people can often experience an overload of grief.

Other losses: Other than bereavement, there are a number of other losses that older people can experience. These include: loss of independence; loss of looks; loss of health; loss of status; loss of being valued; loss of mobility; and loss of family home.

Depression: Depression is a common late life experience. Both major and minor depression are reported in 13 per cent of community dwelling older adults. Many older people can experience feelings of isolation. They can feel "cut off" from society and think that they are completely alone.

Anxiety: Older people often have concerns regarding their own health and well-being. They may also become anxious about practical and financial issues. Many older people worry about how they will cope on a day-to-day basis.

Loneliness: Many older people can experience intense feelings of loneliness. This can happen particularly when an older person remains living in their own home after the death of a spouse.

Fears about the future: Some older people have fears and anxieties about their future and whether or not they can remain living independently in their own homes.

Awareness of own mortality: Often when older people have experienced the loss of a spouse, friends and family, they have a greater sense of their own mortality. Clinicians who do not fully understand the effects of ageing often confuse signs of normal ageing with symptoms of disorders.

Correlates of Ageing

Mental health: As the world's population is ageing rapidly, older people face special physical and mental health challenges which need to be recognized. Over 20 per cent of adults aged 60 and over suffer from a mental or neurological disorder and 6.6 per cent of all disability among over 60s is attributed to neurological and mental disorders. The most common neuropsychiatric disorders in this age group are dementia and depression. Research studies reveal that there is a prevalence of depression, lower life satisfaction and more adjustment problems among elderly. Anxiety disorders affect 3.8 per cent of the elderly population, substance use problems affect almost 1 per cent and around a quarter of deaths from self-harm are among those aged 60 or above. Substance abuse problems among the elderly are often overlooked or misdiagnosed. Mental health problems are under-identified by health-care professionals and older people themselves, and the stigma surrounding mental illness makes people reluctant to seek help. Researchers find a large number of people are getting affected by mental health problems. Physical health and mental health are often intertwined; the physical changes experienced by the elderly can create stress and uncertainty which can in turn cause mental illness, i.e. older adults experience unique physical, psychological and social changes that individually and together may challenge their mental health, sometimes resulting in mental illness. It is estimated that 1 in 5 persons aged over 65 years has a mental health disorder (Jeste, Alexopoulos, Bartels, Cummings, Gallo, Gottlieb, *et al.*, 1999). The World Health Organization has defined mental health as a state of well-being in which the individual realizes his or her own potential, can cope with the normal stresses of life, can live productively and fruitfully, and is able to make a contribution to her or his own community (WHO, 2002). Mental health can be promoted and supported (or neglected and undermined) wherever the individual is situated on the continuum. Good mental health enables seniors to realize their fullest potential and to cope with life transitions and major life events, while poor mental health has the opposite effect. Multiple social, psychological, and biological factors determine the level of mental health of a person at any point of time. As well as the typical life stressors common to all people, many older adults lose their ability to live independently because of limited mobility, chronic pain, frailty or other mental or physical problems, and require some form of long-term care. In addition, older people are more likely to experience events such as bereavement, a drop in socio-economic status with retirement, or a disability. All of these factors can result in isolation, loss of independence, loneliness and psychological distress in older people. In a qualitative study on elderly of Goa, Indira Patel and Prince (2001) reported that depression was a common presentation in primary care, but infrequently diagnosed. Both late-life mental disorders were attributed to abuse, neglect, or lack of love on the part of children towards a parent.

Mental health of older adults can be improved through promoting active and healthy ageing. Healthy ageing has been described as "the ideal situation in which people survive to an advanced age with their vigour and functional independence maintained, and morbidity and disability compressed into a relatively short period before death" but there is still little understanding of the constituent components of healthy ageing and how these differ between social, cultural, economic and traditional contexts. Healthy ageing requires good objective function physically, cognitively, and socially and having a positive state of mind. Mental health-specific health promotion for the older adults involves creating living conditions and environments that support well-being and allow people to lead healthy and integrated lifestyles. Promoting mental health depends largely on strategies which ensure the elderly have the necessary resources to meet their basic needs, such as:

- providing security and freedom;
- social support for elderly populations and their caregivers;
- health and social programmes targeted at vulnerable groups such as those who live alone;
- rural populations or who suffer from a chronic or relapsing mental or physical illness;
- violence or older adults maltreatment prevention programmes; and
- community development programmes.

Well-being: Mental health and emotional well-being are as important in older age as at any other time of life. In our Indian society old age has always been a concern due to lack of power in social, economic and professional spheres; and its closeness to death, but with changed family patterns and value system there is a drastic change in the lifestyle and living standards in the society as well as at home front. As population ageing becomes more and more pronounced, the concern for Mental Health and Well-being of older people is also increasing. With the unprecedented increase in the number of oldest adults, several studies have paid attention to centenarians and their lives exploring factors related to longevity, such as health, generic influences, general lifestyle etc. However, till date in India, research on ageing was primarily confined to socio-demographic profiles, problems of and services to the aged etc. As a result certain issues related to the problems of elderly have received insufficient attention to the scholars and one such area is elderly Well-being, and Mental Health. Even speculation about the nature of the problem has been difficult because of invisibility and sensitiveness of the problem.

In general, well-being shows some degree of positive correlation with positive qualities of life and negative correlation with neuroticism, psychoticism and other such variables. Some determinants of good quality old age positive self concept, a favourable perception of one's capacity to manage affairs, a favourable perception of interrelationship with family, a belief in *karma* and philosophy and a flexible outlook and habits.

Well-being is particularly important as people grow older, since it may contribute to resilience (defined as the ability to cope with and flourish under adversity) in the face of stress and ill-health (Ong, Bergeman and Boker, 2009). World Health Organization defines health as "a state of complete physical, mental and social well-being and not merely the absence of disease or infirmity". Well-being is a multi-dimensional concept that has an affective or feeling component (how happy or unhappy the person is), and a reflective, judgemental component (how satisfied people are with their lives). Well-being also incorporates the notion of functioning effectively and general quality of life, involving issues such as realising one's potential, having some sense of control over one's life and having a sense of purpose (Ryan and Deci, 2001). Understanding well-being at older ages therefore, requires a multi-dimensional approach. Well-being has become an important focus for health and social policy in general, and in relation to older people in particular. Well-being has been linked to ideas about 'active ageing'. Some research and policy appears to assume that well-being is a quality of individuals and can be produced through individual effort. Others have argued that an emphasis on the individual does not sufficiently take into account the importance of relationships between people and that, rather than measuring individual well-being. Well-being is consistently found to be higher in later life than among young or middle aged adults. Among older people (65 and over), the pattern of well-being can be further divided and suggests high levels of well-being in the early post-retirement years, followed by lower levels of well-being in later old age (75 and over).

Health behaviours and well-being: There was a graded association between self-reported health and well-being. Affective, eudemonic and evaluative well-being all predict future subjective health, suggesting that impaired well-being is not just a product of poor health, but it is also systematically associated with the development of poor health.

Engageing in physical activity is paramount to ageing well. Being physically active is inextricably linked to independent living and other factors such as social support, both of which are crucial aspects for well-being in older adults. Regular physical activity is also linked to improvements in immune function and resistance to illness.

Loneliness also has significant detrimental effects on older people's well-being. Older people who are carers can experience lower levels of well-being due to feeling isolated, lacking in social activities and difficulty leaving the house as they cannot leave the person they care for alone. Older carers also neglect their own health as they focus on the person they are caring for.

Thus, in nutshell, physical, social and emotional health are all important aspects of our overall health and well-being. Keeping active in older age is vital for each of these aspects of our well-being. This may mean being physically or socially active, or keeping the mind active.

Quality of Life: Quality of Life (QoL) as an eternal quest for human beings and is conceptualized as a generic, multi-dimensional construct that describes an individual's subjective perception of his or her physical and psychological health, as well as his or her social functioning, environment, and general life status. Health status is an important indicator of the Quality of Life of the elderly. Increasing numbers of older people, demands on health and social care services, and higher expectations for 'a good life' have led to a greater interest in improving and measuring quality of life in older age. The research indicates that the main drivers of quality of life in older age are psychological (social comparison and expectations, an optimistic or pessimistic outlook on life); health (good health and mobility, physical functioning); social (social participation and support); and neighbourhood social capital (local facilities and sense of security). These factors contribute far more to perceived quality of life than objective indicators of material circumstances, such as actual level of income, education, home ownership, or social classes. The World Health Organization defines the Quality of Life (QoL) as "an individual's perception of his/her position in life in the context of the culture and value systems in which he/she lives, and in relation to his/her goals expectations, standards and concerns. It is a broad-ranging concept, incorporating in a comparing way the person's physical health, psychological state, level of independence, social relationships, and their relationship to salient features of their environment."

For old aged quality of life is more than rating their physical health status; emotional and social health are also recognized as very important factors for their well-being. An individual Quality of Life perception, in socio-cultural reality, according to the value system in which the person is inserted, as described by World Health Organization (WHO), expresses a position related to one's goals, expectations, patterns and worries. Quality of life is a holistic approach that not only emphasizes on individuals' physical, psychological, and spiritual functioning, but also their connections with their environments; and opportunities for maintaining and enhancing skills. Ageing, along with the functional decline, economic dependence, and social cut off, autonomy of young generation, compromises quality of life. Reluctance in caring of elderly and concept of QoL is not yet popular in India.

Conclusion

Mental health awareness needs to be integrated into all aspects of health and social policy, health-system planning, and delivery of primary and secondary general health care. The WHO proposition that there can be "no health without mental health" has also been endorsed. Despite all efforts leading to some progress in caring elderly, much needs to be done towards training, research, and providing clinical services to promote mental health in elderly. There is a need to raise awareness about mental disorders in late-life in the community and among health professionals, and to improve access to appropriate health care for the elderly with mental illness to improve the quality of life.

References

Akman, J.S. (2004). The Developmental Psychology of Aged Persons. Psychology (Vol. II) *Encyclopedia of the Life Support System (EOLSS).*

Ageing Well (2004). A Compendium of Factsheets: Well-being across the Life Course, Department of Health. Retrieved from http://www.gov.uk.

Allen, J. (2008). *Older People and Well-being.* London: Institute for Public Policy Research, 2008.

Brar, R., Kaur, J., and Sharma I. (2013). Mental health of elderly as related to their well-being and self-esteem. *International Journal of Humanities and Social Science Invention, 2* (11), 54-57.

Butler, R.N. (1974). Successful ageing and the role of the life review. *Journal of the American Geriatrics Society, 22*, 529-535.

Dhara, R.D., and Jogsan, Y.A. (2013). Depression and psychological well-being in old age. *Journal of Psychology and Psychotherapy, 3*(117), 2161-0487.

Dubey, A., Bhasin, S., Gupta, N., and Sharma, N. (2011). A study of elderly living in old age home and within family set-up in Jammu. *Studies on Home and Community Science, 5*(2), 93-98.

Gupta, I., Dasgupta, P., and Sawhney, M. (2003). Health of the Elderly in India. *Institute of Economic Growth Discussion Paper*. New Delhi: Institute of Economic Growth.

Helen, K.O., Mehta, K.K. and Merg, K.S. (2006). *Understanding and Counselling Older Persons: A Handbook.* Armour Publication Private Ltd.

Lakshmi, S.D. and Roopa, K.S. (2013). Quality of Life of Elderly Men and Women in Institutional and Non-institutional Settings in Urban Bangalore District. *Research Journal of Family, Community and Consumer Sciences. Vol. 1* (3), 7-13.

MacCourt, P. (2004). Seniors mental health policy lens: An instrument for developing policy, legislation, programmes and services that promote and support the mental health of older adults. *British Columbia Psychogeriatric Association.*

Menec, V.H. (2003). The relation between everyday activities and successful ageing: A 6-year longitudinal study. *The Journals of Gerontology Series B: Psychological Sciences and Social Sciences, 58*(2), S74-S82.

Patel, V., and Prince, M. (2001). Ageing and Mental Health in a Developing Country: who cares? Quality studies from Goa, India. *Psychological Medicine, 31*, 29-39.

Raju, S. (2000). Ageing in India: An Overview. In M. Desai and S. Raju (Eds.) *Gerontological Social Perspectives*. New Delhi: BR Publishing.

Raju, M.V.R. (2009). *Health Psychology and Counselling*. New Delhi: Discovery Publication House.

Singh, A., Sahai D., Mathur, N. (2014). A study on prevailing malnourishment among elderly population of Lucknow City. *International Journal of Agriculture and Food Science Technology, Vol. 5*, 35-40.

Tornstam, L. (1989). Gero-transcendence: A reformulation of the disengagement theory. *Ageing Clinical and Experimental Research, 1*(1), 55-63.

Ward, Y.L., Barnes, M., and Gahagan, B. (2012). *Well-being in old age: Findings from participatory research*. University of Brighton and Age Concern, Brighton, Hove and Portslade.

Watt, L.M., and Cappeliez, P. (2000). Integrative and instrumental reminiscence therapies for depression in older adults: Intervention strategies and treatment effectiveness. *Ageing and Mental Health, 4*(2), 166-177.

Well-being in Older age. Department of Communities (2008). Retrieved from http://www.communities.gov.au.

Wong, P.T., and Watt, L.M. (1991). What types of reminiscence are associated with successful ageing? *Psychology and Ageing, 6*(2), 272.

17

Paid for Life

Relational World of FSW (Female Sex Workers)

Archana Shukla and *Deepti Mehrotra*

> "*Prostitution is the business or practice of engageing in sexual relations in exchange for payment.*"—Merriam-Webster Dictionary (2013).

Though India is a very socially conservative country where women and men marry very early, and divorce is rare, prostitution is still a booming, but at the same time neglected industry in the country. A number of studies on individuals both male and female working in other organized sectors have been conducted, but the industry of sex work is ignored.

Prostitution is sometimes described as commercial sex. Each country has its own legal status on prostitution from being permissible, but unregulated, to an enforced or unenforced crime or to a regulated profession. The Fondation Scelles (2012) has released its latest report on Sexual Exploitation which states that at this given moment there are 40-42 million prostitutes at work, which is more than the population of Australia and Canada. A cursory glance at the Indian scenario showed that presently there are an estimated 3 million women working as prostitutes in India. 1.2 million of the sex workers are under the age of 18. The average age that a girl enters the sex trade in India is reported to be between 9 and 12 years old. The human trafficking industry in India is estimated to generate $4 Billion a year (MacAskill and Pradhan, 2013).

Sex work in India is neither legal nor illegal it is tolerated since prostitutes can practice their trade privately, but cannot legally solicit customers in public. Brothel ownership and pimping is illegal. They come across problems in all walks of life as they are being abused physically and mentally. Sex workers are unable to get help from police in situations where they are victims of violence.

Sex workers in India are discriminated against within public services and subjected to violence from clients, brokers, brothel owners, family members and police. The situation is exacerbated by laws that criminalize sex work that push them on the streets, into unsafe and violent situations.

Prostitution History Revisited

The profession of prostitution is one of the oldest in almost all the countries since long in every type of society. In the ancient history of India, the prostitution was present as an organized and established institution and it was also referred in our *Vedas*. In the earlier Indian mythology, there were many instances of high class prostitution in form of very beautiful demigods showing as prostitutes. They are called to as Menaka, Rambha, Urvashi, and Thilothamma (Jaishankar and Haldar, 2006). These are very beautiful, charming and are very perfect in giving attractive dance and musical performances. These prostitutes are used in heaven for amusement of guest in the court of Lord Indra, the Lord of Hindu Gods. These prostitutes were used as to test the zeal and devotion of the '*tapasya*' of the great saints.

In the rule of historian Indian rulers Pandavas and Kauravas, indulging with prostitutes were common. They were an important part of the court and both dynasties possessed harems of aristocracy in Brahmanic India.

In the third century A.D. in the Sanskrit works of Mahakavi Kalidas, religious prostitutes were attached to the famous temples of Mahakala of Ujjain and the system of holy prostitutes became common. This was related to the girls who had been offered by their parents to perform these services of the god and their religion; these types of girls are known as *Devadasi* in South India and as *Mukhies* in North India.

In the period of Mughal Empire, the great importance was given to women and wine, except of Aurangazeb the other Muslim rulers have recognized prostitution and this profession flourished under their eye. During the period of the British regime, the place of women in India was the same. Position of the female sex workers continued to become more and more vulnerable.

The scenario remains the same even in this twenty first century, here one needs to be sensitive to the issue of commercial sex where the self is at jeopardy at every night with every customer but still they are compelled as it is what they have paid for life. How is this self? What is this relational world? Who are these people in this relational world? What they paid for being an FSW? These are some questions which intrigued the researcher to pick up this study.

Review of literature brought to fore a pathetic picture where there was paucity of researches on FSW with psychological orientation in Indian perspective. In the present study relational world comprises relationship with self and significant others (who play a crucial role in one's life), before moving on to relational world an understanding of self is essential.

Self

According to Allport (1965): "The self is something of which we are immediately aware. We think of it as the warm, central, private region of our life. As such it plays a crucial part in our conscious (a concept broader than self), in our personality (a concept broader than consciousness) and in our organism (a concept broader than personality). Thus, it is some kind of core in our being. And yet it is not a constant core. Sometimes, the core expands and seems to go completely offstage, leaving us with no awareness whatsoever of self."

Central to Rogers' personality theory is the notion of self or *self-concept*. This is defined as "the organized, consistent set of perceptions and beliefs about oneself".

The self is the humanistic term for who we really are as a person. The self is our inner personality, and can be likened to the soul, or Freud's psyche. The self is influenced by the experiences a person has in their life, and out interpretations of those experiences. Two primary sources that influence our self-concept are childhood experiences and evaluation by others.

According to Rogers (1959), we want to feel experience and behave in ways which are consistent with our self-image and which reflect what we would like to be like, our ideal-self. The closer our self-image and ideal-self are to each other, the more consistent or congruent we are and the higher our sense of self-worth. A person is said to be in a state of incongruence if some of the totality of their experience is unacceptable to them and is denied or distorted in the self-image.

The popular view of self can be further collaborated with eastern thinkers; self from eastern perspective is best understood in *Vedas*. Life is easier to understand by understanding and analyzing the term death. An organism is said to be dead when it completely stop to respond to external objects. In other words, death is a state of cessation of experience.

Life is, therefore, a continuous series of experience which is known as "*Anubhava Dhara*".

There are three major concepts:

- Experiencer
- He is the subject
- The experienced is the object and the experiencing is the relationship between subject and the object

According to Chinmayanand, human personality comprises the divine spark of light called '*Aatman*' or the self have five layers of matter.

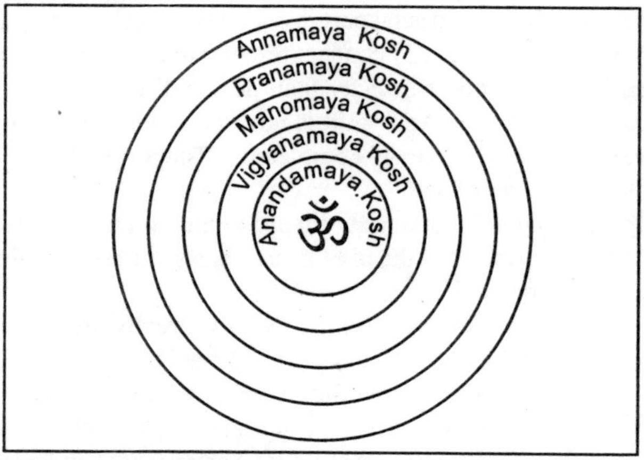

Fig. 17.1: Five Layers of Matter

Relational World of FSW: Explored through Draw A Person Test (DAPT)

Draw a person test was first given by Goodenough in 1926. It is a projective test which is used for the purposes of diagnosis and prognosis. It provides a great deal of information about self-concept, personality style, orientation and concerning areas. The personality traits can be anything from aggressiveness, to homosexual tendencies, to relationships with their parents, to introversion and extroversion (Machover, 1949). There are many versions of the test, but the one discussed in detail here is the version by Machover in 1949. Since 1926, the clinical use of DAPT has increased dramatically. Indeed, in 1961 Sundberg reported that the DAPT was the second most frequently used psychological test in hospitals, clinics and counselling centres throughout the country. Other surveys of psychological testing practice (Crenshaw, Bohn, Hoffman, Matheus and Offenbach, 1968; Lubin, Wallis and Paine, 1971) indicate that DAPT continues to be used with a majority of cases in a variety of clinical settings, it is among the five most frequently used projective tests in research situations. As discussed earlier, DAPT is a projective technique, in which a plane sheet of paper is given to the respondent and is being told: "I would like you to draw a picture of the person. When the first complete drawing is finished, the researcher puts another sheet of paper and told; now I'd like you to draw a person of the opposite sex."

***Analysis*:** DAPT drawings are analyzed by utilizing the structural and content variables. The structural variables concern the style in which the drawing was executed. The content variables concern the type of person drawn, the facial expression, the postural tone and the subtle nuances which communicate to the analyst the emotional tone of the patient who executed the drawing.

***Structure Variables*:** Size, Pencil Pressure, Line Quality, Lack of Detail, Placement on the page, Erasure, Shading, Distortions and Omissions, Transparency, and Sex of First Drawn figure.

The interpretation of drawing also concerns about the body parts of the drawing and how they have been drawn.

***Body Parts*:** Head, Facial Features, Eyes, Nose, Mouth, Chin, Neck, Shoulders, Breasts, Waistline, Trunk, Genitalia, Arms, Hand and Fingers, Hands, Legs, and Feet.

***Identification of Theme*:** Some common themes are drawn to identify the common patterns of behaviour occurring among the Female Sex Workers regarding their physical self, self-concept, significant others, their goals and social self.

The present research comprised of 50 FSW (aged between 20-30 years). A one to one interview was taken after which each response given by them was carefully analyzed and content analysis brought to fore the present picture.

Size

The size of the drawing in DAPT tells about the self-esteem and the manner in which the individual deals with self-esteem (Newmark, 1985). 60 per cent of the sex worker respondents have drawn tiny figures thereby directly indicating inadequacy feelings and withdrawal. The reason behind the tiny drawings is considered to be the feeling of worthlessness and dependent on others. 13 per cent of the respondents have made the drawings covering the entire page reacting with self-expansiveness in order to cover up the inadequate feelings by resorting to compensatory action or fantasy. The probable reason found is in the personality theories which describe that individual to hide his/her shallowness portrays himself/herself as a complete and healthy individual with a large discrepancy in the external and internal self whereas 27 per cent of the respondents have accepted the fact of being a sex worker or leading this life permanently thereby making the drawings of appropriate size.

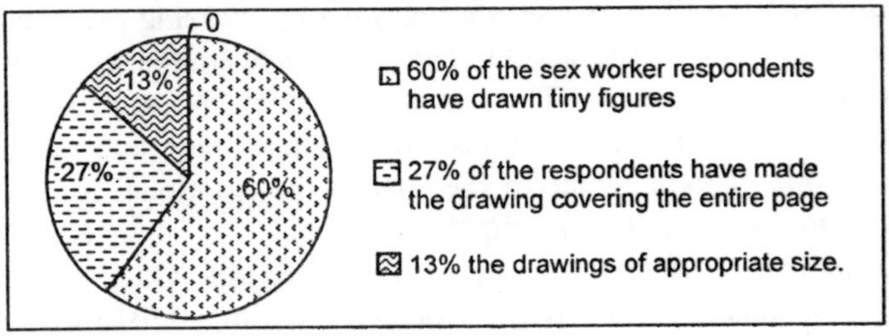

Fig. 17.2: Size

Stroke and Line Quality

Long pencil strokes indicate controlled behaviour, perhaps even inhibition in the extreme; short strokes are said to indicate impulsive behaviour and excitation (Newmark, 1985).10 per cent of the population's drawings appear as a series of disconnected dashes showing problems with reality contact and may have confused bizarre thoughts. 60 per cent of the population has drawn drawings using straight lines which indicate rigidity while 30 per cent of the respondents have curved lines in their drawings which suggest flexibility in their behaviour.

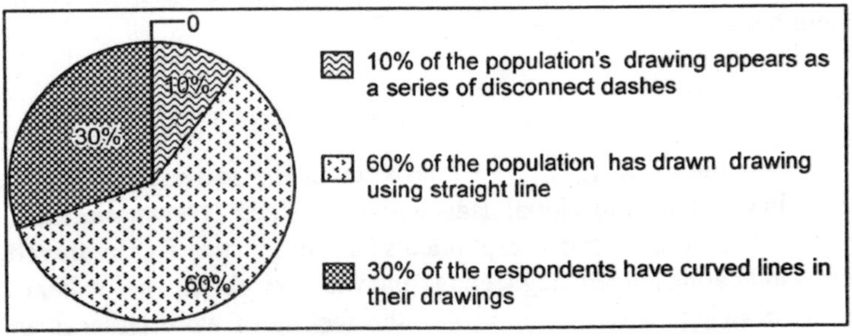

Fig. 17.3: Stroke and Line Quality

Lack of Details

60 per cent have lack of details in their drawings indicating withdrawal tendencies with an associated reduction of energy (Newmark, 1985). At times lack of acceptance of self (as they being FSW) could be a probable reason for above finding.

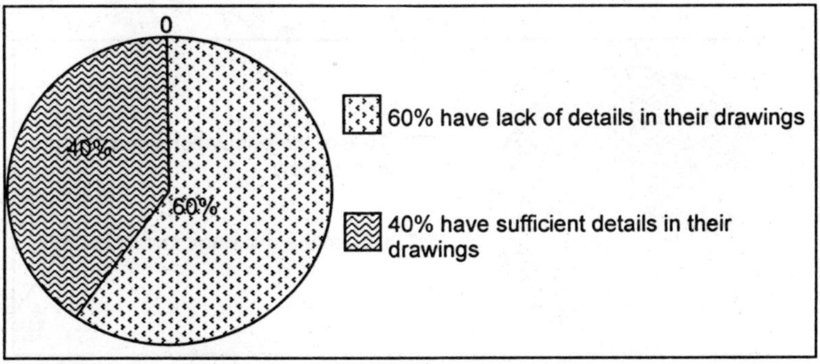

Fig. 17.4: Lack of details

Placement

77 per cent of the respondents have placed their drawings roughly in the middle of the page which is typical in most of the population. 7 per cent of the population has placement on the right side of the page indicating introversive tendencies: negativism and rebellious tendencies while 17 per cent have placement of their drawings on the left hand side of the page indicating impulsive acting out behaviour; a tendency towards immediate, frank and emotional satisfaction of motives; extroversion; preoccupation with one's changing needs; a self-centred approach to life and orientation and concern with the past (Newmark, 1985).

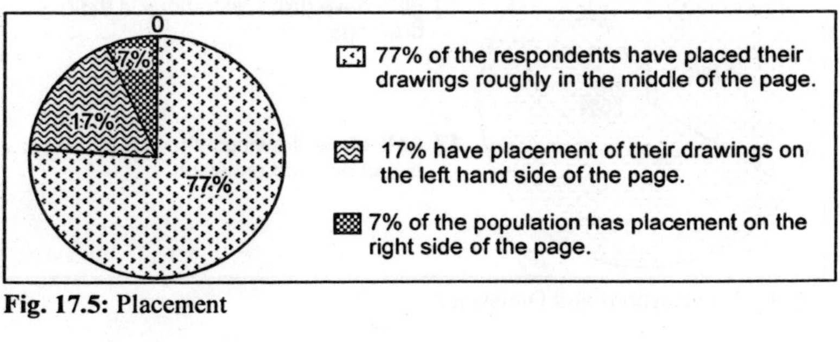

Fig. 17.5: Placement

Erasure and Shading

Excessive use of erasure and shading indicates uncertainty; anxiety and conflict (Newmark, 1985). However, in most of the drawings erasure and shading is found which according to Handler and Reyher (1964, 1965, 1966) is an attempt to give the drawing a sense of three-dimensionality revealing uncertainty, anxiety and conflict.

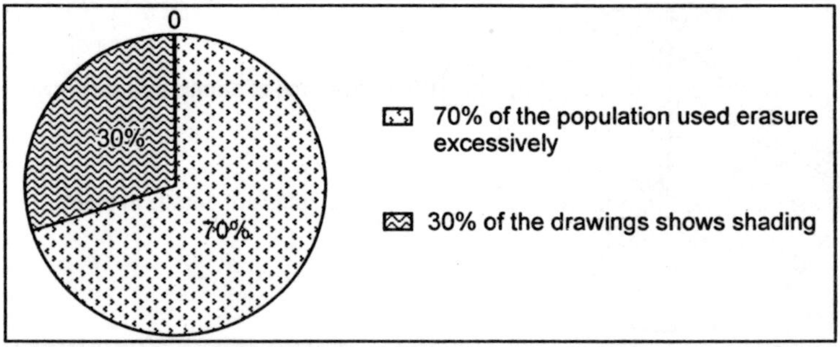

Fig. 17.6: Erasure and Shading

Distortions and Omissions

Gross distortion indicates poor reality contact and negative self-concept (Newmark, 1985). 66 per cent have gross distortions in their drawings showing poor reality contact and negative self-concept. 34 per cent of the drawings showed moderate distortion and omission which indicates conflict and anxiety. The omissions of body parts have been mentioned in the analysis of body parts.

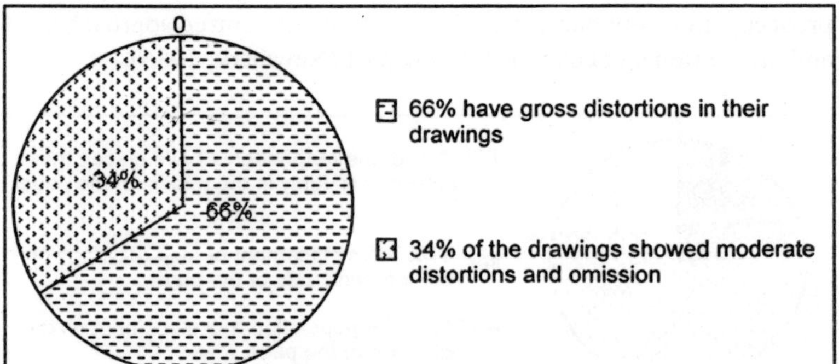

Fig. 17.7: Distortions and Omissions

Transparency

Transparency here can be understood as poor reality ties (Newmark, 1985). 70 per cent of the participants have presence of transparency in their drawings suggesting poor judgement; sexual disturbance and conflict which is an obvious finding with this population.

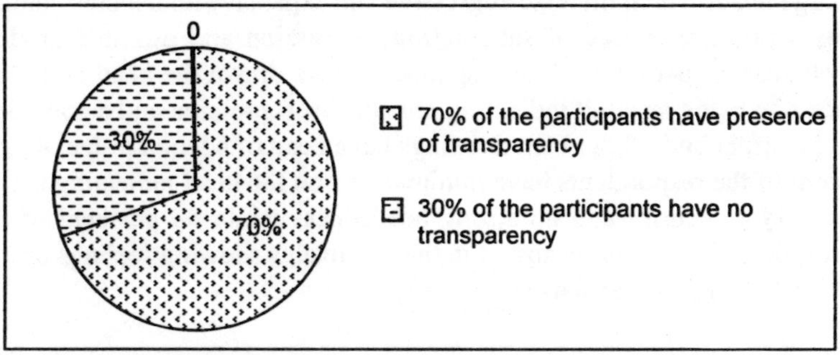

Fig. 17.8: Transparency

Sex of First Drawn Figure

33 per cent of the respondents in their drawings have drawn the opposite sex studies which interprets strong attachment or dependence on a person of the opposite sex, poor self-concept, or greater interest and/or awareness of the opposite sex compared with the same sex while 60 per cent of the respondents have drawn female sex first showing identification with their sex while 7 per cent have denied about drawing the female sex (Newmark, 1985).

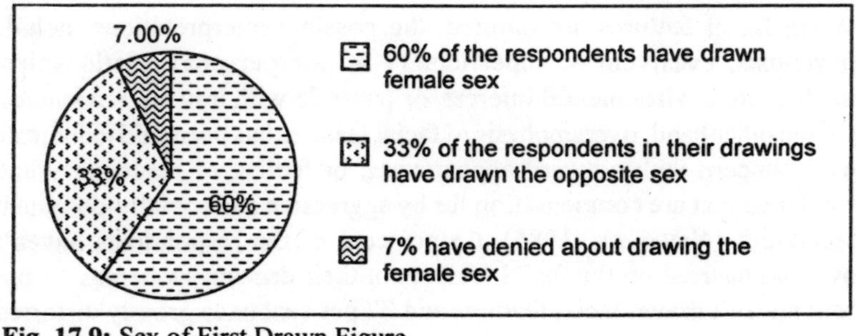

Fig. 17.9: Sex of First Drawn Figure

Body Parts

Head

Head is the symbol of intellectual and fantasy activity and symbol of impulse-control and the site of socialization and communication (Newmark, 1985). 27 per cent of the respondents have made unusually large heads which indicate aggressive and expansive tendencies, fantasy as a primary source of satisfaction, regression and possible anxiety whereas 53 per cent of the respondents have drawn the head child like despite being an adult indicating immaturity, repression and a good deal of conflict and 20 per cent drawings have head of adequate size. 47 per cent of the respondents have minimal hair on the head indicating a high need for security and no strong headedness while 53 per cent of the respondents have hairs absent in their drawings showing feelings of low physical vigour and sense of security.

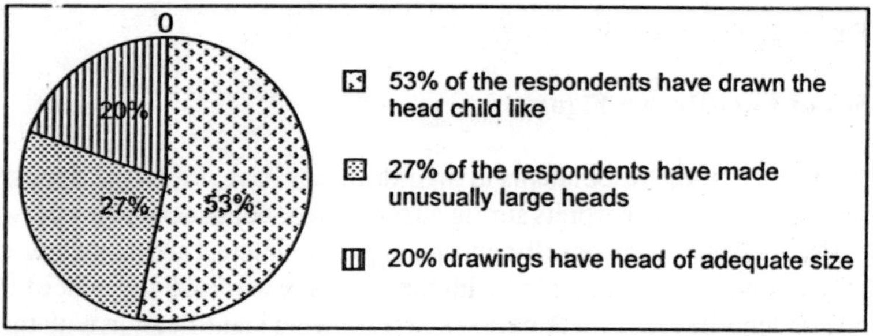

Fig. 17.10: Head

Facial Features

When facial features are omitted, the possible interpretations include psychosis, evasiveness, superficiality in interpersonal relationships, inadequate environmental interest, or possible withdrawing tendencies. On the other hand, overemphasis of facial features has been said to indicate over-concern with outward appearances; or feeling of inadequacy and weakness that are compensation for by aggressive and socially-dominant behaviour (Newmark, 1985). 63 per cent of the respondents haven't overemphasized on the facial features in their drawings whereas 10 per cent haven't drawn facial features and 27 per cent have grossly distorted facial features drawn in their drawings indicating conflict and a feeling of negativity towards their body.

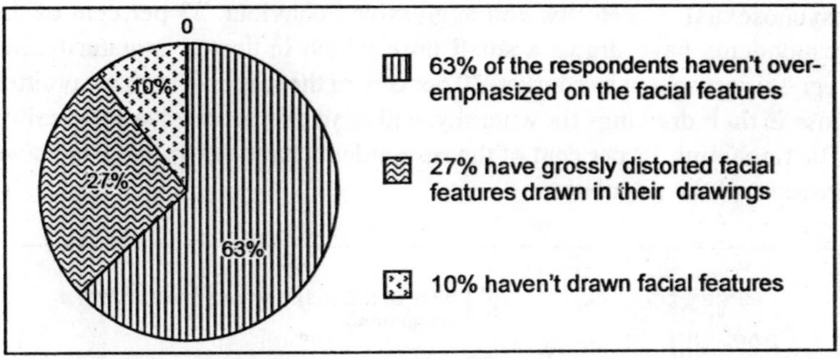

Fig. 17.11: Facial features

Eyes

33 per cent of the respondents have drawn dotted eyes, whereas 10 per cent of the respondents have drawn unusually large or strongly reinforced eyes, which indicate suspiciousness, hypersensitivity to social opinion and the remaining 37 per cent of the respondents have drawn the eyes with the pupil omitted or empty eyes that indicate introversion, self-absorption and not interested in perceiving their environment 20 per cent drawings show eyes omitted from the drawings showing tendency not to perceive themselves and the environment as well as communication difficulties (Newmark, 1985).

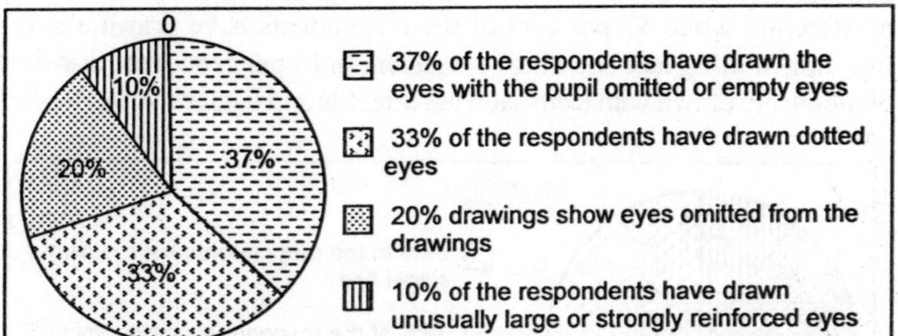

Fig. 17.12: Eyes

Nose

Nose is said sometimes to be a phallic symbol or symbol of power motive (Newmark, 1985). Large noses have been found in drawings of 7 per cent of respondents which indicates sexual difficulties including psychosexual immaturity, and aggressive behaviour. 53 per cent of the respondents have drawn a small nose which indicates immaturity and regressive response to conflict. 30 per cent of the respondents have omitted nose in their drawings showing shy, withdrawn or depressive personality. The remaining 10 per cent of the respondents have drawn nose as drawn by most of the population.

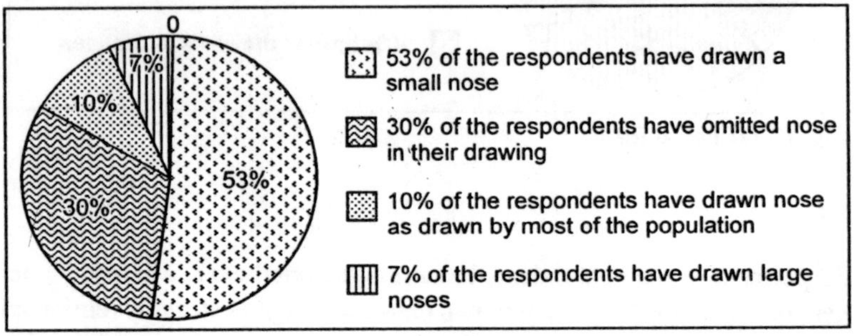

Fig. 17.13: Nose

Mouth

Newmark (1985) indicates that mouth depicts regressive defences, oral emphasis in the personality. 33 per cent of the respondents have omitted mouth in their drawings. Omission interprets oral aggression, depressive tendencies, difficulties in the communication and rejection for the need of affection while 57 per cent of the respondents have drawn a single line, non-smiling face showing depression. In 10 per cent of the drawings of mouth are drawn with teeth showing infantile and aggressive tendencies.

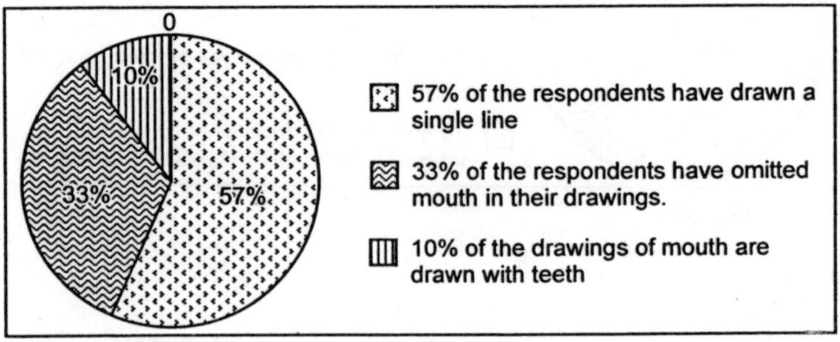

Fig. 17.14: Mouth

Ears

Ears have been omitted by 70 per cent of the respondents which are seen normally in the population, whereas 30 per cent of respondents show large ears which indicate hypersensitivity to criticism, idea of reference, paranoid tendencies or possible auditory hallucinations (Newmark, 1985).

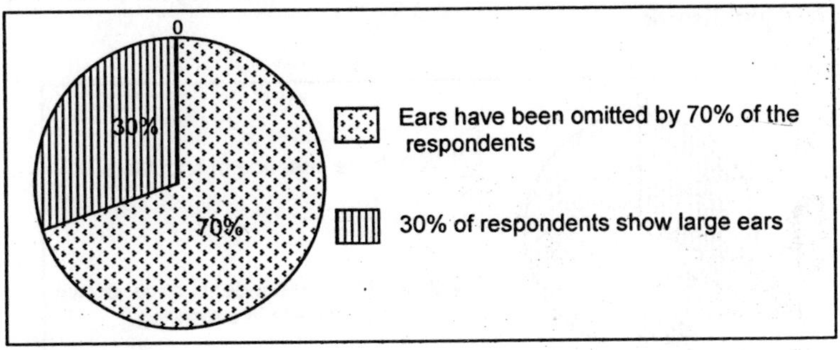

Fig. 17.15: Ears

Neck

The neck is typically regarded as the link between intellectual life (symbolized by head) and the affect (basic body impulses). The neck represents ego control and id impulse (Newmark, 1985). The short neck comprises 43 per cent in the drawings indicate tendencies to be gruff, stubborn and rigid in their behaviour but they consider psyche and soma same. 50 per cent have drawn long necks showing the difference between the intellect and emotions and rigid and socially and culturally stiff. The neck is omitted by 7 per cent of the respondents showing impulsivity.

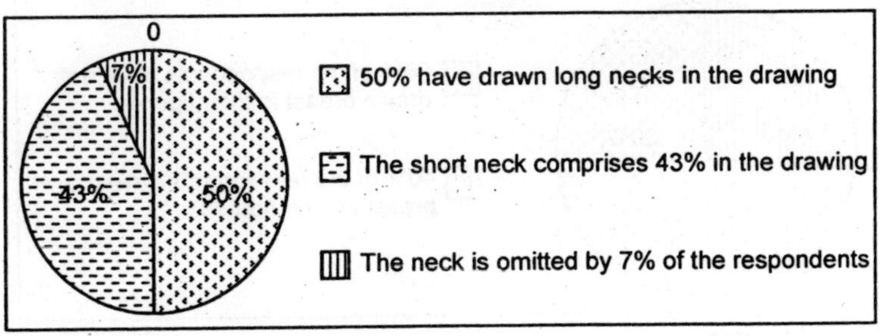

Fig. 17.16: Neck

Shoulders

Well-drawn and neatly rounded shoulders have typically been said to be normal, indicating adequate, well balanced control of impulses and behaviour (Newmark, 1985). 30 per cent of the respondents have drawn broad shoulders in a drawing which typically indicate a need for physical power. 70 per cent have absence of shoulders suggesting the presence of a thought disorder.

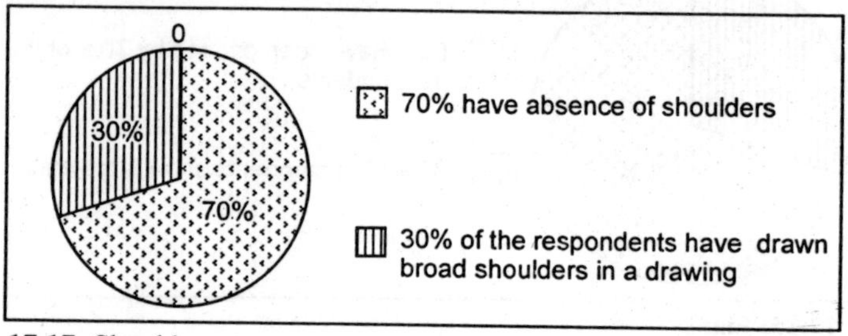

Fig. 17.17: Shoulders

Breasts

40 per cent of the respondents have drawn breasts in their figures. Tiny breasts drawn by the respondents show lack of nurturance and a need to be the mother, while large or decorative drawn breasts show sexual fantasy, exhibitionism and sexual confusion; unusually large breast drawn by females may indicate identification with a dominant mother, exhibitionism or narcissistic problems (Newmark, 1985).

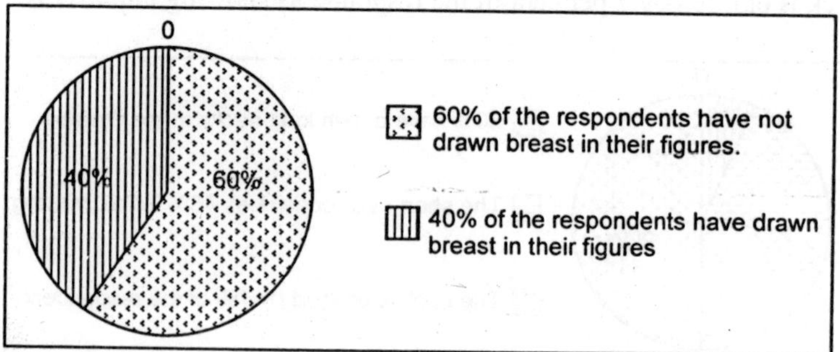

Fig. 17.18: Breast

Arms, Hands and Fingers

7 per cent of the respondents have drawn long and outstretched hands showing acquisitive and compensatory ambition, a need for physical desire, a desire for interpersonal contact and a desire for help and affection. 13 per cent of the respondents have drawn short hands indicating a lack of ambition, feelings of inadequacy, passivity or possible castration fears. 20 per cent of the respondents have omission of fingers which indicate a feeling of difficulty in interpersonal relationships or masturbation guilt (Newmark, 1985).

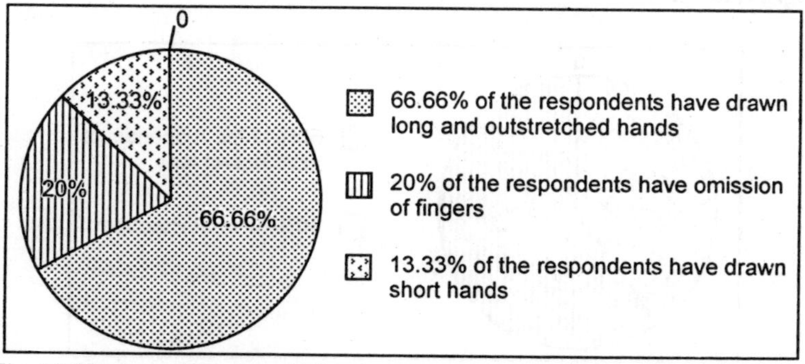

Fig. 17.19: Arms, Hands and Fingers

Legs and Feet

Legs or feet are typically symbolic of security feelings and/or feelings concerning mobility (Newmark, 1985). 40 per cent have drawn short legs a strong need for autonomy, whereas 47 per cent have drawn short legs showing feelings of immobility and constriction. 40 per cent have omitted feet which suggest a feeling of constriction with lack of independence, loss of autonomy and feeling of helplessness whereas 60 per cent of the respondents have drawn feet showing goal clarity and orientation and 13 per cent of the drawings have legs missing in their drawings showing needs of security and mobility.

Findings emerged from drawn a person test—

- Majority of the sex worker respondents has drawn tiny figures thereby directly indicating inadequacy feelings and withdrawal. The reason behind the tiny drawings is considered to be the feeling of worthlessness and dependent on others.

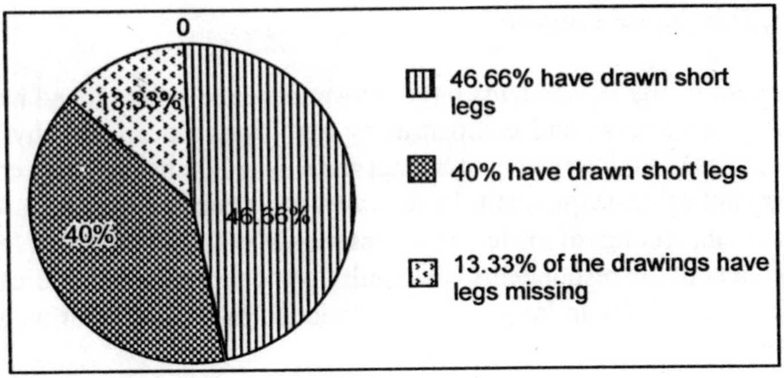

Fig. 17.20: Legs

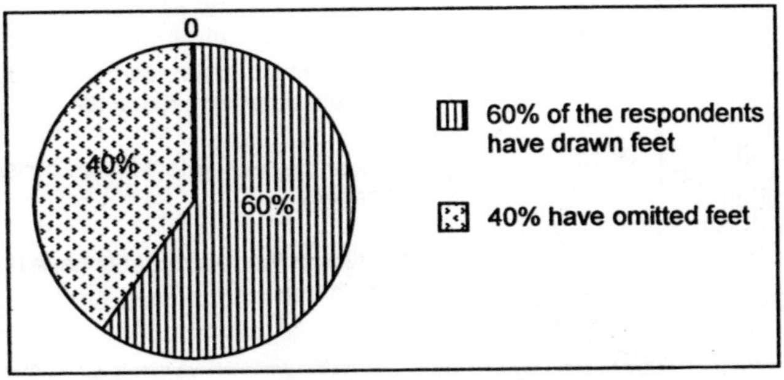

Fig. 17.21: Feet

- Most of the population has drawn drawings using straight lines which indicate rigidity.
- Gross distortions in their drawings were present which shows poor reality contact and negative self-concept.
- Respondents have drawn the head child like despite being an adult indicating immaturity, repression and a good deal of conflict.
- Majority of female sex workers has drawn the eyes with the pupil omitted or empty eyes that indicate introversion, self-absorption and not interested in perceiving their environment.
- Large noses found in drawings indicate sexual difficulties including psychosexual immaturity, and aggressive behaviour.
- The respondents have omitted mouth in their drawings. Omission interprets oral aggression, depressive tendencies, difficulties in the communication and rejection for the need of affection.
- The respondents have drawn long and outstretched hands showing acquisitive and compensatory ambition, a need for

physical desire, a desire for interpersonal contact and a desire for help and affection.

- Legs or feet are typically symbolic of security feelings and/or feelings concerning mobility, majorities have drawn short legs showing feelings of immobility and constriction.
- The drawings have legs missing in their drawings showing needs of security and mobility.

Conclusion and Implications

On the basis of above findings one can aptly say that what they have paid for life in becoming female sex workers is much more that what they got in return. As they seemed to be seriously threatened in many aspects like health problems, abused physically and mentally, social stigma and discrimination.

Majority of the sex worker respondents has drawn figures directly indicating inadequacy feelings, withdrawal, and feeling of worthlessness. Dependency on others hand has emerged in addition with rigidity, poor reality contact, negative self-concept, immaturity and good deal of conflict. Besides introversion, self-absorption, not interested in perceiving their environment, psychosexual immaturity, aggressive behaviour, difficulties in the communication has emerged as dominating features in their responses. To add more it is rejection for the need of affection, a need for physical desire, desire for interpersonal contact, needs of security and mobility that ruled the profile.

The above findings were indicative of the fact that the self of FSW is at challenge in their relational world. The time, energy and emotions they have invested/paid in becoming FSW has resulted into desertedness, isolation, stigmatized, they being considered as marginalized, and unworthy of respectful life. This study is a small attempt to bring to for some basic realities of FSW. Yet a great deal remains to be explored as enormous amount of knowledge about prostitution was gained during the course of working in this area, but what becomes most clear during this effort is the vast amount that remains unknown, undocumented and unspoken.

The exact number of female sex workers in India is open to dispute, the exact number of sex workers is unknown and calculating the number of female sex workers is very difficult as sex work is mostly hidden and the population is transient, with people moving in and out of sex work constantly.

Despite tall talks of social welfare, women empowerment and

community development female sex worker is the grassroots reality. An effort must be done to bring them into mainstream, to build a platform where one can uncover the crude realities existing in society.

References

Allport, G.W. (1961). *Pattern and Growth in Personality.* New York: Holt, Rinehart & Winston.

Charpenel, Fondation Scelles (2012), Sexual exploitation, *Economica.*

Crenshaw, D.A., Bohn, S., Hoffman, M.R., Matheus, J.M., and Offenbach, S.G. (1968). The use of projective methods in research: 1947-1965. *Journal of Projective Techniques and Personality Assessment, 32*(1), 3-9.

Goodenough, F.L. (1926). *Measurement of Intelligence by Drawings.* NewYork: Harcourt Brace,

Handler, L. and Reyher, J. (1966). Relationship between GSR and anxiety indexes in projective drawings. *Journal of Consulting and Clinical Psychology, 30*, 605-607.

Handler, L. and Reyher, J. (1965). Figure drawing anxiety indexes: A review of the literature. *Journal of Personality Assessment, 29*, 305-313.

Handler, L. and Reyher, J. (1964). The effect of stress on the Draw-A-Person Test. *Journal of Consulting Psychology, 28*, 259-264.

Jaishankar, K., and Haldar, D. (2006). Prostitution in India: Issues and Trends. European & International Research Group on Crime, *Ethics and Social Philosophy*, (3)2.

Lubin, B., Wallis, R.R., and Paine, C. (1971). Patterns of psychological test usage in the United States: 1935-1969. *Professional Psychology, 2*(1), 70.

Macaskill, A. and Pradha, B. (1998). Sold for Sex at Puberty Village Girls' Fate in India. *Bloomberg Business Week*, Retrieved 19 September, 2013.

Machover, K. (1949). *Personality Projection in the drawings of human figure.* Springfield, IL: Charles Thomas, Publisher.

Newmark, C.S. (1985). *Major Psychological Assessment Instruments*, (Volume 1): Allyn & Bacon.

Rogers, C. (1959). A Theory of Therapy, Personality and Interpersonal Relationships as Developed in the Client-centred Framework. In S. Koch (ed.), *Psychology: A Study of a Science.* Vol. 3: *Formulations of the Person and the Social Context.* New York: McGraw Hill.

Sundberg, N.D. (1961). The practice of psychological testing in clinical services in the United States. *American Psychologist, 16*(2), 79.

http://www.thekundaliniyoga.org/vedanta/pancha_kosha_five_layers_of_human_existence.aspx

http://www.bhakti-yoga-meditation.com/hindu-maya-suffering.html

18

Impact of Peer Pressure and Parenting Behaviour on Adolescents' Cigarette Smoking Tendency

An Overview

Purnima Awasthi, Ravi P. Pandey and *Saroj Verma*

Peer pressure has been widely identified as an influential component of adolescents' development. In spite of advances in tobacco control, adolescents' cigarette smoking tendency remains a serious health problem for them. The smoking status of friends has been indicated to be one of the highest associates of adolescents' smoking tendency in various studies. Adolescents may acquire tendency of cigarette smoking due to either peer pressure, where adolescents acquire the same act of their friends or peer selection, where adolescents choose friends based on their cigarette smoking status. Another important aspect for understanding peer group influences on adolescents' cigarette smoking tendency is school environment. Thus, it becomes important to come across the reasons of smoking tendency that may affect an adolescent's social and personal growth and functioning. Another important aspect of adolescents' initiation towards smoking cigarette is the parenting behaviour. Studies reveal greater chances of acquisition of cigarette smoking tendency among adolescents where their parents and friends smoke. The present review focuses on peer group influences and parenting behaviour on adolescent cigarette smoking tendency with particular focus on published studies that have investigated these aspects. Specifically, we examine the theoretical explanations for how social influences work in relation to adolescents' cigarette smoking tendency; discuss the association between peer and adolescent smoking tendencies; consider peer socialization and friends selection processes with respect to smoking; investigate the characteristics of best friends, and close friends that may increase cigarette smoking tendency among adolescents.

Smoking is considered as one of the most common health impairing behaviours involving recreational drug use, in which tobacco is burned and smoke is tasted or inhaled. Health professionals have identified cigarette smoking (in which the active drug is nicotine) as one of the most serious preventive health problems of youth (Erickson, Gotham, Sher, & Wood, 1996). Tobacco kills up to half of its users, it kills nearly 6000000 (six million) people each year, more than 5000000 (five million) of those deaths are result of direct tobacco use while more than 600000 (six lakh) are the result of non-smokers being exposed to second-hand smoke, unless urgent action is taken the annual death is expected to rise more than eight million by 2030 (Beaglehole, Detels, Gulliford, & Lansang, 2011).

Smoking is estimated to cause about 71 per cent of lung cancer, 42 per cent of chronic respiratory disease and nearly 10 per cent of cardiovascular disease. The report suggests that deaths due to use of tobacco will increase to 7.5 million by 2020 and may account for 10 per cent of all deaths. Surprisingly, nearly 80 per cent of these preventable deaths will be among people living in low and middle-income countries, contrasting the notion that people from high income countries are at higher risk. Over 80 per cent of cardiovascular and diabetes deaths, and almost 90 per cent of deaths from chronic obstructive pulmonary disease occur in low and middle-income countries due to health impairing behaviour (Ezzatt & Lopez, 2003).

According to the WHO Global Report on "Tobacco Attributable Mortality" (2012), 7 per cent of all deaths (for ages 30 and over) in India are attributable to tobacco. The most prevalent form of tobacco is smokeless tobacco and 206 million users consume the same. Smokeless tobacco usage in India is the highest in the world with 25.9 per cent of the adults—32.9 per cent of men and 18.4 per cent women—use it (Global Adult Tobacco Survey, 2012). Within communicable diseases, the deaths attributed to tobacco use account for 5 per cent of all deaths caused by lower respiratory infections and 4 per cent of tuberculosis deaths. The Report on Tobacco Control in India (2004) estimated that nearly 8-9 lakh people die every year in India due to diseases related to tobacco use. It was assumed that up to one in five deaths from tuberculosis (TB) could be avoided if TB patients did not smoke.

Numerous factors are found to be responsible for adolescents smoking behaviour in which peer pressure/influence and parenting behaviour has been identified as the most important factors that leads to adolescents' smoking. Adolescents have very strong needs to be liked and accepted by friends and the larger peer group, which can result in enjoyable feelings when accepted or extreme stress and anxiety when excluded and disparaged by peers. For many adolescents, how they are seen by peers is the most important aspect of their lives (Santrock, 2007). Peers, as members of the same age cohort may play an important role in process of adolescents' personal and social positive growth related development.

Theories of Smoking

Smoking is an extremely complex practice involving a combination of biological, psychological and social processes. Theories of smoking and smoking cessation differ in their conceptualizations of the relative importance and interrelationships among three aspects, with some variation in how they deal with the psychological factors.

Cognitive-behavioural theories often have distinct sub-theories that hypothesize the relationships between cognitive aspects and factors influencing habituated and reactive behaviours. One sub-set of expectancy value theories focus on rational appraisals of costs and benefits. These are purely or largely cognitive in focus and include such theories as the theory of planned behaviour (Ajzen, and Fishbein, 2010), the health beliefs model (Rosenstock, 1988), the rational addiction model (Becker, and Murphy, 1988) and the trans-theoretical model (DiClemente & Prochaska, 1983). Behavioural theories focus on how people learn to behave in particular ways. Behaviourists believe people learn to behave through mechanisms such as conditioning, and positive and negative reinforcement. They respond to stimuli in their environment and establish an association or linkage between two events. In the context of smoking, a person learns to associate smoking with other feelings and events (e.g. being in a stressful situation or having a coffee) and these continue to 'cue' their smoking behaviour.

The most and frequently used psychological model of smoking is based on learning theory. Basically, it argues that people become smokers because of the positive reinforcements they obtain from smoking. Initially smoking is physically unpleasant, but this is overruled because of the social reinforcement from peers (Pomerlau, 1979).

Social theories consider smoking as a social activity. Even when the smoker smokes alone he or she still smokes in a society where cigarettes are widely available and promoted. Murray *et al.* (1988) suggested that smoking is given different meanings in different settings. For example, at workplace going for a cigarette provides an opportunity to escape from the everyday routine. Outside work, smoking may be perceived as a means of reaffirming social relationships. For young people who generally go to pub, the sharing of cigarettes may be the mean of initiating, maintaining and strengthening social bonds.

Peer Pressure

The relationship process that has spawned the most persistent interest among youth is peer pressure or, more generally, peer influence. Peers are children or adolescents who are about the same age or maturity level (Santrock, 2007). Peer pressure has been defined both as a part of the normal process of psychological development, and a major contributor to the development of risk-taking behaviours (Jessor & Jessor, 1977). Peer pressure that a peer group observes or individual maintains that encourages changing their attitudes values or behaviours to conform the group norms (Brown, 2004). Researchers sometimes use peer pressure but most of the time use the term peer influence, which is simply assumed to exist on the basis of a statistical association between the smoking behaviour of adolescents and their friends.

Theories of Peer Pressure

Numerous theoretical frameworks have been used to explain the process by which social relationships affect individuals' health-risk behaviours, such as drug, alcohol and tobacco use. Social learning theory (Akers, 1977, 1998; Bandura, 1977) consider both social processes and cognitive meditation as important in the attainment and maintenance of behaviour, such as smoking. According to this perspective, behaviours are learned through the observation of others engaged in a behaviour and subsequent modelling of this behaviour, as well as the rewards/punishments and favourable/unfavourable definitions associated with the behaviour. The extent to which individuals are influenced by models' behaviour depends on the characteristics of models, the attributes of observers and the perceived consequences of adopting similar behaviour (Bandura *et al.*, 1963).

Social learning principles underlie primary socialization theory (Donnermeyer & Oetting 1998; Oetting, *et al.*, 1998), Primary socialization theory places emphasis on the relational bonds that exist between teenagers and their family, peers and school, as such bonds serve as channels through which information about norms and behaviours are transmitted. Similar to the view of relational bonds, social bonding theory proposed by Hirschi (1969), this perspective holds that when the bonds between youth and others in their lives are strong and the direction of influence is pro-social, youth are not expected to engage in behaviours such as drug, alcohol and tobacco use. A theory which emphasizes social pressures to adopt unhealthy behaviour is that of Social inoculation theory (Duryea, 1991; McGuire, 1968, 1974). Premised on the belief that young people lack the negotiating skills to resist unhealthy behaviour arising from peer pressure and other influences, the theory proposes a range of techniques which is claimed that it can 'inoculate' young people from such pressure. Social identity theory (Terry *et al.*, 2000) suggests that adolescents try on several identities and adopt the norms that are central to the social identity of the peer group to remain in good standing. Similarly, social exchange theory (Kelley & Thibaut, 1985) argues that friendships and group membership requires fair exchanges (reciprocity), leading to conformity of behaviour between friends and group members.

Parenting Behaviour

A great deal of research indicates the significance of parental influences on many types of adolescent behaviour. However, inconsistencies in findings have been found that examined the relationship between parent and adolescent smoking behaviour. Findings reveal that parental influence may be relatively modest. As primary socializing agents, parents can maintain an important influence on their offspring's smoking behaviour. In some studies, role of parents in the development of adolescents' smoking have concentrated on parents' anti-smoking socialization practices (Chassin *et al.*, 2005; Harakeh *et al.*, 2005; Henriksen & Jackson, 1997). Communication about smoking-related issues is one of the important aspects of anti-smoking socialization. Through conversations, parents cannot only explain the house rules (Clark *et al.*, 1999), but also can discuss reasons for not smoking, which is related to a lower risk of adolescent's smoking (Chassin *et al.*, 1998). Nevertheless, whether conversations are effective or not seems to depend on the quality of the parent-child communication. A protective factor that comes in light is the quality of communication, which indicates that parents who discuss smoking-related issues in a constructive and respectful manner with their children can prevent adolescents from smoking (Harakeh *et al.*, 2005).

Methodology

Inclusion Criteria

The review focuses on the findings based on peer pressure, parental influence and adolescents smoking tendency. Studies generally include adolescents and youth belonging to age group of 11 to 23 years, and youth consuming any kind of tobacco products. The review highlights published empirical and theoretical studies based on peer pressure, parental influence, and adolescents' smoking tendency.

Search Strategy and Selection of Article

Published empirical and theoretical studies were reviewed using a standard review methodology. Science direct, Sage, Springer, PubMed, Google scholar and different organizations survey research have been included. Issues such as peer pressure and smoking, role of peer pressure on adolescents' smoking behaviour, smokers' role model, peer group influence on adolescents' smoking behaviour, quality of peer relations among adolescents smoking cigarettes etc. have been thoroughly described.

Results

After thorough literature review, some relevant studies implicated world-wide from 1980 onwards have been selected, which explored the peer pressure/influence and parental influence on adolescents' smoking tendency. Constructs like friendship selection, quality of peer relations, parent-child communication, parenting style and adolescents smoking etc. were assessed. Key findings of studies regarding peer and parental influence are summarised.

Sample

The sample size of reviewed studies related to adolescents' smoking tendency, peer pressure, and parental influence ranged from 165 to 2520. The samples were collected from several schools of North Carolina, Norvey, Australia, Britain, and India. The sample represented different socio-demographic categories of urban and rural areas.

Method and Measures

Out of all included studies some studies were longitudinal and some were cross-sectional. Both quantitative and qualitative comparative studies have been found relevant to peer pressure and adolescents smoking. The measures used by researchers in these studies were self-administered questionnaire and interview schedule. It appeared to be difficult to illustrate a broad inference for the adolescents' smoking tendency due to distinction in research methodologies and tools employed in the studies reviewed. For example, some studies used non-standardized measurement scales and tools with small sample size. Some have compared peer pressure and smokers' tendency with inappropriate control groups having incongruous sampling methods and sampling biases. The present review also highlights in-depth qualitative interviews as well as quantitative assessment of psychological constructs by several researchers.

Peer Selection and Influence

Peer selection is the tendency to choose friends who are more alike in certain characteristics, while social influence implies one changes his or her opinions, attitudes, behaviours in response to that of others (Aseltine, 1995). The majority of research suggests that peer influence may be an important factor, as found in early cross-sectional studies showing significant correlations between adolescents' cigarette smoking tendency and the smoking behaviours of friends (Bauman, Bryan, Chenoweth, Fisher, 1984; Cleary, Leventhal, 1980). Longitudinal data also shows increased risks of cigarette smoking among those whose friends are smokers (Aloise-Young, Hansen, Graham, 1994; Flay, Hu, Siddiqui, *et al.*, 1994). The degree to which peer influence is responsible for adolescent substance use is currently in doubt. Similarity between adolescents and their friends are usually been used as evidence of peer influence. However, many studies comparing the effects of peer selection and influence have found selection effects to be more powerful than influence effects in accounting for similarity among adolescent and friend in cigarette use (Bauman and Ennett, 1994) and other problem behaviours (Billy and Udry, 1985; Danish and Farrell, 1993).

Despite the consistency of results in many studies, some have indicated that peer influence has been overestimated, because much of the research fails to address projection and selection effects (Bauman, and Ennett, 1994). For example, many studies rely on adolescents' perception of peers' behaviour in spite of the peers' own reports of their behaviour to assess similarity in smoking between friends (Bentler, Huba, 1980; Degirmencioglu, Pilgrim, and Urberg, 1997; Flay, Hu, Siddiqui, *et al.*, 1994; Chassin, Montello, Presson, *et al.*, 1986). If adolescents incline to project their own smoking behaviour onto their friends, the similarity in smoking between adolescents and peers will be inflated when perceived reports are used.

Peer Pressure and Adolescents' Smoking Tendency

Studies reveal peer influence to be one of the strongest factors that led to the acquisition of smoking tendency among adolescents (Conrad, Flay, & Hill, 1992; Kobus, 2003). However, adolescent smoking is most often a social behaviour, they fequently smoke in the presence of others (Biglan, Friedman, and Lichtenstein, 1995) and they smoke it as a way to achieve social belonging (Kobus, 2003; Mermelstein, 1999) and are more likely to smoke if their close friend smoke (Chassin, Presson & Sherman, 1984; Flay *et al.*, 1995).

Researchers found adolescents' perceptions that smoking is prevalent among their same age peers have been linked to their own smoking behaviour (Botvin *et al.*, 1992; and Sussman *et al.*, 1999). Adolescents rarely report direct pressure from peers to smoke, but rather, the pressure to smoke may be implied by being with others who are smoking and their need to achieve a sense of acceptance or belonging (Mermelstein, 2003; Nichter *et al.*, 1997). Evidence suggests that affective experiences (i.e. positive or negative emotions, feeling stressed) and social situations (i.e. being in the company of others, with smokers present, while eating and/or drinking) can elicit urges to smoke amongst the adolescents (Baer, Lichtenstein, 1988; Burger, Gochfeld, 1990). Some work has supported and extended this point, showing that friends play an important role in both harmful and positive activities (Berndt, 1999; Mounts and Steinberg, 1995; Urberg, 1999; Wentzel, 1999). The prevalence of smoking increases dramatically during adolescence (Johnston *et al.*, 2007). Though not all experimental users increase their uptake over time (Abroms *et al.*, 2005; Tucker *et al.*, 2004), early initiation increases the likelihood of habituation, leading to a host of negative outcomes (Gilpin and Pierce, 1995).

A review of peer group influences on adolescents' smoking based on longitudinal studies available from 1999 explored the extent to which peer smoking predicts adolescent smoking (Farhat, and Simons-Morton,

2010). The authors acknowledged 40 prospective studies linking peer group smoking or measures of substance use, including smoking and future adolescents' cigarette use. All but one of the studies reported positive relations between peer use at baseline and adolescent smoking at follow-up. The review also highlighted the difference of peer influence on adolescent smoking by socio-demographic characteristics, including gender differences and less clear effects of age group and ethnicity. Social bonds (e.g. with school and family) and individual characteristics such as genetics and personal attributes were also found to moderate peer smoking (Farhat *et al.*, 2010).

A longitudinal analysis based on a nationally representative sample of US adolescents followed for eight years from high school to adulthood tried to empirically quantify the role of peer social networks in explaining smoking behaviour (Ali & Dwyer, 2009). Researchers controlled for potential biases in the data: parental characteristics (such as parent smoking status and education) and other socio-demographic factors (e.g. age, grade level, gender, access to cigarettes at home). They estimated that a 10 per cent increase in the proportion of classmates who smoke would increase the likelihood of smoking by more than 3 per cent, while an increase in smoking rates of 10 per cent among an individual's close friends would increase the likelihood of smoking by 5 per cent. They concluded that peer effects are significant factors of smoking, which persist into adulthood (Ali and Dwyer, 2009).

Similarly, recent Australian study examined peer effects in smoking for 75000 adolescents aged 15-16 years across 26 European countries (McVicar, 2011). It was based on international school survey data, which was highly similar across countries due to common sampling frames. Methods and questionnaires were statistically significant and large peer effects were observed in almost all cases. It was estimated that, on average across countries, a one percentage point increase in the proportion of smoking classmates would be associated with an increase of 0.31 to 0.38 per cent in the probability that a 'typical' adolescent smokes, a range that varied between countries (McVicar, 2011).

Qualitative research from Western Australia found that some adolescent experimenters and smokers saw trying a cigarette in the spirit of 'joining in' or 'giving it a go'. However, the same research found that young people of indigenous or lower socio-economic status background were much more likely to describe overt peer pressure or encouragement to try smoking (Coase, Lang, and Wood, 2005 and Leavy, Phillips, Rosenberg, and Wood, 2010).

Socializing processes that facilitate smoking can also disappoint the use of cigarette smoking (Farhat, and Simons-Morton, 2010). For example, being 'cool' is important to teenagers (Clarkson, Corti-Giles Donovan, and Watson, 2003), although what is believed to be cool also changes across time, peer groups and social contexts. Smoking has traditionally been viewed as one of the symbols of 'coolness' among teenagers (Danesi, 1994). While 'coolness' is still recognized by young people as one of the reasons why some of their peers smoke (Eureka Strategic Research, 2005), research undertaken in Western Australia for the Smarter than smoking project suggests that the inverse is increasingly true, with those who smoke often regarded as 'losers' or 'trying too hard to be cool' (Lang, Coase and Wood, 2005). Refusing an offer of cigarettes or declaring that 'I don't smoke' is increasingly socially acceptable and normative among many youth cohorts (Lang *et al.*, 2005). Among groups with a negative prevailing attitude to smoking, peer influence may of course deter uptake of smoking (Farhat *et al.*, 2010; Kobus, 2003; Mermelstein, Flay and Turner, 2004).

A study on British population has indicated that forming romantic attachments ('dating') at an earlier age is a predictor for becoming a smoker later, independent of other possible confounding factors. Researchers speculated that dating and smoking behaviours may be connected by a desire to appear to be more grown up (Fidler, Jarvis, West, and Wardle, 2006), which is consistent with tobacco industry advertising linking its products with sex appeal and popularity (DiFranza, and Wellman, 2006).

Social norms need only to be perceived to influence behaviour (Farhat *et al.*, 2010), young smokers tend to collect together and also overestimate the extent of smoking in their own age group, and giving them a distorted sense of what is normal behaviour (Farhat *et al.*, 2010; Pederson and Tyas, 1999). The National Drug Strategy Household Survey for 2004 (Australia) reported that about two-thirds (64%) of recent smokers aged 12-15 said that 'all or most' of their friends and acquaintances were smokers as well. A further 20 per cent said that 'about half' of their peer group were smokers. Only 1 per cent of smokers in this age group said that none of their friends and acquaintances smoked. The effect declined with increasing age, with 28 per cent of smokers aged 20 years or older reporting that 'all or most' of their friends and associates were smokers, 32 per cent saying 'around half were', and 39 per cent saying only a few of their peer group smoked. Adolescents who think that smoking is normative and that most of their peers smoke are more likely to start smoking (Flay, Mermelstein, and Turner, 2004; DiFranza, and Sargent, 2003).

Susan *et al.,* (1993) conducted a study in University of North Carolina on peer group structure and adolescents' cigarette smoking by using cross-sectional design. 165 to 292 ninth grader students of different schools of North Carolina were selected for the study. They were assessed using some self-administered questionnaire. In this study, researchers found that, social network concepts were focus to the consideration of adolescents smoking such that isolated adolescents might smoke while group members and associates might choose not to smoke. It has been suggested that parents are more important at the preparation stage while peers become more important as the adolescent begin to experiment with cigarettes.

Alexander and associates (2001) conducted a study on peer school and adolescents' cigarette smoking by using longitudinal design with quantitative analysis and selected 2525 adolescent age grade 7 to 12 years. Adolescents smoking were assessed from in school questionnaire and in home interview; adjusting for age, gender, socio-economic status, parent education, school and availability of cigarettes in the home, the risk of current smoking was significantly associated with peer networks in which at least half of the members smoked.

Rebecca and others (2008) carried out a study on parental smoking-specific communication, adolescents smoking behaviour and friendship selection by using cross-sectional design with quantitative analysis selected 428 full families (14 to 17 years, 13 to 15 years). All these assessed on self-administered questionnaire related to parental smoking, best friend smoking, adolescents smoking quality of smoking-specific communication. Result shows that a high quality of parental smoking-specific communication reduces the likelihood of adolescents' smoking. Both the quality and frequency of parental smoking-specific communication were found to be adolescents' selective affiliation with non-smoking friends.

Wiium *et al.* (2006) study on smoker's role models and intention to smoke among adolescents, selected nationally representative sample of 15 year old 1670 adolescents from Norvey. Longitudinal design with quantitative analysis was employed. Intention to smoke was assessed by some self-administered questions, like "Do you smoke daily in two year's time?" In this study researchers provided evidence that the smoking behaviour of role models were related to adolescents' intention to smoke and this relationship is partly mediated by intra-personal factors such as attitude, subjective norms and perceived behavioural control regarding smoking.

Parenting Behaviour and Smoking Tendency

Adolescents generally more likely to start smoking if their parents smoke; if they belong to lower class; if they feel social pressure to smoke; and if there has been major stressors in the family member's job loss (Bauman, and Foshee, 1992; Casas, Oetting, Swaim, and 1996; Hamilton, Sussman, and Unger, 2004). Adolescents are also at increased risk to start smoking if their parents separate. These effects are partly due to the increase in stress and depression that may result from separation (Kirby, 2002). In Indian family, parents play a key role in initiation of tobacco use by a young child or adolescent. Tobacco use by parents or an elder sibling increases the likelihood that a child begins smoking (Anand, Kapoor, and Kumar, 1995; Gulati, Gadre, and Notani, 1991). However, it seems essential to examine the protective effects of other anti-smoking practices and family influences, which may protect against smoking in different SES samples (Simons-Morton, 2004; Skinner *et al.*, 2009) in preparation for family-based smoking prevention interventions.

Stronger family attachment and ties, communication, and parental respect have been shown to be protective against smoking initiation in different SES level (Berenson, Croft, Hunter, and Vizelberg, 1987; Ellickson and Morton, 1999; Ellickson *et al.*, 2003; Freeberg and Stein, 1996; Headen *et al.*, 1991). Research evidenced that parent adolescent discussions about rules on smoking and drinking and parent control increased the use of these substances (Andrews, Ary, Hops, Harris and Tildesley, 1993; Bee-Gates, Henriksen, and Jackson, 1994). On the other hand, some studies also revealed family communication and communication style to be associated with reduced substance use (Bouris, Dittus, Jaccard and Guilamo, 2008; Dittus, Gordon, Jaccard, 1998).

Chassin *et al.* (1985) found that parental smoking was associated with early onset among teenagers, escalation to heavy smoking, and persistence over time. Various indicators of poor social attachment with parents have been found to be associated with increased risk of smoking. Strong attachment with parents enhances sense of well-being and capacity to handle stressful events. It has been suggested that teenagers with poor social attachment have a weaker self-image and a greater need to portray themselves to their peers as tough or cool, for example, smoking cigarettes (Cleary and Leventhal, 1980). In a longitudinal study of Scottish adolescents Glendinning *et al.* (1997) found that perceptions of family support were inversely related to smoking, and this effect was raised when there was evidence of fewer parental controls.

Studies reveal that most adolescents maintain close relations with their parents despite the "minor perturbations" accompanying this transition (Steinberg, 1993). Parents play an important role in determining adolescent involvement in risk behaviours. Adolescents may "learn" to engage in risk-taking behaviour by observing their parents' behaviour. Parental modelling and permissive attitudes towards smoking and substance use have been implicated in the initiation of substance use in early adolescence (Fitzgibbon and Hawkins, 1993; Werner, 1991). Parental monitoring has been widely studied as an important correlate of adolescents' risk-taking behaviour (Dittus and Jaccard, 1991).

Some studies reveal that adolescents living with both biological parents have reduced risk of smoking as compared to adolescents living in single parents or reconstituted families (Bjarnason *et al.*, 2003; Fidler *et al.*, 2008; Griesbach *et al.*, 2003; Isohanni *et al.*, 1991; Otten *et al.*, 2007; Patton *et al.*, 1998a). Interestingly this association has been found to be very consistent across countries (Bjarnason *et al.*, 2003; Cumsille and Darling, 2003). A review of studies assessing the association between adolescent smoking and parent and sibling smoking behaviours showed that across studies sibling smoking was found to be a stronger and more consistent predictor of adolescent smoking than parent smoking (Avenevoli and Merikangas, 2003).

Conclusion

Smoking tendency of adolescents seems to be an interesting topic of research in the field of Health Psychology. Many researchers are trying to understand the causes of smoking, but still there is a need to accomplish empirical and systematic research to assess psychological and social factors responsible for smoking.

Peer pressure is one aspect of peer socialization, in which adolescents are influenced by their friends (Farhat *et al.*, 2010); just how influential it remains has been a matter of debate. Some researchers have argued that the importance of peer influence has been overestimated, and that the clustering of smoking behaviour within peer groups could be because adolescents seek out friendships with individuals who share similar interests, of which smoking may be just one signifier (Candel, de Vries, Engels, Mercken, 2006; Candel, de Vries, Mercken, van Osch, 2011; Degirmencioglu, Pilgrim, Urberg, 1997).

Michell (1996) concluded that the effect of peer pressure as an influence on adolescent health behaviour is not proven, and is in practice very complex to interpret. It is important to understand that young people are not a similar group, and that there are distinct peer clusters that smoke and do so for different reasons. It is probable that peer influences both interact with and are compounded by a host of other predictive factors (Holliday, Moore, and Rothwell, 2010) in which selection and socialization processes may operate independently, but may also have reciprocal effects. Both processes—selection and influence—supported by studies, but relative importance is strong matter of debate (Farhat *et al.*, 2010).

It seems that both peer influence and parental influence play an important role in determining the adolescents' smoking tendency and other type of risk taking behaviour. Peer influence is traditionally studied explicitly by asking adolescents whether their smoking was influenced by peers. Such type of direct questioning on the source of smoking not only leads to results that are subjective and difficult to verify, but more seriously tends to overestimate peer influence. However, researchers should re-examine their beliefs and assertions about the role of peer influence in adolescent smoking tendency.

Despite the large number of studies identifying an association between adolescent peer relationships and smoking, researchers' understanding of how peers contribute to this behaviour remains limited. For example, the processes by which teenagers are socialized to smoke, including both being influenced by and influences on their friends, is unclear. Similarly, the extent to which cigarette smoking or variables related to smoking is involved in youths' decisions to select into or select out of relationships with peers is unknown. Even less is known about the complementary process of selection, where youth are selected by peers to enter friendships or are excluded from such relationships based on smoking.

Most importantly more attention may be given to the social processes operating in the peer context. In spite of making assumptions about those processes on the basis of factors associated to smoking behaviour between adolescents and their friends, a more valid understanding of the sources of smoking initiation is important for the development of more effective interventions to prevent smoking. If smoking is surely a factor of peer influence and peer selection, then prevention programmes must emphasize refusal skill efficacy while also encourageing adolescents to select friends based on interests other than smoking. Negative peer influences are the main risk factors related with anti-social development among children and adolescents.

To understand adolescents smoking tendency and develop effective preventive interventions, it is important that the factors such as nature of relationships with peer, parental monitoring, school and neighbourhood environment, self-control, self-regulation, relationship to parents and some demographic factors like parent's education, residence, etc., that may moderate peer influence can be identified. Such moderating variables may reveal detrimental impact of peer influence as well as the social and familial impact that may buffer the negative impact of peer and parental influence.

References

Aloise-Young P., Graham, J.W., and Hansen, W.B. (1994). Peer influence on smoking initiation during early adolescence: A comparison of group members and group outsiders. *Journal of Applied Psychology, 79,* 281-287.

Ali, M. and Dwyer, D. (2009). Estimating peer effects in adolescent smoking behaviour: A longitudinal analysis. *Journal of Adolescent Health, 45*(4), 402-408.

Akers, R.L. (1977). *Deviant Behaviour: A Social Learning Approach* (2nd ed.). Belmont, CA: Wadsworth.

Ajzen, I. and Fishbein, M. (2010). *Theo:y of Planned Behaviour: Predicting and Changing Behaviour:* The reasoned action approach. New York: Psychology Press.

Alexander, C., Piazza, M., Mekos, D., and Valente, T. (2001). Peers, schools, and adolescent cigarette smoking. *Journal of Adolescent Health, 29*(1), 22-30.

Andrews, J.A., Hops, H., Ary, D., Tildesley, E., and Harris, J. (1993). Parental Influence on Early Adolescent Substance use: Specific and Non-Specific Effects. *Journal of Early Adolescence, 13*, 285-310.

Aseltine, R.H. (1995). A reconsideration of parental and peer influences on adolescent deviance. *Journal of Health and Social Behaviour, 36*, 103-121.

Bandura, A. (1977). Social learning theory. New York: *General Learning Press.*

Becker, G., and Murphy, K.A. (1988). Theory of rational addiction. *The Journal of Political Economy, 96*(4), 675-700.

Billy, J.O.G., and Udry, J.R. (1985). Patterns of adolescent friendship and effects on sexual behaviour. *Social Psychology Quarterly, 48*, 27-41.

Bjarnason, T., Davidaviciene, A.G., Miller, P. (2003). Family structure and adolescent cigarette smoking in eleven European countries. *Addiction, 98*(6), 815-24.

Chassin, L., Presson, C.C., Pitts, S.C., and Sherman, S.J. (2000). The natural history of cigarette smoking from adolescence to adulthood in a Midwestern community sample: Multiple trajectories and their psychosocial correlates. *Health Psychology, 18*(3), 223-231.

Chassin, L., Presson, C.C., Rose, J., Sherman, S.J., Davis, M.J., and Gonzalez. J.L. (2005). Parenting style and smoking—specific parenting practices as predictors of adolescent smoking onset. *Journal of Paediatric Psychology; 30*, 333-344.

Chassin L. *et al*., (1986). Changes in peer and parent influence during adolescence: Longitudinal versus cross-sectional perspectives on smoking initiation. *Developmental Psychology, 2*, 327-342.

Clark, P.I., Scarisbrick-Hauser, A., Gautam, S.P., and Wirk, S.J. (1999). Anti-tobacco socialization in homes of African-American and white parents, and smoking and non-smoking parents. *Journal of Adolescent Health, 24*, 329-339.

Conrad, K.M., Flay, B.R., and Hill, D. (1992). Why children start smoking cigarettes: predictors of onset. *British Journal of Addiction, 87*, 1711-1724.

Darling, N., and Cumsille, P. (2003). Theory, measurement, and methods in study of family influences on adolescent smoking. *Addiction, 98* (Suppl. 1), 21-36.

De Vries H., Candel, M., Engels, R., and Mercken, L. (2006). Challenges to the peer influence paradigm: Results for 12-13 years olds from six European countries from the European Smoking Prevention Framework Approach study. *Tobacco Control, 15*(2), 83-89.

Detels, R., Beaglehole, R., Lansang, M.A., and Gulliford, M. (2011). *Oxford Textbook of Public Health.* Oxford University Press, New York, 234-238.

Dittus, P., and Jaccard, J. (1991). *Parent-teen Communication: Towards the prevention of unintended pregnancies.* New York: Springer, Verlag., 121-142.

Duryea, E.J. (1991*)*. Principles of non-verbal communication in efforts to reduce peer and social pressure. *Journal of School Health, 61*, 5-10.

Ellickson, P.L. and Morton, S.C. (1999). Identifying adolescents at risk for hard drug use: Racial/ethnic variations. *Journal of Adolescent Health, 25*, 382-395.

Ellickson, P.L., Orlando, M., Tucker, J.S., and Klein, D.J. (2004). From adolescence to young adulthood: Racial/ethnic disparities in smoking. *American Journal of Public Health, 94*, 293-299.

Ellickson, P.L., Perlman, M., and Klein, D.J. (2003). Explaining racial/ethnic differences in smoking during the transition to adulthood. *Addictive Behaviours, 28*, 915-931.

Ennett, S.T., and Bauman, K.E. (1994). The contribution of influence and selection to adolescent peer group homogeneity: The case of adolescent cigarette smoking. *Journal of Social Psychology, 67*, 653-663.

Ezzati, M., and Lopez, A.D. (2003). *Estimates of Global Mortality Attributable to Smoking, 362*, 847-852.

Farrell, A.D. and Danish, S.J. (1993). Peer drug associations and emotional restraint: Causes or consequences of adolescents' drug use? *Journal of Consulting and Clinical Psychology, 61*, 327-334.

Fishbein, M. and Ajzen, I. (1975). *Belief, Attitude, Intention, and Behaviour: An Introduction to Theory and Research.* Reading, MA: Addison Wesley.

Flay, B.R., Hu, F.B., Siddiqui, O. *et al.*, (1994). Differential influence of parental smoking and friends' smoking on adolescent initiation and escalation of smoking. *Journal of Health and Social Behaviour, 35*, 248-65.

Foshee, V., Bauman, K. (1992). Parental and peer characteristics as modifiers of the bond-behaviour relationship: An elaboration of control theory. *Journal of Health and Social Behaviour, 33*(1), 66-76.

Freeberg, A.L., and Stein, C.H. (1996). Felt obligation towards parents in Mexican-American and Anglo-American Young Adults. *Journal of Social and Personal Relationships, 13*, 457-471.

Griesbach, D., Amos, A., Currie, C. (2003). Adolescent smoking and family structure in Europe. *Journal of Social Science and Medicine, 56*, 41-52.

Guilamo, V., Bouris, A., Dittus, P., and Jaccard, J. (2008). Mother adolescent communication about tobacco use in urban Puerto Rican and Dominican Families. *Youth and Society, 40*, 86-113.

Hawkins, J.D., and Fitzgibbon, J.J. (1993). Risk factors and risk behaviours in prevention of adolescent substance abuse. Adolescent medicine state of the art reviews: *Adolescent Substance Abuse and Addictions, 4*(2), 249-262.

Harakeh, Z., Scholte, R.H.J., Vermulst, A.A., de Vries, H., and Engels, R.C.M.E. (2010). The Relationship between parents' smoking, general parenting, parental smoking communication, and adolescents' smoking. *Journal of Research on Adolescence, 20*, 140-165.

Hamilton, L.C., Hamilton, L.R., Duncan, C.M., and Colocousis, C.R. (2008). Place matters: challenges and opportunities in four rural Americas. *Carsey Institute Reports on Rural America, Vol. 1*, No. 4.

Hetherington, R., Baistow, K., Katz, I., Trowell, J. (2001). *The Welfare of Children with Mentally Ill Parents: Learning from inter-country comparisons.* Wiley and Sons; Chichester, UK.

Hirschman, R.S., Leventhal, H., and Glynn, K. (1984). The development of smoking behaviour: Conceptualization and supportive cross-sectional survey data. *Journal of Applied Social Psychology, 14*, 184-206.

Hirschi, T. (1969). *Causes of Delinquency.* Los Angeles, CA: University of California Press.

Hoffman, B.R., Monge, P.R., Chou, C.P., and Valente, T.W. (2007). Perceived peer influence and peer selection on adolescent smoking. *Addictive Behaviours, 32*(8), 1546-1554.

Huba, G.J., and Bentler, P.M. (1980). The Role of Peer and Adult Models for Drug Taking at Different Stages in Adolescence. *Journal of Youth Adolescence, 9*, 449-465.

Hunter, S.M., Croft, J.B., Vizelberg, I.A., and Berenson, G.S. (1987). Psychosocial influences on cigarette smoking among youth in a southern community: The Bogalusa Heart Study. *Morbidity & Mortality Weekly Report, 36* (Suppl. 4), 17S-23S.

Isohanni, M., Moilanen, I., Rantakallio, P. (1991). Determinants of teenage smoking, with special reference to non-standard family background. *British Journal of Addiction, 86*, 391-8.

Jackson, C., and Henriksen, L. (1997). Do as I say: Parent smoking, anti-smoking socialization, and smoking onset among children. *Addictive Behaviours, 22*, 107-114.

Jaccard, J., Dittus, P.J., and Gordon, V.V. (1998). Parent-adolescent congruency in reports of adolescent sexual behaviour and in communication about sexual behaviour. *Child Development, 69*, 247-261.

Jayant, K., Notani, P.N., Gulati, S.S., and Gadre, V.V. (1991). Tobacco use in school children in Bombay, India. A study of knowledge, attitude and practice. *Indian Journal of Cancer, 28*, 139-147.

Jessor, R., and Jessor, S.L. (1977). *Problem behaviour and psychosocial development: A longitudinal study of youth.* (pp. 224-245), New York: Academic Press.

Johnston, L.D., O'Malley, P.M. and Bachman, J.G. (2007). Monitoring the Future National Survey results on drug use, 1975-1999. Volume I: Secondary school students (NU4 Publication No. 00-4802). *National Institute on Drug Abuse.*

Kapoor, S.K., Anand, K., and Kumar, G. (1995). Prevalence of tobacco use among school and college going adolescents of Haryana. *Indian Journal of Paediatrics, 62*, 461-466.

Kobus, K. (2003). Peers and adolescent smoking. *Addiction, 98* (Suppl. 1), 37-55.

Leventhal, H., and Cleary, P.D. (1980). The smoking problem: A review of the research and theory in behaviour risk Modification. *Psychological Bulletin, 88*, 370-408.

Leavy, J., Wood, L., Rosenberg, M., and Phillips, F., (2010). Try and try again: Qualitative insights into adolescent smoking experimentation and notions of addiction. *Health Promotion Journal of Australia, 21*(3), 208-14.

McGuire, W.J. (1974). Communication persuasion models for drug education: Experimental findings. In Goodstadt, M. (ed.), *Research Methods and Programmes of Drug Education.* Addiction Research Foundation, Toronto.

McGuire, W.J. (1968). The nature of attitudes and attitude change, *Handbook of Social Psychology, Vol. 1*, Addison-Wesley, Reading, pp. 136-314.

McVicar (2011). Estimates of peer effects in adolescent smoking across twenty six European Countries. *Social Science and Medicine, 73*(8), 1186-93.

Mermelstein, R. (1999). Explanations of ethnic and gender differences in youth smoking: A multi-site, qualitative investigation. The Tobacco Control Network Writing Group. *Nicotine & Tobacco Research*, 212-18.

Mercken, L., Candel, M., van Osch, L., and de Vries H. (2011). No smoke without fire: The impact of future friends on adolescent smoking behaviour. *British Journal of Health Psychology, 16*(1), 170-88.

Murrey, M., Jarett, L., Suian, A.V., and Rumun, R. (1988). *Smoking Among Young Adults*. Aldershot: Gower.

Nichter, M., Nichter, M., Vuckovic, N., Quintero, G., and Ritenbaugh, C. (1997).

Smoking experimentation and initiation among adolescent girls: Qualitative and quantitative findings. *Tobacco Control, 6*(4), 285-95.

Oetting, E.R., and Donnermeyer, J.F. (1998). Primary socialization theory: The etiology of drug use and deviance. *Journal of Substance Use and Misuse, 33*(4), 995-1026.

Patton, G.C., J.B., Carlin, C. Coffey, *et al.*, (1998). Depression, anxiety and smoking initiation: A prospective study over 3 years. *Journal of Public Health, 88*(10), 1518-1522.

Pierce, J.P., Gilpin, E.A. (1995). A Historical-analysis of tobacco marketing and the uptake of smoking by youth in the United-States—1890-1977. *Health Psychology, 14*, 500-508.

Pollard, M.S., Tucker, J.S., Green, H.D., Kennedy, D., and Go M-H. (2010). Friendship networks and trajectories of adolescent tobacco use. *Addictive Behaviours, 35*(7): 678-85.

Prochaska, J.O., DiClemente, C.C. (1983). Stages and processes of self-change in smoking cessation towards an integrative model of change. *Journal of Consulting and Clinical Psychology, 51*(3), 390.

Rebecca, N.H. *et al.*, (2008). Parental Smoking-specific Communication, Adolescents' Smoking Behaviour and Friendship Selection. *Journal of Youth Adolescence, 37*, 1229-1241.

Rosenstock, I.M., Strecher, V.J., and Becker, M.H. (1988). Social learning theory and the health belief model. *Health Education and Behaviour, 15*(2), 175-183.

Santrock, J.W. (2007). *Adolescence* (11th ed., p. 311). New Delhi: Tata McGraw Hill.

Scott, J. (2000). *Social Network Analysis: A Handbook.* London, UK: Sage Publications.

Simons-Morton, B. and Farhat, T. (2010). Recent findings on peer group influences on adolescent smoking. *Journal of Primary Prevention, 31*(4), 191-208.

Sher, K.J., Gotham, H., Erickson, D., and Wood, P.K. (1996). A prospective, high-risk study of the relation between tobacco dependence and alcohol use disorders. *Alcoholism: Clinical and Experimental Research, 20*, 485-492.

Simons, M.B. (2007). Social influences adolescent substance use. *American Journal of Health Behaviour, 31*(6), 672-684.

Terry, D.J., and Hogg, M.A. (2000). *Attitudes, Behaviours, and Social Context: The role of norms and group membership.* Lawrence Erlbaum Associates. 1, 91-S98.

Tucker, J.S., Klein, D.J., and Elliott, M.N. (2004). Social control of health behaviours: A comparison of young, middle-aged, and older adults. *Journal of Gerontology: Psychological Sciences and Social Sciences, 59B*, 147-150.

Urberg, K.A., Degirmencioglu, S.M., and Pilgrim, C. (1997). Close friend and group influence on adolescent cigarette smoking and alcohol use. *Developmental Psychology, 33*, 834-44.

World Health Organization, (2009). Report on the global tobacco epidemic, implementing smoke-free environments. WHO, Geneva.

WHO, (2008). Report on the global tobacco epidemic, 2008. The MPOWER package. WHO, Geneva.

Wood, L., Lang, A., and Coase P. (2005). Smarter than Smoking Qualitative Research. A Research Report. West Perth, Australia: *TNS Social Research*.

19

Cognitive Competence of the Tribal Children of South Kamrup District

Rita Rani Talukdar

Cognition is broadly the power of thinking in human mind. Cognitive development is defined as thinking, problem solving, concept understanding, and information processing overall intelligence. Cognition means to learn, perceive or understand. Learning a word, explaining its meaning, naming, describing an object, specifying its user and predicting what would happen if the object is lost. The process of cognition is brought about by a number of abilities called cognitive skills like synthesis, analysis, reasoning, evaluation, induction, deduction, generalization etc. cognition is a term used to describe the psychological process involved in the acquisition, organization and use of knowledge emphasizing the rational rather than emotional characteristics. Cognition refers to the processing of information about the environment that is received through the senses.

Cognitive abilities are the function of brain and develop with age. As the brain matures more and more abilities develop, not only in number, but also in quality. The infant initially can only take in the information but gradually he develops the ability to process this information and use it for his own benefit. It is this growth and refinement of cognitive abilities which is referred to a cognitive development.

The main objective of this investigation was to study the cognitive competence among the tribal children. The study was conducted in the south Kamrup area of Assam. The tribal children belonged to two groups, the Boro and Rabhas. There were 120 tribal and 120 non-tribal children. Two tools were used to collect the data. The Embedded Figure Test and a semi-structure interview schedule for the general information. The result showed that the tribal children performed poorer in comparison to the non-tribal children. The male children are found to be more field independent than the female children among both the groups. The overall performance indicated that the tribal children have poor cognitive competence. They are poor in non-embedding task. However, further research needs to be conducted before drawing generalization.

Introduction

Human Cognition, from a developmental perspective, is the result of a long history of growth beginning at the earliest stages. Our perceptions, memories, and language and thought processes are governed by the basic genetic structure we inherit and the changes we experience in response to the demands made during our long and varied interaction with the physical and social environment. The critical feature is that cognition develops—that is, cognition and thinking emerge—in an orderly fashion as individuals progress from infancy to adulthood, and then some cognitive skills may decline in old age. These changes may be caused by—

- Neurological and physical maturation (or deterioration) of the person.
- The family, social, and educational milieu in which the person lives.
- The interaction between a physically challenging person and his or her environment.

Cognitive development over the lifespan of people has been approached from several independent perspectives: developmental psychology, neuron-cognitive development and cognitive development. Cognitive development takes place over the entire lifespan of human beings and other creatures from before birth to death; however, in this study we are concentrating on cognitive development during the early part of life.

Interest in the development of cognitive psychology, throughout a person's lifespan was initially stimulated by the seminal work of Jean Piaget of Switzerland and the theoretical legacy left by the thoughtful works of Lev S. Vygotsky of Russia. Much has been written and is generally available about the life and times of Piaget but less is none of the life and theories of Vygotsky. These two theories are important in terms of establishing a general framework, recent ideas and data have contributed significantly and to our current understanding of the forces implicated in cognitive development. Cognitive development is the study of cognition as it unfolds throughout the lifespan of a human being.

Each and every culture adopts its own rearing practices and thus it varies from culture to culture. The natural and cultural components predominate cognition among children. The cultural components are inherited from our ancestors and are practiced in our day-to-day life and these are experimented on the parameter of scientific utility by our social scientists, anthropologists and psychologists. Therefore, there is a need to concentrate on such social issues, which influence the behaviour phenomena.

The study of differences between cultural groups in cognitive processes and cognitive competence is one of the basic areas in cross-cultural psychology. The interest lies in assessing the generalized ability of principles of cognitive behaviour and in understanding how culture influence learning, thinking, problem-solving and memory.

Objectives of the Study

1. To study the cognitive abilities of the tribal children.
2. To develop an understanding about the culture of these two groups and its relating features like the skills and competence among the children.
3. To explore the psychological processes which differentiate the tribal children from the non-tribal children?

Hypothesis of the Study

1. Tribal children perform low score on Embedded Figure Test tasks than non-tribal children, indicating that tribal children show poor perceptual capacity.
2. Tribal children are lower on field independence than non-tribal children who are higher on field independence.
3. Male children are more field independent than female children among both the groups.

Methodology

Sample: The sample consisted of 120 tribal children and 120 non-tribal children within the age group of 6 years and 11 years. They are selected randomly from different schools of South Kamrup District of Assam.

Two tribes were taken—Boro Kachari and the Rabha (60 + 60 = 120). In both the groups 50 per cent were male and 50 per cent were female. Thus, the sample was matched on age, sex and education (2×2 factorial design was used).

Materials: The tools used in the present investigation were—

1. Semi-Structured Interview Schedule,
2. The Embedded Figures Test, originally developed by Witkin

A pilot study was initially conducted with 30 tribal and 30 non-tribal children to establish the reliability and validity of the tools developed and used in the present study.

A semi-structured interview schedule was prepared by the Research Scholar to collect information related to the subjects Age, sex, educational qualification, type of family, social stratification, use of drug in the family, animal husbandry etc.

The Embedded Figures Test is a perceptual test in which the subject has to locate a previously seen simple figures within a large complex figure. The scores on EFT reflects extent of competence at perceptual and intellectual (i.e. cognitive) tasks may serve in the assessment of broad, salient dimension of personal functioning is a longstanding one in the history of psychological testing. Ever since, the introduction of intelligence tests, patterns of abilities revealed in test performance have been used in clinical appraises of ego functioning. The specific rationale for using EFT to assess broad dimensions of personal function comes from cognitive style theory and the evidence accumulated in the course of its extensive research application. Cognitive styles are the characteristic, self-consistent modes of functioning which individuals show in their perceptual and intellectual activities. These cognitive styles are manifestations in the cognitive sphere of still broader dimensions of personal function which cut across diverse psychological areas.

The simple and complex figures which make up the EFT are modification of figures selected from those used by Gottshaldt (1926). After extensive studies with a large series of figures and a variety of different colour arrangements, 24 complex figures and 8 simple figures are selected. Each of the simple figures was embedded in several different complex figures. Two main criteria were used in selecting the complex figures. First, it was necessary to produce a series of figures graded in difficulty of disembedding depending on the structure of the complex figure, the detection of the simple figure may be easy or difficult, second, it was desirable to have a variety of simple figures, so that no one of them would be encountered a great number of times. This was intended to reduce the role of practice. The set of 24 cards was divided into two sets. The first set of 12 cards called Form A was used for this study.

Procedure: For the purpose of assessment of Embedded Figure Test performance, the data were collected from the school going children, the age ranging from 6 years to 11 years. The general information about the subject was collected through a semi-structural questionnaire prepared by the Researcher. While administrating EFT a total of 3 minutes time was allowed to the subject for each card to search the simple figure embedded in the complex figure. If the subject fails to do so he gets zero. If he is successful then 1 (one) mark is assigned to him. If a child fails to perform the task continuously for three times then the test is stopped. The information obtained from the subjects were systematically placed and analyzed.

The two groups were compared on various measures. They are tribal, non-tribal and male, female. The sample was matched on age, sex and education. The 2×2 factorial design was used. The parametric test like mean, SD, t-test and ANOVA were worked out to see the differences amongst groups.

Results and Discussion

Cognitive abilities are the function of brain and develop with age. As the brain matures more and more abilities develop, not only in number, but also in quality. The infant initially can only take in the information, but gradually he develops the ability to process this information and use it for his own benefit. It is this growth and refinement of cognitive abilities which is referred to a cognitive development. The main objective of this study was to study the cognitive competence of the tribal children and to develop an understanding about the culture of these two groups and its relating features like the skills and competence among the children. The researcher also wanted to explore the psychological processes which differentiate the tribal children from the non-tribals.

From the data obtained for this study, it is evident that the non-tribal children have performed significantly better than the tribal children in identifying the simple figures hidden in the complex figure cards.

Table 19.1: The Scores of the Two Groups and the t-test

Group	*Mean*	*S.D.*	*SEM*	*Mean Difference*	*SEM D*	*t*
Tribal	4.308	2.495	.326			
Non-Tribal	7.890	2.502	.326	3.582	.460	7.785

Table 19.2: The scores of the two groups on Embedded Figures Test (12 Tasks) (N-120)

Task	*Tribal Children*		*Non-Tribal Children*	
	Mean	*S.D.*	*Mean*	*S.D.*
1.	0.2916	0.4545	0.65	0.4769
2.	0.5166	0.4997	0.9	0.3
3.	0.4916	0.4999	0.7916	0.4061
4.	0.5916	0.4915	0.9166	0.2763
5.	0.0916	0.2885	0.675	0.4683
6.	0.0166	0.1280	0.1	0.3
7.	0.5416	0.4982	0.875	0.3307
8.	0.0333	0.1795	0.325	0.4683
9.	0.5583	0.4965	0.741	0.4377
10.	0.9	0.3	0.991	0.0909
11.	0.275	0.4965	0.833	0.3726
12.	0	0	0.0916	0.2885

The mean score of non-tribal is 7.89 as compared to that of tribal is 4.308. The S.D. was found to be 2.502 and 2.495 respectively. Out of the 12 cards none of the tribal subjects could perform all the 12 tasks successfully whereas 3 of the non-tribal subjects performed all of them successfully. 8 of the tribal subjects have total failure, scoring no marks at all. The highest score obtained on EFT was 10 out of 12 among the non-tribal children, that also scored by only one subject. Whereas among the non-tribal, a number of subjects have obtained this score (Table 19.1) The tribal and non-tribal children differ significantly in EFT test (Table 19.2). The obtained result of EFT supports the hypothesis that tribal children perform low score on EFT tasks than non-tribal children indicating.

The tribal children show poor perceptual capacity. Table 19.2 shows the scoring of the total sample on all the 12 tasks respectively.

Those subjects who have better non-embedding quality performed better on cognitive task and are more field independent. The non-tribal

Table 19.3: The t-test scores on the Embedded Figures Test for various groups

Sl. No.	*Group*	*N*	*t*
1	Tribal *vs.* Non-Tribal	120	11.21**
2	Male Tribal *vs.* Female Tribal	66	1.13
3	Male Non Tribal *vs.* Female Non-Tribal	60	1.28
4	Male Tribal *vs.* Male Non-Tribal	60	8.40**
5	Female Tribal *vs.* Female Non-Tribal	60	7.55**
6	Male Tribal *vs.* Female Non-Tribal	60	6.75**
7	Female Tribal *vs.* Male Non-Tribal	60	9.38**

Note = $P < 0.01$** $P < .05$*

subjects have better non-embedding quality and they are more field independent as shown in Table 19.2.

There is no significant difference between male subjects and female subjects. But significant differences have been found between male tribals and male non-tribals as well as between female tribals and female non-tribals.

The mean and SD scores of tribal subjects and non-tribal subjects were worked out. The female subjects performed poorer than the male subjects in both the groups. The mean and S.D. for the tribal females is 4.05 and 2.5588 and that of non-tribal female subjects in 7.6 and 2.634. Since male subjects have performed better than the female subjects in 7.6 and 2.634. Since, male subjects have performed better than the female subjects, male children are more field independent. But the differences between male and female children within the groups do not exist significantly. The t-test values (Table 19.3) indicate significant differences between tribal *vs.* non-tribal, female tribal *vs.* female non-tribal, male tribal *vs.* female non-tribal, and female tribal *vs.* male non-tribal. Differences between male tribal *vs.* female tribal and male non-tribal *vs.* female non-tribal was found to be non-significant. The performance of the tribal subjects *vs.* non-tribal subjects was compared in all the 12 tasks of EFT. Significant differences were found in tests 1, 2, 3, 4, 5, 6, 7, 8, 9, 11 and 12. The difference was found not significant in test 10.

In one of the studies Sinha (1980) tested four cultural groups—nomadic Birhors, transitional sedentary Birhors, agricultural Oraons and sedentarised urban school children. Male-Female differences were found to be not significant among transitional Birhors and agricultural Oraons. Urban boys were, however, significantly higher on field independence than girls.

Table 19.4: Summary of Analysis of Variance for the scores obtained by various groups (N-120)

Source of variance	*Sum of Square*	*df*	*Mean Squares or Variance*	*F*
Among all groups	788.633	3	262.877	41.890**
Within groups	1480.966	236	6.275	NS
Between culture A_1 & B_1	770.416	1	770.416	122.77**
Between Sex B_1 & B_2	18.15	1	18.15	NS
Interaction A × B	0.067	1	0.067	NS
Within treatments	1480.966	236	6.275	
Total	2269.60	239		

Chatterjee and Bhaskar (1982) found that urban subjects were more field independent than the field dependent subjects. Jahoda and Gustar (1979) found ethnic and sex difference in spatial perceptual tasks but there was no significant sex differences on mental rotation or shape assemble. Laosa and De Avila (1979) reported from their study that traditional community subjects were relatively field independent. Field independence increased progressively with age. Huss, Eric-T and Kayson, Wesley (1985) found that sex and age were significant. Boys found the hidden figures faster than the girls and older subjects faster than the younger ones, providing that boys are more field independent than the girls.

A semi-structured interview schedule prepared by the Research Scholar was used as a tool to collect information related to the subjects. Ecological factors and cultural factors like settlement pattern, system in the society, social stratification, animal husbandry and environmental factors like family organization, relationship between parents and children and drug use in the family were found to play important role in the development of cognition in children. Most of the tribal children belonged to disgruntled families with least interaction between parents and children. Due to lower interaction with parents, the children fail to develop intellectual and perceptual capacity. It was also found that the parents of the tribal children have the regular habit of consuming home-made alcohol and tobacco. There was difference observed in the child rearing practices also among the tribal families. The women spent most of their time in household and animal husbandry.

The Embedded Figures Test responses revealed that what it assesses most of all is the ability to break-up an organized visual field in order to keep a part of it separate from that field. In a field dependent mode of perceiving perception is strongly dominated by the overall organization of the surrounding field and parts of the field are experienced as fused. In a field independent mode of perceiving, parts of a field are experienced as discrete from organized ground. Extremely high correlation has been found between the (visual) EFT situations and both tactile and auditory non-embedding tasks (Axelrod & Chohen, 1961; While, 1954, Witken Lomonaco, Birnhaum & Herman, 1968). Sex differences have been found. Boys and men tend to be more field independent than girls and women.

The tribal children's performance on EFT was poorer than the non-tribal. This has indicated that the tribal children have poor perceptual capacity, i.e. they are poor in disembedding tasks. The non-tribal subjects have performed significantly better compared to the tribal subjects indicating that they are field independent and have better disembedding capacity. This accepts the hypothesis that Tribal children perform low score on Embedded Figure Test tasks than non-tribal children, indicating that tribal children show poor perceptual capacity.

There were no significant differences between the males and females within the groups. But significant differences among the male tribal and male non-tribal groups and female tribal and female non-tribal groups. Male have shown better disembedding quality among both the groups indicating themselves to be more field independent as compared to females who are more field dependent. There are 12 tasks in the EFT out of which the tribal children could perform only 10 tasks successfully whereas the non-tribal children could perform all the 12 tasks successfully. Many of the tribal children failed to perform even a single task. The highest score obtained by the tribal children was 10 out of 12 whereas in non-tribal children it was 12 out of 12. The scoring is based on time taken to complete the task. The tribal children took more time to complete the task and gave wrong responses many times. The non-tribal children could find the hidden figures faster and traced the figures correctly.

The performance of the non-tribal children is better on the Embedded Figures Test. The inability to identify the simple figures indicates poor perceptual capacity and the result indicates that the tribals have poor perceptual capacity in comparison to the non-tribals.

Those subjects who performed better on embedded figure test are found to be field independent and possess better disembedding qualities. The non-tribal children who have performed better than the tribal children are more field independent. This accepts the hypothesis that tribal children are lower on field independence than non-tribal children who are higher on field independence.

The result predicted that the male children are more field independent than female children among both the groups. Male children have performed better than the female children among both the groups, but the difference between male and female children within the groups do not exist significantly. Thus, the hypothesis that male children are more field independent than female children among both the groups is rejected.

Thus, culture of the social groups shows significant differences in various areas of human potentialities and cognitive abilities. The results of this study provide valuable information about the performances of tribal and non-tribal children of Assam. It has been found from the discussion of the above findings that tribal children showed poor cognitive competence than the non-tribal children. The tribal children possess low disembedding quality and perceptual ability. These tribal children are found to be low on field independence as compared to non-tribal children.

References

Beiri, J., (1966). Cognitive complexity and personality development. In O.J. Harvey (ed.) *Experience Structure and Adaptability*, (pp. 13-37). New York, Springer.

Chatterjee, R.G. and Bhaskar, P. (1982). Field Independence, Intelligence, Ecology and Geometrical Figure Recognition. *Journal of Social Psychology, 118* (1), 133-34.

Huss, E.T. and Kayson, W. (1985). Effects of Age and Sex on Speed of finding Embedded Figures. *Perceptual and Motor Skills, Vol. 61* (2), 591-94.

Jahoda, G. (1970). A Cross Cultural Perspectives in Psychology. *Advancement of Science, 27*, 1-14.

Jatin Mipun (2008). *The Mising (Miris) of Assam: Development of a New Life Style*.

Mishra, R.C. and Chaubey, A.C. (2002). Acculturation Attitudes of Kharwar and Agaria Tribal Groups of Sonebhadra. *Psychology and Developing Societies, 14*(2), 201-220.

Sinha, D. (1989). *Perceptual Style among Nomadic and Transitional Agricultural Birhors.* Paper presented at the 4th International Conference of Cross Cultural Psychology, Munich, 1989.

Solso, L.R. (2001). *Cognitive Psychology*, Pearson Education (Singapore) Pvt. Ltd. Indian Branch, 482 F.I.E. Patparganj, Delhi, 2001.

Solso, L.R. (2006). *Cognitive Psychology*, Pearson Education in South Asia, Sixth Edition, published by Dorling Kindsley (India), 2006.

Witkin, H.A., Lewis, H.B., Hertzman, M., Machover, K., Meissner, P.H. and Wapner, S. (1972). *Personality Thought Perception*, New York: Harper, 2954, (Republished, Westport, Conn. Green Wood, 1972).

Witkin, H.A. (1969). Social Influence in the Development of Cognitive Style, pp. 687-706. In D.A. Goslin (ed.) *Handbook of Socializations: Theories and Research*, Chicago, R. and McNally.

Saikia, Y. (2004). *Assam and India: Fragmented Memories, Cultural Identity and the Tai-Ahom Struggle, 2004.*

20

Promoting Marital Life

Comparison of Capital and Non-Capital Region

Megha Kharkwal and *Aradhana Shukla*

In these days considerable attention is being made to study the life of professional women and their psychosocial profile. It has also been noticed that since these women perform successfully in both fields of life like home and organization so they feel more problems than those women who do not have any job. It impacts on their mental and physical health. In this study an attempt will be made to seek out the psychophysical health of professional women with special reference to marital adjustment affected by their age and residential variation. The delineation of concepts is as follows:

Marital Adjustment

One of the most important relationships between a man and woman is marriage. It involves emotional and legal commitments which is quite important in any adult life. Moreover, selecting a partner and entering into a marital contract is considered both maturational milestone and personal achievement. There is no doubt that the choice of marital partner is one of the most important decisions one makes in his/her lifetime. People marry for many reasons, like: love, happiness, companionship and the desire to have children, physical attraction, or desire to escape from an unhappy situation (Bernard, 1984). Marriage is a commitment with love and responsibility for peace, happiness and development of strong family relationships. Marriage is "*socially legitimate sexual union, begun with a public announcement and undertaken with some ideas of permanence; it is assumed with more a less-explicit marriage contract, which spells out the reciprocal rights and obligations between the spouses and future children*" (Balack, 1990).

Marital adjustment is "the state in which there is an overall feeling in husband and wife of happiness and satisfaction with their marriage and with each other" (Thomas, 1987). All the marriages are aimed at happiness in one or another way. Most couples marry filled up with expectations. Some of the expectations will be realistic while others unrealistic. This is due to the complex nature of marriage and each individual is as complex as a universe. Therefore, in marriage two universes close together (Veenboven, 1983). Marital adjustment calls for maturity that accepts and understands growth and development in the spouse. If this growth is not experienced and realized fully, death in marital relationship is inevitable. A relationship between couples is not instantaneous rather a slow progress. "*It is like the undetected cancer that kills silently and softly.*" A study on 581 couples and 25 per cent of them disclosed that at some time in the adjustment process, they discussed discovering and 18 per cent had seriously considered it (Left Court, 1976).

There is a list of six areas of marital adjustment, which is defined by the psychologist, such as, religion, social life, mutual friends, in laws, money and sex (Lazarus, Delingis, 1985). Another psychologist defines ten areas of marital adjustment, i.e. values, couple growth, communication, conflict resolution, affection, roles, cooperation, sex, money and parenthood (Margalin, 1980). A study on marriage and marital adjustment in USA presents social activities and recreation, training and disciplining of children, religion, in law relationship, financial matters, sexual relationship, communication, mutual trust and companionship as the areas of marital adjustment (Smith, 1961).

Comprehensive study of husbands and wives investigated some of the factors that contributed to marital satisfaction. Some of their findings revealed existing social, cultural, educational level the greater satisfaction. Occupation and income, which are often thought to be associated with levels of satisfaction, have no relationship with it. The number of children too affects marital satisfaction (Parron, 1982). There is evidence that the pressures of manageing multiple roles in women are the greatest, and the psychological benefits of employment are the least, under conditions of heavy family responsibilities that is, when young children are at home (Blood, 1960). However, beyond specific factors such as these, what is important to marital satisfaction over the course of marriage is the ability of partner to adjust to a variety of changes and to cope with a number of stresses. Marital role can be defined as set of attitudes and behaviours a spouse is expected to demonstrate in the context of the marriage relationship (Gore, Manigione, 1983). A marital role comprises cultural expectations associated with the husband or with a wife. A husband is expected to provide divorce, court cases for alimony, physical abuses and single parents; it does seem as if handling a relationship can be a tricky and often taxing issue. The possible causes can be endless. More often than not, stress arising from marital relationships is manifested in chronic disorders such as depression, insomnia and hypertension. Since, a relationship depends on the nature of the persons involved, it helps to seek the middle path when the inherent individual differences surface. It often helps to change one's attitude, go for counselling or talk openly with your spouse about problems facing your relationship (Weiten, 1996).

This study is divided into two subsequent sub-studies. In study one, an attempt had been made to trace the pattern of professional quality of life and marital adjustment. In study two, counselling devices were suggested to promote quality of life and minimizing adjustment problems. The description of studies is as follows:

STUDY ONE

Impact of Age, Professional Level and Residential Setting on Professional Quality of Life and Marital Adjustment

The aim of this study was to find out the developmental impact of professional level and residential setting on professional quality of life and marital adjustment, the objectives and hypothesis were as follows:

1. The first objective of the study was to find out the impact of chronological age on professional quality of life and marital adjustment. It was contended that variation in chronological age would cause variation in the magnitude of the marital adjustment and professional quality of life.
2. The second objective of the study was to ascertain the pattern of the professional quality of life and marital adjustment as influenced by the professional level. It was hypothesized that professional difference would lay its impact on professional quality of life and marital adjustment.
3. The third objective of the study was to ascertain the impact of the residential locale on professional quality of life and marital adjustment. It was assumed that participants living in different residential setting would evince difference in the scores of professional quality of life and marital adjustment.

Keeping these views in consideration this study was planned.

Method

Sample: Three hundred sixty women ranging between 25-50 years served as participants. They hailed from capital regions of (Delhi, Lucknow and Dehradun) and non-capital regions of (Almora, Nainital and Haldwani) and belonged different strata, namely high (Doctors, Engineers, University/Degree College Teachers, Bank Managers) middle (Inter-College Teachers, Bank Clerks and Nurses) and low (Peons and Maids). In this way twenty participants were taken in each cell and data were arranged according to the requirement of 3-way factorial design with 3 age groups (25-30, 35-40 and 45-50 years), 3 professional types (high, middle and low) and 2 residential locale.

The systemic presentation of experimental design is as follows:

Table 20.1: Schematic Presentation of experimental Designs

	A								
	A1			A2			A3		
	B1	B2	B3	B1	B2	B3	B1	B2	B3
C1									
C2									

Legends:

A=Chronological age	***B= Professional Type***	***C= Residential Setting***
A1=25-30 Years	B1= High Level Professional	C1= Capital Region
A2= 35-40 Years	B2= Middle Level Professional	C2= Non-Capital Region
A3=45-50 Years	B3=Low Level Professional	

Tools

Marital Satisfaction Scale: As the psychology of women, whether married or unmarried revolves around the family, it was considered as the important determiner of quality of life. Therefore, this scale was constructed (Shukla and Kharkwal, 2013). This scale is constructed in five points mode and consists of 45, five point items dealing with various situations as determiners of marital adjustment. Score ranges between 45-225. Low score indicates high satisfaction and high score *vice versa.* Spirit half reliability of the scale is .69.

Procedure

Data collection was done individually and best efforts were made to avoid external distractions.

Results

Impact of Chronological age, professional type and residential setting on marital satisfaction: The marital adjustment was measured by marital satisfaction scale and analysis of variance was used to analyze the data. Finding are given below:

Table 20.2: Summary table of analysis of variance showing the impact of chronological age, professional type and residential setting on marital adjustment

Sources of variation	*SS*	*df*	*MS*	*F*
A	2.56	2	1.28	1.19
B	2.50	2	1.25	1.16
C	1.17	1	1.17	1.09
AB	8.76	4	4.38	4.06
AC	11.20	2	5.60	5.19
BC	7.78	2	3.88	3.60
ABC	22.29	4	5.57	5.16
Errors(within)	371.52	344	1.08	
		359		

Table 20.2 reveals that the main effect of chronological age was insignificant (*F, 2, 359 = 1.19 P >.05*). It was found that the level of marital satisfaction varied with increase in chronological age, but the difference was not so high. The professional level effect was also insignificant (F, *2,359 = 1.16 P >.05*). It was noted that variation in professional type caused variation in the score of marital satisfaction scale but the discrepancy was meagre. The residential setting was also insignificant. (*F, 2, 359=1.09 P >.05*) but it was found that capital and capital discrepancy was not pronounced.

The two-way interaction of chronological age and professional type was significant (*F, 4, 359= 4.06 P < .05*) as shown in Figure 20.1.

The chronological age and residential setting interaction was significant (*F, 2, 359= 5.19 P <.01*) and it is presented in Figure 20.2.

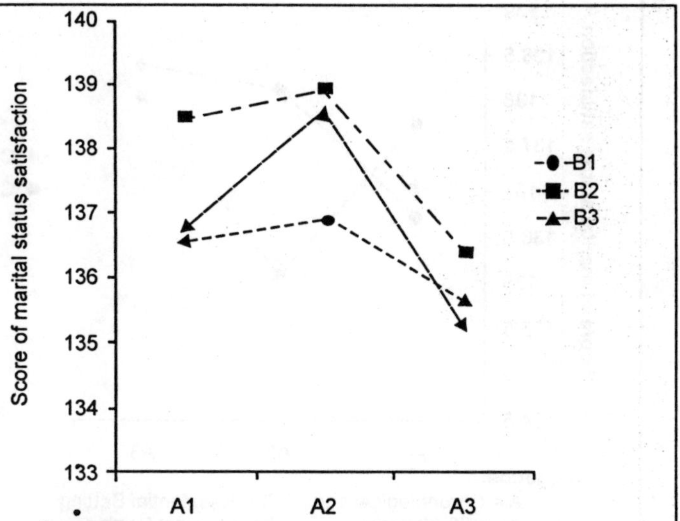

Fig. 20.1: Impact of Chronological age and professional type on marital status satisfaction

The professional level and residential interaction was also significant (*F, 2, 359= 3.60* $\underline{P}$ *< .05*) and it is presented in Figure 20.3.

The three-way interaction of chronological age, professional level and residential setting was significant (*F, 4, 359= 5.16* $\underline{P}$ *< .01*) and it shows that all variable laid their impact on marital satisfaction as shown in Fig. 20.4.

STUDY TWO

Promoting Quality of Life in Professional Women

The aim of this study was to promote the quality of life in the women, so an attempt was made to trace out least satisfied participants and the aspects of their worries and problems. After this, the intervention list was suggested to them. They are follows and they can follow it to make their life full of quality.

Yoga: Yoga is sense of control and full concentration over the task.

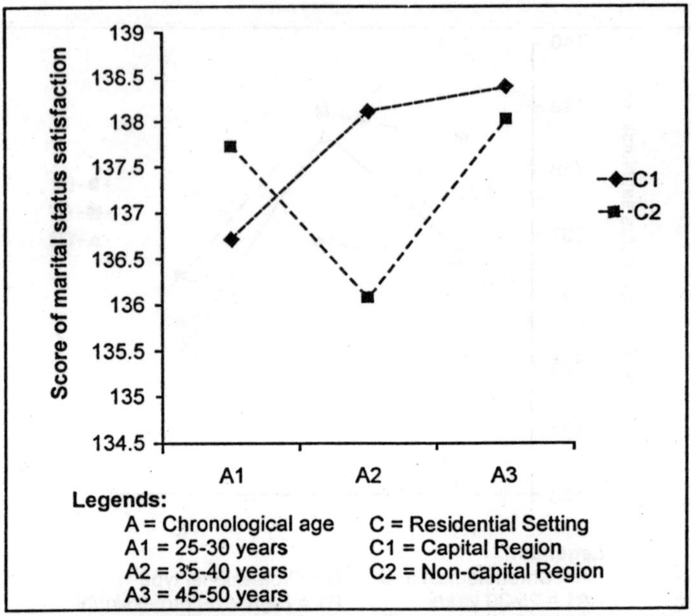

Fig. 20.2: Impact of chronological age and residential setting on martial status satisfaction

It makes a person fit and fine psychophysically as well as mentally. If people perform yogic exercise and concentrate well in their work, they can enhance positivity in themselves.

Sharing: Sharing deals with the intake or discharge of one's and other's pleasure and pains. It is essential for a normal and healthy life. Therefore, we can exchange our views with some personal relations so that normality could be established.

Caring: Every person wants to be cared by the other one so it will be a helpful tool for them to care their spouse.

Relationship satisfaction: Relationship satisfaction is a very important tool for the betterment of quality of married life. Partners effects have been studied to evaluate the perspective that there are burdens associated with being in a relationship with someone with mental health problems and that these burdens may result in lower relationship with the partner (Chakrabarti, Kulhara, and Verma, 1993; Coyne *et al.*, 1987).

Marital Adjustment: It can be seen that the phenomenon of marital adjustment is given a priority in all cultures, as marriage is one of the most important commitments of an individual makes in his or her life. A

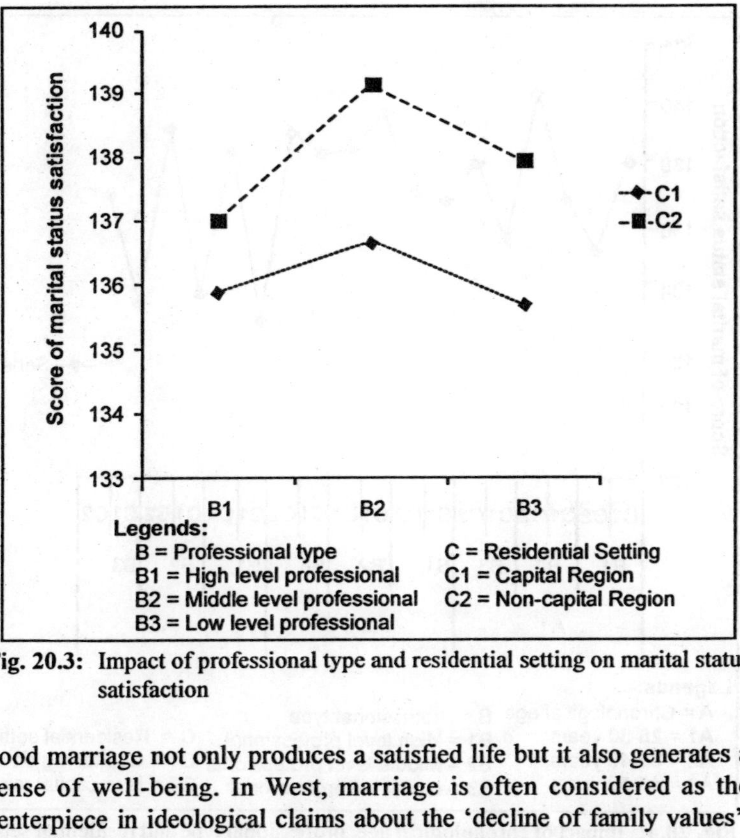

Fig. 20.3: Impact of professional type and residential setting on marital status satisfaction

good marriage not only produces a satisfied life but it also generates a sense of well-being. In West, marriage is often considered as the centerpiece in ideological claims about the 'decline of family values'. Marital adjustment has been related to personality, job and home stresses, mental illness, depression, education, sex role attitude, happiness and success in life.

Sinha and Mukherjee (1990), define marital adjustment as, "*the state in which there is an overall feeling between husband and wife, of happiness and satisfaction with their marriage and with each other.*"

All the marriages are aimed at happiness in one or another way. Most couples marry filled up with expectations. Some of the expectations will be realistic while other are unrealistic. Marital adjustment calls for maturity that accepts and understands growth and development in the spouse. If this growth is not experienced and realized fully, death in marital relationship is inevitable. A relationship between couples is not instantaneous rather it is a slow progress.

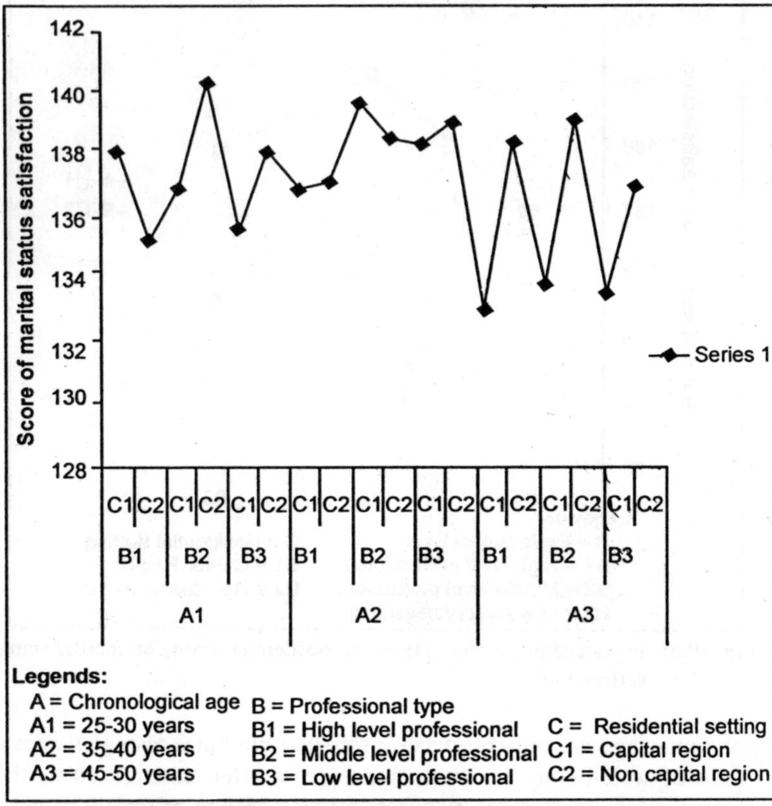

Fig. 20.4: Impact of chronological age, professional type and residential setting on marital status satisfaction

Emotional Adjustment: Emotional behaviours expressed by couples differed as a function of age, gender, and marital satisfaction. The intensity of the middle-age intimacy crisis depends on the need-satisfaction of the relationship and particularly on the success achieved in the previous stages of intimacy. Older adults are biased towards the positive aspects of close relationships (Story, Nathan T. *et al.*, 2007), emotionally positive and responsive listening is one of the keys to successful conflict resolution in marriage (Pasupathi, Monisha *et al.*, 1999).

In other couples, the resolution of conflict was less emotionally negative and more affectionate than in middle-aged marriages. Differences between husbands and wives and between happy and unhappy marriages were also found. Wives were more affectively negative than husbands, whereas husbands were more defensive than wives, and unhappy marriages involved greater exchange of negative affect than happy marriages.

Couples engage in naturalistic discussions about important topics related to their relationship. These interactions are studied to determine if there are signs in emotional experience, behaviour, language, and physiology that can be used to discriminate between the interactions of couples who are satisfied and dissatisfied with their relationship, to discriminate between couples at different stages of the life span, and to predict what will happen to the level of couples relationship satisfaction over time. What kinds of couples fare well as they cope with these transitions and what kinds of couples fare poorly.

Unlike many other aspects of human functioning which show pronounced declines with age (e.g., memory, psychomotor skills), many aspects of emotional functioning appear to be relatively spared as the age, and some even show signs of continuing improvement and positive development in late life.

Discussion and Conclusion

Findings generally are revealed that although married life is considered as the flowery path of life, yet it demands many sufferings, pains and compromises as well. Unfortunately, it becomes even more when the females go out from home, i.e. she is professional. To manage the both platforme of life is very difficult for her. Sometimes, she adjust with these sufferings and sometimes it becomes a challenge for her.

Working females have to play dual roles as they are employed outside house. They shoulder more responsibilities than males, adjust their time and energy for children, spouse, and household activities and make adjustment accordingly. Barling (1986) in his study on *"inter-role conflicts and marital function"* found that conflict regarding work and family roles was associated with lower levels of marital adjustment among dual earner couples.

In contrast, males are more mentally healthy than females. A balance of psychic force in the males shows sound mental health. Ability to understand and to share other people's emotions, the ability to concentrate at work and interest in several activities in middle aged males result in good adjustment with spouse and with the family members. They always have an inner feeling to spend quality time with their spouse, take care of and satisfy sexual needs of the partner. They have concern and feel responsible for needs of the family members and for smooth functioning of the family, they are able to make equal role distribution among the family members. They try to maintain balance between family and society. During middle age, the males have less family responsibilities (as the children are grown up or settled down) and would also desire to spend some time for social work or welfare activities. It leads to their overall life satisfaction. Hill (2005) conducted a study on 1,314 individuals and found that work to family facilitation was positively related to job satisfaction and negatively related to individual stress. Family, the work facilitation was positively related to organization commitment. Working fathers reported long work hours (49 hours/week), major involvement in household responsibilities (46 hours/week), and a work culture less supportive of their family life than working mothers reported. However, working fathers reported less individual stress, and greater family satisfaction than working mothers did. In addition to this, some informed devices were also suggested for them to minimize their stress and make a promotion to raise their quality of life. For this, they were suggested for tolerance, a sense of positivism, friendliness with the spouse and the family members' responsibility tendency to give, regard to elders and last but not least the conversion of ego into "identity feel".

References

Balack, G.W. (1990): Perspective on the Relationship between Cardiovascular Disease and Affective Disorder. *The Journal of Clinical Psychology. S1*, 4-9.

Benard, J. (1984): *Work and Family: Changing rules of Men and Women*. Palo Alto, CA: Mayfield.

Blood, R.O., Wolfe, D.M. (1960): *Husband and Wives*. New York.

Thomas, E.I. (1997): *Marital Communication and decision making*. New York, Free Press.

Gore, S., Manigione, T.W. (1983): Social roles and Sex roles and Psychological distress: Additive and interactive models of sex differences. *Journal of Health and Social Behaviour*, *24*:300-12.

Lazarus, R.S. and Delingis, A. (1985): Psychological stress and coping in ageing. *American Psychologist*, *38*: 245-54.

Leffcourt, H.M. (1976): *The Locus of Control: Current Trends in Theory and Research*. New York: Wiley.

Margolin, G. (1980): Behaviour exchange in happy and unhappy marriages. A family life cycle perspectives. *Behaviour Therapy, 12*:329-43.

Parron, E.M. (1982). Golden Wedding Couples: Lessons in Marital Longevity. *Generations*, *7*: 14-6

Smith, H.C. (1961): *Personality adjustment,* New York: McGraw-Hill.

Story, T.N. Berg. C.A., Smith, T.W., Beveridge, R. Henry, N.J., and Pearce, G. (2007): Age, Marital Satisfaction and optimism as Predicators of Positive sentiments override in middle aged and older married couples. *Journal Articles Psychology and Ageing*, *22* (4), 719-727.

Veenboven, R. (1983): The growing impact of marriage, *Social Indicators Research, 12*:49-63.

Weiten, W. (1996): *Psychological applied to modern life Adjustment in the 80s* (2nd edition). California: Wordsworth.

21
Cultivating New Resources
Increasing Strength in Human Life

Aradhana Shukla

In these days researchers and health care professionals are paying attention on positive topics and use of personal strength is becoming increasingly more attractive (Aspin Well & Staudinger, 2003; Peterson and Seligman, 2004). Researches on "positive psychotherapy" suggest that the nurturance of strength in the client is very necessary and positions outcomes are very possible to come. Fluckinger and Groose (2008) have stated that nurturing strength in client produces therapeutic bonding mastery experience and decline in the symptom of disorder. Resources done on educational setting suggest that students having more personal strength are associated with more work strength (Hayes *et al.*, 2006; Louis, 2009; Bowers and Lopez, 2010).

It has been observed that strengths are associated with a wide range of positive and desirable outcomes like subjective well-being (Govindji and Linley, 2007; Proctor, Maltby and Linley, 2009), stress management (Wood, Linley, Maltby, Kashdan and Hurling, 2011) and satisfaction of obtaining goal (Linley, Neilson, Wood, Gillett and Biwa's Diener, 2010). Some researchers suggest that psychological strength can be considered as important tool in person's development.

Strength as a Personality Variable

Dealing with the notion of strength one can also think about its development. Many scholars have defined it as a behaviour while some others have stated it as personality variable. Numerous definitions of strength exist and they define it as:

- A capacity for feeling, thinking and behaving in a way that allows optimal function in the pursuit of valued outcomes (Linley and Harrington, 2007).

- A combination of talents (naturally recurring pattern of thoughts, feelings and behaviour), knowledge (facts and lessons learned), and skills (the steps of an activity) (Buckingham and Clifton, 2001).
- The psychological ingredients—process or mechanisms—that define morally valued virtues (Peterson and Seligman, 2004).
- The advocates of strength psychology usually think strength as a natural/genetic process which makes a distinction between good and/or bad and behave accordingly.

Clifton and Harter (2003) have acknowledged the role of personality in the foundation of strength, "The findings of high composition may hint that how people most efficiently grow and develop in dynamically related to who they are begin with—people can change the changeable (satisfaction, subjective well-being, engagement, performance etc.), but most efficiently through who they are to begin with their (inherent talents)".

Indicators of Human Strengths

It is true that strengths energize the person and enable him to make a distinction between good-bad, acceptable-unacceptable, desirable-undesirable and favourable-unfavourable. However, we can judge a person having high mental strength if he/she, at least following traits, like well-being, gratitude, forgiveness, optimism, good personality, spirituality, good and well knitted society, good company, constructive use of time, attachment, commitment, caring, empowerment, support, boundary, social competence and most important among all positive orientation towards life. They minimize negative resources and feel strength and positive outlook in the life.

Positive Psychological Capital: Determinants of Strength

When we think strength as a capital we think that it is comprised with psychological attributes. These attributes are acquired and developed with age, social demands and the passage of time. Luthans (2004) and Luthans and Youssef (2004) have comprised four positive psychological variables (Fig. 21.1). These variables involve Bandura's (1997) efficacy (confidence on one's ability to reach a desired goal), hope (the capacity to find pathways to desired goal with motivation or energy), optimism (the ability to attribute good outcomes to internal, stable and pervasive causes) and resiliency (the capacity of endurance). The pathways of positive psychological capital are shown in Fig. 21.1.

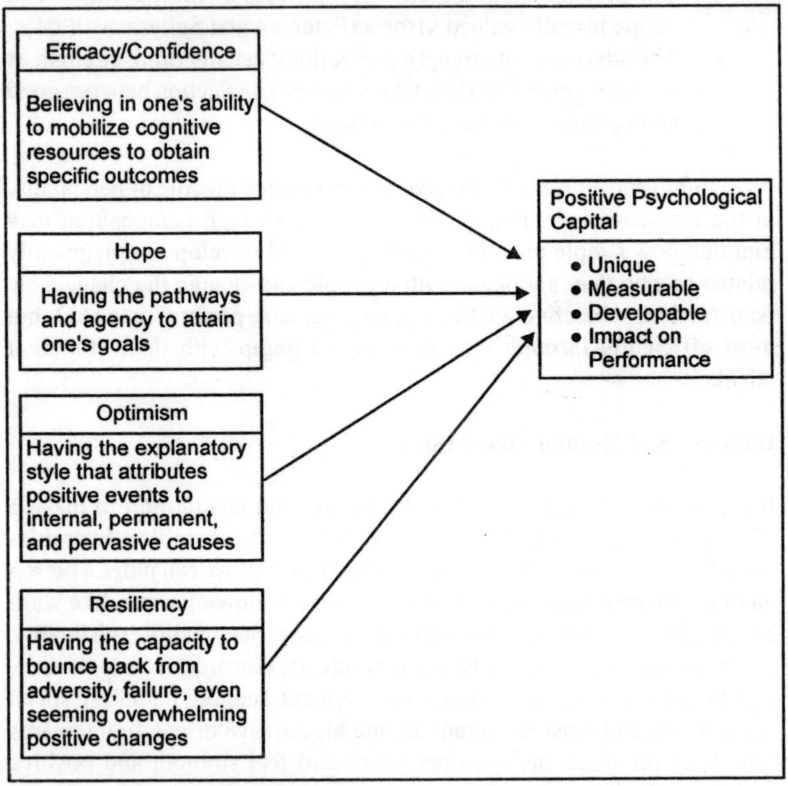

Fig. 21.1: Determinants of strength

Getting Mental Strength: A person, in case, who wants to get rid of from mental ill-health he can easily do it. Actually, feeling of mental health (physical health too) as an "internally felt process" one can do it after a proper exercise. However, these strategies are as follows:

(i) ***Satisfaction:*** Satisfaction is an internal process and it facilitates mental health. When a person is aware about his/her capabilities and limitations he/she can develop a feeling of satisfaction and recover his/her mental health.

(ii) ***Self-Actualization:*** Self-Actualization is a process of self-awareness which helps a person to know his good/bad qualities and limits. It makes a person efficient to perceive the world in real way. Then it makes a person mentally healthy.

(iii) ***Will-Power:*** Firm determination, confirmed will-power and ability to do things construct will-power. On the basis of internal voice a person can become mentally healthy and can get stable personality.

(iv) ***Spiritual Exercise*:** Here the importance of Yoga cannot be denied. It helps a person to reach towards eternity.

On the basis of this discussion, it can be opined that mental health is a process that carries a person towards perfection.

Minimizing Stress and Gaining Strength: There are many visions following which one can minimize stress and gain strength. They are as follows:

- There is no use of regret on the past. Strength can be acquired at any time.
- Supporting others is highly needed to nurture strength and for capacity-building.
- Faith on oneself and others is essential to build strength.
- Endeavour, goal setting and working accordingly, goal orientation and satisfaction are the important and significant determinants of psychological strength.
- Believing in oneself and knowing one's capacities are the strong pillars of strength.
- Some help from counsellors and healthcare professionals can also be taken time to time.
- Enjoy good company and be with the people of positive orientations.

Hazards of Mental Strength

If we want to gain mental strength, at first we have to give up the things/ideas given below because they serve as the hazards of human strength:

(i) ***Wasting Time and Feeling Sad for Them:*** We do not see mentally strong people feeling sad for their circumstance or dwelling on the way they have been maltreated. They learn to take the responsibility for their actions and results and they have an inherent capacity on the basis of which they think that the course of life is not always very fair, so they try to solve the problem on the basis of their own.

(ii) ***Give Up Their Power:*** Mentally strong people really avoid giving others the power to make them feel inferior. They understand that they are in the control of their action and emotions. They know their strength very well and know the device of their management.

(iii) ***Shy Away from Change:*** Mentally strong people embrace change. They welcome and appreciate change. They fear from becoming co-placement and stagnant.

(iv) ***Waste Energy on Things They Can't Control***: The people having strong mental strength do not waste their time, idea or money on the people, event or circumstance on which they do not have any control.

(v) ***Worry About Pleasing Others:*** People having strong mental strength try their best to give happiness to the society but they do it in true condition. They do not make false strategies to give praise to the unworthy people.

(vi) ***Fear Taking Calculated Risk***: A mentally strong person is willing to take calculated risk. With the consistent development of mental strength an individual can weigh the risk and benefits thoroughly and wilfully assess the potential downfall and even the worst scenario prior to the taking of action.

(vii) ***Dwell on the Past:*** There is strength in acknowledging past experiences and the things learned from past experiences but a mentally strong person is able to avoid miring their mental energy in past disappointment or in fantasies of the "glory days" gone by. They invest their energy in optimal present and future.

(viii) ***Make the Same Mistakes By and By:*** A person having strong mental health accepts full responsibility of his all deeds (whether good or bad, acceptable or unacceptable). He is self-reflective in nature.

(ix) ***Resent other People's Success:*** It is the sign of a person of high mental strength that he should be happy on the success of others. He does not become jealous or resentful when he sees other one climbing on the ride of success.

(x) ***Giving up the Job after Failure***: Every failure is a chance to improve. Therefore, mentally strong people have to try their best endeavour even after consistent failure. It has also been stated in Sanskrit:

Prarabhyate na khalu vighna bhayena neechaiyah
Prarabhya vighna vihita viramanti madhyah
Vighnaih pura punrapi pratihanyamana
Prarabhya chottam janah na parityajanti

Bhartrihari *(Nitishataka)*

(xi) ***Fear Alone Time:*** Mentally stray people enjoy and sometimes treasure their solitude. They use their down lane to reflect to plan and to be productive. Most importantly, they do not depend on others to share their happiness and mood.

(xii) ***Feel the World Owes as Them Anything:*** Mentally strong people enter in the world prepared to work and succeed on their merits at every stage of the game.

(xiii) ***Expectation of Immediate Result***: Whether it is a workout plan or starting a business mentally strong people expect immediate and better result. They have "staying power" and they understand that genuine changes take time.

Surfing Mental Strength

We should encourage our own strength and to share it with our friends and society. For this we have to make following arrangements:

- ***Getting to Know Our Friend's Weakness and Strength:*** We should at first observe the weakness of our friend's and then ask them to reveal their weakness. If they are able to get them revealed we should suggest them to minimize them.
- ***Discovering Our Own Strength:*** We can also indent by our own weakness and after knowing them, we can also reduce them. Also, we can take a help from *www.strengthsfinder.com*
- ***Capitalizing Our Own Strength:*** There are numerous strategies for capitalizing our strength. We can consult www.reflectivehappiness.com to go deeper.
- ***Strength Enhancing Exercise:*** Although, strength is a personality variable and it is embedded in the person yet better attempts are warranted to make it more powerful. Hereunder, are some strategies that are essential to enhance the magnitude of strength?

- ***Evaluation of Core Belief:*** It is our concern that we should develop conduct core for ourselves and allow our emotions, thoughts and ideas to do only such work. Also, there is a need to judge the significance, applications and authencity of our thoughts.
- ***Expansions of Mental Energy:*** Although, it is a rather difficult task yet it produces a lot while fostering mental strength. In spite of gossiping, watching TV or peeping in the lives of others, one should consume his energy in productive task and it will become a habit later on.
- ***Replacement of Negative Thoughts with Productive Thoughts:*** If someone always feels negativity and surrounded by negative events he becomes "mental looser". So, negative thoughts should always be converted into positive thoughts. We should be optimistic by nature and we should realize that we are the products of strength as well as of weakness.
- ***Practice of Tolerating Discomfort:*** Strength, not only fosters, but also teaches us to widen our comfort zone. *"Self-centredness"* hampers strengths and tolerance of discomfort, well-acquaintance with our emotions, understanding our controlled and uncontrolled feelings and expand our comfort zone in contradictory situations are the indicators of our strength.
- ***Evaluation of Everyday Progress:*** If we can develop a habit of self-critic or self-evaluator we will be self-actualizer later on. We have to make a critical evaluation of our everyday progress.

If we make it our mission to obtain mental strength we should know that this can be obtained through:

- Curing mental illness.
- Making the lives of people more comfortable and fulfilling.
- Identifying human strength.
- Use of strength.
- Appreciating positive works so that they could be followed.
- Nurturing the genius and trained professionals for health care and building support.

References

Aspinwall, L. and Staudinger, U.M. (2003). *A Psychology of Human Strength:*

Fundamental Questions and Future Directions for Positive Psychology. Washington, DC:

Bowers, K.M. and Lopez, S. (2010). Capitalizing on personal strengths in college, *Journal of College and Character, 11*, 1-11.

Bandura, A. (1997). *Self-efficacy: The Exercise of Control.* New York: Freeman.

Baumeister, R.F., Bratslavsky, E., Finkenhaur, C. and Vohs, K.D. (2001). Bad is Stronger than Good. *Review of General Psychology, 5*, 323-370.

Bradburn, N.M. (1996). *The Structure of Psychological well-being.* Chicago: Aldine.

Bryant, F. B., and Veroff, J. (1982). The structure of psychological well-being: A socio-historical analysis. *Journal of Personality and Social Psychology, 43*, 653-673.

Costa, P.T. and McCrae, R.R. (1988). Personality in Adulthood. A six year longitudinal study of self reports and spouse ratings of the NEO Personality Inventory. *Journal of Personality and Social Psychology, 54*, 853-863.

Csikszentmihalyi, M., (1990). *Flow: The Psychology of Optimal Experience.* New York: Harper & Row.

Csikszentmihalyi, M., (1975/2000). *Beyond Boredom and Anxiety.* San Francisco: Jossey-Bass.

Clifton, D. and Harter, J.K. (2003). Investing in strengths. In K. Cameron, J.E. Dutton, and R. Quinn (Eds.). *Positive Organizational Scholarship: Foundation of a New Discipline.* San Francisco, CA: Barrett-Koehler.

Diener, E. (1984). Subjective well-being. *Psychological Bulletin, 95*, 542-575.

Diener, E. (2000). Subjective well-being: The science of happiness and a proposal for a national index. *American Psychologist, 53*, 34-43.

Diener, E. and Biswas-Diener, R. (2002). Will money increase subjective well-being. *Social Indicators Research, 57*, 119-169.

Diener, E. and Diener, M. (1995). Cross-cultural correlates of life satisfaction and self-esteem. *Journal of Personality and Social Psychology, 68*, 653-663.

Diener, E., Diener, M., and Diener, C. (1995). Factors predicting the well-being of nations. *Journal of Personality and Social Psychology, 69*, 653-663.

Diener, E. and Emmons, R.A. (1984). The independence of positive and negative affect. *Journal of Personality and Social Psychology, 47*, 1105-1117.

Emmons, R.A. (1986). Personal strivings: An approach to personality and subjective well-being. *Journal of Personality and Social Psychology, 51*, 1058-1068.

Fluckinger, C. and Grosse Holforth, M. (2008). Focusing the therapist's attention on the patient's strengths: A preliminaty study to foster a mechanism of change in outpatient psychotherapy. *Journal of Clinical Psychology. 64*, 876-890.

Fordyce, M.W. (1997). Development of a programme to increase personal happiness. *Journal of Counselling Psychology, 24*, 511-520.

Fordyce, M.W. (1983). A programme to increase happiness: Further studies. *Journal of Counselling Psychology, 30*, 483-498.

Govindji, R. and Linley, A. (2007). Strengths use, self concordance and well-being: Implications for strengths coaching and coaching psychologists. *International Coaching Psychology Review, 2*, 143-153.

Hayes, S.C., Luoma, J.B., Bond, F.W. Masuda, A., and Lillis, J. (2006). Acceptance and commitment therapy: Model, processes and outcomes. *Behaviour Research and Therapy. 44*, 1-25.

Linley, P.A. and Harrington, S. (2007). Playing to your strengths. *The Psychologist, 19*, 85-89.

Linley, P.A. and Harrington, S. (2006). Playing to your strengths. *Psychologist, 19*, 86-89.

Linley, P.A., Joseph, S. and Wood, A.M. (2006). Positive psychology: Past, present, and (possible future). *Journal of Positive Psychology, 1*, 3-16.

Linley, P.A. Nielsen, K.M., Wood, A.M., Gillett, R., and Biswas-Diener. R. (2010). Using signature strengths in pursuit of goals: Effects on goal progress, need satisfaction, and well-being, and implications for coaching psychologists. *International Coaching Psychology Review, 5*, 6-15.

Louis, M.C. (2009). A summary and critique of existing strengths-based educational research Utilizing the Clifton Strengths Finder. Internal paper, The Gallup Organization.

Peterson, C. and Seligman, M.E.P. (2004). *Character Strengths and Virtues: A Handbook and Classification.* Washington, DC: American Psychological Association Press and Oxford University Press.

Proctor, C. Maltby, J. and Linley, P.A. (2009). Strengths use as a predictor of well-being and health-related quality of life. *Journal of Happiness Studies, 10,* 583-630.

Seligman, M.E.P. and Csikszentmihalyi, M. (2000). Positive psychology: An introduction. *American Psychologist, 55*, 5-14.

Wood, A.M., Linley, P.A., Maltby, J., Kashdan, T.B., and Hurling, R. (2011). Using psychological strengths leads to less stress and greater self-esteem, vitality, and positive affect: Longitudinal examination of the strengths use questionnaire. *Personality and Individual Differences, 50*, 15-19.

Wood, A.M. and Tarrier, N. (2010). Positive clinical psychology: A New vision and strategy for integrated research and practice. *Clinical Psychology Review, 30*, 819-829.

Index